T0331897

Handbook of the Hemopoietic Microenvironment

Contemporary Biomedicine

Handbook of the Hemopoietic Microevironment
    Edited by *Mehdi Tavassoli,* 1989
The Red Cell Membrane
    Edited by *B. U. Raess and Godfrey Tunnicliff,* 1989
Leukolysins and Cancer
    Edited by *Janet H. Ransom and John R. Ortaldo,*
    1988
Methods of Hybridoma Formation
    Edited by *Arie H. Bartal* and *Yashar Hirshaut,*
    1987
Monoclonal Antibodies in Cancer
    Edited by *Stewart Sell* and *Ralph A. Reisfeld,* 1985
Calcium and Contractility: *Smooth Muscle*
    Edited by *A. K. Grover* and *E. E. Daniel,* 1984
Carcinogenesis and Mutagenesis Testing
    Edited by *J. F. Douglas,* 1984
The Human Teratomas: *Experimental and Clinical*
    Biology
    Edited by *Ivan Damjanov, Barbara B. Knowles,*
    and *Davor Solter,* 1983
Human Cancer Markers
    Edited by *Stewart Sell* and *Britta Wahren,* 1982
Cancer Markers: *Diagnostic and Developmental*
    Significance
    Edited by *Stewart Sell,* 1980

Handbook

of the
Hemopoietic Microenvironment

Edited by

Mehdi Tavassoli

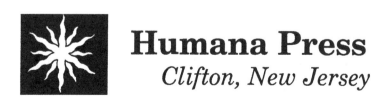

Humana Press
Clifton, New Jersey

Library of Congress Cataloging-in-Publication Data

Handbook of the Hemopoietic Microenvironment / edited by Mehdi Tavassoli
      p. 453 cm.–(Contemporary biomedicine)
      Includes bibliographies and index.
      ISBN 0-89603-147-0
      1. Hematopoiesis I. Tavassoli, Mehdi, 1933– . II. Series
      [DNLM: 1. Bone marrow—cytology. 2. Bone marrow—physiology.
      3. Hematopoiesis. 4. Hematopoietic System—cytology.
      5. Hematopoietic System—physiology. WH 140 H236]
      QP92.H36 1989
      612.4'91—dc20
      DNLM/DLC
      for Library of Congress   89-15497
                                                     CIP

Preface

In 1868, Ernst Neumann recognized that blood cells require continuous replenishment during postnatal life. Before him, the assumption was that cells of the blood, like nerves once formed in the embryo, remain in the body throughout life. Neumann also recognized that this process occurred within the bone marrow, because this tissue provided a favorable environment for proliferation and differentiation of blood cell precursors.

Vera Danchakoff, the Russian embryologist working in the US, in 1916 made an analogy to the soil and the seed. Bone marrow forms the soil, providing a favorable environment for the growth of seed, the hemopoietic stem cell, and other progenitor cells.

> Imagine in the remote past a heap of similar tree seeds. These seeds develop in our moderate climate into a tall and many branched tree. Suppose the wind bears a part of the seeds away and brings them to a land possessing different environmental conditions, we will say the arctic lands. There the seeds may develop but they may produce trees no higher than our moss.

Some 50 years later, the advent of bone marrow transplantation techniques proved her to be correct: in 1961, Till and McCulloch developed their celebrated spleen colony technique, and shortly after, Trentin and coworkers found that the difference in the differentiation pathways of these colonies is determined by the differences in the environmental "niches" in the stroma of hemopoietic tissues. Simultaneously, many other techniques were used to gain further insight into cellular components of stroma and extracellular matrix and the nature of their interactions with hemopoietic stems cells and progenitor cells.

A quarter of a century has passed since this area of research opened, and it has now blossomed. Yet, surprisingly, no volume has been devoted to a synthesis of this field. In this volume, which is devoted to the treatment of "soil," some of the leading authorities in the field have undertaken this synthesis. John Trentin provides a historical perspective, as well as a definition. He critically reviews the evidence for the presence of hemopoietic microenvironments. Marshall Lichtman and coworkers deal with the structural analysis of bone marrow and, particularly, the relevance of this structure to the last stage of hemopoiesis, i.e., the egress of mature cells into the circulation. Robert McCuskey, one of the few who uses the exacting technique of in vivo microscopy, describes the contribution of this unique method to our understanding of the hemopoietic microenvironment. Fatty involution of marrow and the role of adipose tissue, the strange bedfellow of hemopoietic tissue, is the subject of another chapter. A cellular ester membrane model has been useful in elucidating many aspects of microenvironmental control of hemopoiesis. This area will be reviewed by William Knospe.

Three chapters deal with the cellular components of the stroma. In a comprehensive chapter, Mati Shaklai describes cellular components of stroma in vivo at a morphologic level, but also makes a correlative comparison with an in vitro system. Peter Quesenberry discusses the stroma in long-term marrow culture. In the past few years, many of these stromal cells have been cloned, and the study of their structural–functional characteristics are expected to answer certain remaining questions. Dov Zipori will review this area. The interface of immune and hemopoietic systems and the modulation of hemopoiesis by monocytes and T-lymphocytes are treated in a chapter by Joao Ascensao and Esmail Zanjani, who have also considered the immune nature of failure of hemopoiesis. In analogy with "seed" and "soil," we may then speak of the "worm" to identify one pathogenesis of marrow failure.

The role of extracellular matrix is coming into focus, not only in the regulation of hemopoiesis, but also as a regulatory factor in cell biology in general. Renate Gay and colleagues will provide and introduction to this area and will synthesize our knowledge of noncollagenous matrix in the regulation of hemopoiesis. The role of the collagenous matrix will be treated in a different chapter by Kenneth Zuckerman and coworkers. Finally, the development of knowledge generally aims at applications, and thus, N. T. Shahidi will discuss the potential clinical applications of this field.

Therefore, this volume is intended as a reading source for all investigators in experimental hematology, but also provides a reference source for hematologists, cell biologists, experimental pathologists, immunologists, and even biochemists.

Among many, I am grateful to Kenneth Brinkhaus, who appreciated the void of literature in this area and persuaded me to undertake this task, a task that would have been impossible without the dedicated and highly organized administrative assistance of Jackie Davis. I am also indebted to the authors of the individual chapters, many of whom tolerated, with good humor, my frequent and often repetitive vexing requests for revisions. If this volume as a whole is more than the sum of its parts, the credit belongs to them.

Mehdi Tavassoli

References

Tavassoli, M. (1980), *Blood, Pure and Eloquent* (Wintrobe, M. M., ed.), McGraw Hill, New York, pp. 57–79.

Neumann, E. (1968), *Zentralbl. Med. Wissensch.* **6**, 689.

Danchakoff, V. (1916), *Anat. Rec.* **10**, 397–414.

Till, J. E. and McCulloch, E. A. (1961), *Radiat. Res.* **14**, 213–222.

Trentin, J. J. (1970), *Regulation of Hematopoiesis* (Gordon, A. S., ed.), Appleton-Century-Crofts, New York, pp. 161–186.

Dedication

To Marie, Ali, Javad, and Cherine
for their understanding and encouragements.

Contents

Preface v
Contributors xxi

Hemopoietic Microenvironments
Historical Perspectives, Status, and Projections
John J. Trentin

Introduction 1
Definition 3
Radiation Protection by Marrow Transplantation 4
The Spleen Colony Assay 5
Antecedents of the Hemopoietic Microenvironment
   Concept 5
      Homing 5
      Unexplained Failure of Marrow Isografts 7
Spleen Colony Types 9
      Decision 9
Spleen Colony Retransplantation 14
Effect of Erythropoietin Deprivation on Spleen
   Colony Types 18
Visualization of Erythropoietin-Sensitive
   Stem Cell Colonies 20
Decision for Lineage-Specific Differentiation 23
Endoclonal Origin of the Second Line of Differentiation 25
The Working Hypothesis 28
Tests of the Working Hypothesis 29

Bone Marrow Colonies and Characteristics 29
Hemopoietic Colony Characteristics in Transplanted
  Spleen or Bone Marrow Stroma 30
Whole Spleen Stroma Transplant 'Cure'
  of Sl/Sl^d Anemia 33
Effect of Mouse Hemopoietic Microenvironments
  on Rat CFU-S 36
Microenvironmental Control of Eosinophilic
  Granulocyte Response to Tetanus Toxoid 38
Microenvironmental Control of Mast Cell
Differentiation 39
Dissecting the Hemopoietic Microenvironment.....................40
Other Evidence of the Roles of Marrow, Spleen, and Thymus
  Organ Stroma in Hemopoiesis and Lymphopoiesis 41
Hemopoiesis on Intraperitoneal Cellulose Acetate
Membranes 42
CFU-S Heterogeneity 42
Reversible Effect of Marrow and Spleen Microenvironments
  on Thymic Progenitor Cell Differentiation and
  Proliferation..46
Reversible Predisposition of CFU-S for Direction
  of Differentiation 48
Hemopoietic Hormone (Growth Factor) Receptors 50
Pluripotency of Hemopoietic CFU-S for Lymphoid
  Differentiation 51
Lymphoid-Inductive Microenvironments 52
In Vitro Bone Marrow Cultures 55
  Early Methods 55
  The Dexter Method 56
  The Greenberger Modification 57
  B-Lymphocyte Cultures 58
Distinctive Stromal Cells of Erythroid and Granuloid
  Spleen Colonies...59
  Erythroid Colonies 59

Granuloid Colonies 64
Other Candidate for In Vivo Hemopoietic Microenvironment
   Stromal Cells 65
Hemopoiesis 68
   Random or Controlled? 68
Projections 77
Malignancy-Inducing Microenvironments? 77
References 78

Molecular and Cellular Traffic
Across the Marrow Sinuses
Marshall A. Lichtman, Charles H. Packman,
and Louis S. Constine

Introduction 87
Marrow Structure 88
   Arterial and Venous Circulation 88
   Marrow Sinuses 90
   Marrow Nerves 99
Evidence for Discrimination in the Release
   of Marrow Cells 100
Factors Governing Release of Hemopoietic Cells 103
   Biophysical Properties of Developing Hemopoietic
      Cells 104
Cell Releasing Factors 107
   Control of Blood Flow in Marrow 110
The Anatomical Process of Release 110
   Ultrastructural Features of Reticulocyte Egress 111
   Modeling Reticulocyte Egress 117
   Ultrastructural Features of White Cell Egress 121
   Ultrastructural Features of Platelet Release 123
   Release of Immature Cells in Healthy Subjects 130
   Release of Immature Cells in Pathological States 130

Release from and Reentry into Marrow of Stem Cells
    and Progenitor Cells 132
References 133

In Vivo Microscopy of Hemopoietic Tissue
Robert S. McCuskey

Introduction...141
In Vivo Microscopic Methods..142
    Basic Methods 142
    Transillumination Methods 143
    Epi-illumination Methods 146
In Vivo Microscopic Studies of Hemopoietic Tissue 147
References 154

Fatty Involution of Marrow and the Role of Adipose Tissue in Hemopoiesis
Mehdi Tavassoli

Introduction...157
Distribution of Red and Yellow Marrow 159
The Role of Bone 160
Ectopic Implantation of Bone Marrow 163
Marrow Adipocyte 170
    Development 170
    Structure 171
    Function 172
Distinct from Extramedullary Adipocytes 174
    Functional Differences 176
Heterogeneity of Marrow Adipocytes 178
Marrow Adipocytes in Culture 180
Conclusions 182
References 184

Hematopoiesis on Artificial Membranes
William H. Knospe

Hematopoiesis on Flat CEM 190
Hematopoiesis On Stromally-Enriched, IP-Implanted
  Tubular CEM 194
Hematopoiesis and Proteoglycans...201
Role of Bone and Tooth Matrix Proteins
  in Hematopoiesis 202
Irradiation of Stromal Cells...207
Studies of Scraped, Devitalized, and Reimplanted CEM ...209
Overall Perspective and Significance of Hematopoiesis
  on CEM 210
References...216

Cellular Components of Stroma In Vivo in Comparison with In Vitro Systems
Mati Shaklai

Introduction...219
Cellular Components of the Stroma 220
  Reticular Cells In Vivo 220
  Fibroblastic Reticular Cells in Long-Term Cell
    Culture 225
  Macrophages 230
  Macrophages of Bone Marrow Origin in Long-Term
    Culture 244
References...247

Stromal Cells in Long-Term Bone Marrow Cultures
Peter J. Quesenberry

Introduction...253
Cell Types in Adherent Layer...256

Growth Factor Production by Adherent Cells 264
Studies in Other Species Including Human 267
Lymphoid Growth and Long-Term Culture 272
TC-1 Cell Line 274
Hypothesis...278
References 280

Cultured Stromal Cell Lines
from Hemopoietic Tissues
Dov Zipori

The Hemopoietic Microenvironment 287
    Putative Functions...287
    Nature of Stromal Cells 290
    Primary Cultures of Bone Marrow Stromal Cells........293
    The Requirement for Permanent Stromal Cell Lines ..296
Hemopoietic Stromal Cell Lines...297
    Derivation 297
    Growth 303
    Morphology...304
    Adipogenesis...306
    Cytoplasmic Enzymes 307
    Extracellular Matrix 308
    Cell Surface Markers 309
    Classification 309
    Long-Term In Vitro Hemopoiesis 311
    Colony Stimulating Factors (CSF)...................................313
    Differentiation-Restraining Activities 316
    Other Regulators of Hemopoiesis 317
    Leukemia Cell Inhibitory Activity (LCIA)....................317
    Promotion of Leukemia Cell Growth 321
    Promoters of Leukemia Cell Differentiation 323
    Transplantation and Tumorigenesis...............................323
    Modulation of In Vitro Functions 324
    Tissue and Cell-Lineage Specificity 325

Summary 326
References 329

Cellular Interactions in the Regulation of Human Hemopoiesis In Vitro
Joao L. Ascensao and Esmail D. Zanjani

Normal Hemopoiesis 335
    Role of T-Cells 335
    Role of Monocytes 351
    Role of NK Cells 353
Abnormal Hemopoiesis 354
    Aplastic Anemia 354
References 363

The Collagenous Hemopoietic Microenvironment
Renate E. Gay, C. W. Prince, K. S. Zuckerman, and S. Gay

Introduction 369
The Genetically-Distinct Types of Collagen 373
    Type I Collagen 373
    Type II Collagen 378
    Type III Collagen 379
    Type IV Collagen 380
    Type V Collagen 381
    Type VI Collagen 382
    Type VII Collagen 383
    Type VIII Collagen 383
    Type IX Collagen 384
    Type X Collagen 384
    Type XI Collagen 384
Collagenous Bone Marrow Stroma 385
Synthesis of Collagenous Matrix by Stromal Cells
    of the Bone Marrow 388

Bone Marrow Collagen in Hematologic Disorders 389
Myelofibrosis...390
Future Prospects 394
References..394

The Hemopoietic Extracellular Matrix

**Kenneth S. Zuckerman, Charles W. Prince,
and Steffen Gay**

Introduction...399
The Role of the Extracellular Matrix in Regulating
    Cell Growth and Differentiation 401
Characterization of Noncollagenous Extracellular Matrix
    Macromolecules Found in Bone and Bone Marrow........402
        Fibronectin...403
        Laminin 404
        Proteoglycans 405
        Other Extracellular Matrix Proteins of Bone
            and Bone Marrow 408
        Summary of Extracellular Matrix Macromolecules
            Found in Bone and Bone Marrow 410
Identification of Extracellular Matrix Proteins in the Stroma
    of Long-Term Bone Marrow Cell Cultures......................412
        Fibronectin and Laminin 412
        Proteoglycans 414
        Summary of Extracellular Matrix Glycoproteins
            and Proteoglycans Produced in Long-Term
            Bone Marrow Cultures 415
The Role of Extracellular Matrix Components in Regulating
    Hemopoiesis in Long-Term Bone Marrow Cultures.......416
Reconstitution of Bone and Bone Marrow In Vivo by
    Ectopic Implantation of Devitalized, DemineralizedBone
    Matrix 417

Studies of the Abnormal Hemopoietic Microenvironment
   of Sl/Sl^d Mice 421
Summary...426
References 428

Bone Marrow Microenvironment
Clinical Observations
N. T. Shahidi and W. B. Ershler

Clinical Implications 434
Functional Abnormalities of Cellular Components of Bone
   Marrow Microenvironment 435
      T-Lymphocytes 436
      Bone Marrow Macrophages 438
      Bone Marrow Fibroblasts 440
References 442

Index 445

Contributors

JOAO L. ASCENSAO • *Department of Medicine, University of Connecticut Health Center, Farmington, Connecticut*

LOUIS S. CONSTINE • *Department of Radiation Oncology, University of Rochester Medical Center, Rochester, New York*

W. B. ERSHLER • *Department of Pediatrics and Medicine, University of Wisconsin, Madison, Madison, Wisconsin*

RENATE E. GAY • *Department of Medicine and Biochemistry, University of Alabama, Birmingham, Birmingham, Alabama*

STEFFEN GAY • *Department of Medicine and Biochemistry, University of Alabama, Birmingham, Birmingham, Alabama*

WILLIAM H. KNOSPE • *Section of Hematology, Department of Medicine, Rush-Presbyterian-St Luke's Medical Center, Chicago, Illinois*

MARSHALL A. LICHTMAN • *Department of Medicine, University of Rochester Medical Center, Rochester, New York*

CHARLES H. PACKMAN • *Department of Medicine, University of Rochester Medical Center, Rochester, New York*

ROBERT S. McCUSKEY • *Department of Anatomy, College of Medicine, University of Arizona, Tucson, Arizona*

CHARLES W. PRINCE • *Department of Medicine and Biochemistry, University of Alabama, Birmingham, Birmingham, Alabama*

PETER J. QUESENBERRY • *Department of Medicine, University of Virginia School of Medicine, Charlottesville, VA*

N. T. SHAHIDI • *Department of Pediatrics and Medicine, University of Wisconsin, Madison, Madison, Wisconsin*

MATI SHAKLAI • *Division of Hematology, University of Tel-Aviv, Beilinson Medical Center, Petah Tiqvah, Isreal*

MEHDI TAVASSOLI • *Veterans Administration Medical Center, University of Mississippi School of Medicine, Jackson, Mississippi*

JOHN J. TRENTIN • *Baylor College of Medicine, Houston, Texas*

ESMAIL D. ZANJANI • *V. A. Medical Center, University of Nevada, Reno, Nevada*

DOV ZIPORI • *The Weizmann Institute of Science, Rehovot, Israel*

KENNETH S. ZUCKERMAN • *Division of Hematology–Oncology, University of Alabama, Birmingham, Birmingham, Alabama*

Chapter 1

Hemopoietic Microenvironments

*Historical Perspectives,
Status, and Projections*

John J. Trentin

Introduction

The interesting history of over a century of knowledge of the bone marrow as the seedbed of the blood, a seedbed in which migratory stem cells proliferate and differentiate, has been reviewed by Tavassoli[1] up to the concept of hemopoietic microenvironments first formally presented in 1970.[2] The status of studies on hemopoietic microenvironments in 1974 is presented in a report of a workshop[3] and updated in a concise review in 1983.[4] The present chapter deals with the evolution of the concept of hemopoietic stromal microenvironmental subdivisions within the marrow, spleen and thymus, and the advances in technology and knowledge leading to the discovery that:

1. In the mouse, and presumably humans, there exist throughout adult life pluripotent bone marrow stem cells that can

and do self-renew, proliferate, and differentiate into each of the many hemopoietic and lymphocytic cell lines.

2. The bone marrow and the spleen are each subdivided into multiple hemopoietic microenvironments, the relatively radioresistant stromal cells of which somehow control the self-renewal and differentiation of pluripotent hemopoietic stem cells into each of at least four cell lines, erythropoietic, neutrophilic granulocytopoietic, megakaryocytic, and eosinophilic granulocytopoietic, but in ratios different in the marrow than spleen.

3. Self-renewal and proliferation of the pluripotent hemopoietic stem cell (PHSC) occurs in both the erythroid and neutrophilic granuloid splenic hemopoietic microenvironments (colonies), more so in the latter, despite tremendous pressure for differentiation during radiation recovery. (The inability to dissect and transplant bone marrow hemopoietic colonies precludes direct demonstration for marrow colonies, but other evidence indicates that renewal of PHSC is greater in marrow, in which granulopoietic colonies outnumber erythropoietic colonies 2 to 1, than in spleen in which erythropoietic colonies outnumber granulopoietic colonies 3 to 1.)

4. Endoclonal differentiation within a growing spleen or marrow colony can be changed *abruptly* from erythropoiesis to granulopoiesis as it grows from spleen stroma into bone marrow stroma implanted into the spleen, and vice versa, with a line of demarcation exactly at the junction between spleen and marrow stroma.

5. Microenvironments for the differentiation of pluripotent bone marrow stem cells into T-lymphocytes exist in the thymus, and into B-lymphocytes in the bone marrow.

6. Microenvironments for the differentiation of marrow pluripotent hemopoietic stem cells into mast cell clones exist in the caecum, stomach, mesentery, and skin.

7. Long-term in vitro proliferation of the pluripotent bone marrow stem cell, capable of rescuing lethally irradiated mice and differentiating into each of the several hemopoietic and lymphocytic cell lines, occurs only in intimate cell–cell contact with an adherent layer of bone marrow-derived stromal cells. Self renewal, differentiation, proliferation, and maturation along each cell line is driven by a multiplicity of growth factors, rapidly being elucidated.

The original concept of hemopoietic stromal microenvironments arose to rationalize some paradoxical dilemmas of dogma.[2] Despite much early skepticism, the importance of stromal cell-stem cell microenvironmental interactions in stem cell self-renewal, differentiation, and proliferation, in both the hemopoietic and lymphoid systems, is now widely recognized. The remaining differences pertain largely to interpretations of mechanisms of action, based, in part, on differences between in vivo and in vitro systems. Hopefully, this chapter, volume, and, most assuredly, time will contribute toward resolving these matters.

Definition

It became apparent that the same four types of hemopoietic colonies of monoclonal origin occurred in both the spleen and bone marrow of lethally irradiated mice injected with bone marrow cells, but in different ratios of colony types in each organ, and that the sites of origin of the erythroid, granuloid, and megakaryocytic colonies within the spleen were consistently different from each other. Therefore, the term hemopoietic microenvironments was created to distinguish different microgeographic stromal cell influences within an organ on the pluripotent colony forming stem cells, as opposed to whole organ differences, each of which is composed of the sum of its stromal microenvironments.[5,6] The locations of different stromal hemopoietic microenvironments are indicated by the origin sites of the different types of colonies. The number, arrangement, cell types, and functions of the stromal cells that constitute each of the different kinds of hemopoietic microenvironments are not yet known, but are under intensive investigation. Judging by the close proximity of at least four types of intermingled microenvironments, each within the spleen and bone marrow, it seems likely that a single microenvironment may be composed of relatively few stromal cells. It is apparent that the larger spleen colonies must outgrow their original stromal microenvironment and encompass others.

Radiation Protection by Marrow Transplantation

Great impetus to the sciences of experimental hematology, immunology, and radiobiology was given by the pioneer observations of Leon Jacobsen on the radiation-protective effects of shielding certain parts of the body, or exteriorized spleen, against otherwise lethal total-body irradiation,[7] and protection of whole-body irradiated mice by spleen transplantation.[8] Egon Lorenz quickly extended the radiation-protective effect to bone marrow transplantation and correctly deduced that the protective effect was the result of cellular repopulation rather than a humoral mechanism,[9] a fact soon thereafter proven by different kinds of cell marker studies. That cellular repopulation of irradiated mice extended to the lymphoid as well as the hemopoietic system, was deduced by the discovery that the "secondary disease," after protection with nonisologous bone marrow, was the result of a graft vs host reaction, rather than secondary rejection of transplanted marrow,[10,11] and was first proven by cell marker studies.[12]

The Spleen Colony Assay

Introduction of the spleen colony assay by Till and McCulloch as a direct measure of the radiation sensitivity of normal mouse bone marrow cells[13] and the subsequent demonstration by chromosome marker methods that such spleen colonies were clonal in origin,[14] represented a major development in the technology of bone marrow transplantation studies that would both raise and answer many questions. To date, this represents the only direct method for quantitation of the pluripotent bone marrow stem cell, although it was early apparent, but widely overlooked until recently, that not all spleen colony forming cells (CFU-S) are pluripotent.

Antecedents of the Hemopoietic Microenvironment Concept

Homing

Within a decade and a half after the first report of irradiation protection by bone marrow transplantation,[9] the "homing" of several hemopoietic and lymphoid cell types, each to its proper organ or part of that organ, was generally recognized and taken for granted.[15-19] But few people thought about what constituted "home" for each cell type and why, especially after lethal irradiation had emptied all the rooms of the several "homes." When marrow cells are injected intravenously, the first capillary bed they encounter is in the lungs. But the lungs do not become hemopoietic or lymphocytopoietic, nor do the skeletal muscles or many other body parts to which those injected cells that escape the lungs may be shunted next. Only those stem cells that pass through and encounter their proper "homes" become effectively hemopoietic and lymphocytopoietic. Why? It became an effective teaching tool to show a histological section of the normal spleen or bone marrow and then a section of the "empty" spleen (*See* color Fig. 1 of ref. 2) or the "empty" bone marrow cavity a week after lethal irradiation without marrow transplantation. It did not take much imagination to realize that these organs, and the rest of the hemopoietic and lymphoid system, although relatively "empty," still contained a population of relatively radioresistant stromal cells that had participated in a remarkably effective task of removing and/or recycling a graveyard of cellular debris. Nor did it require much stretch of the imagination to realize that these stromal cells and/or their cellular or extracellular products must still constitute "homes," avidly awaiting their next migrating tenants.

Some specific and unique "homing" pathways have been described. Intravenously injected labeled thoracic duct small lymphocytes, but not large lymphocytes, have been found to leave the circulation by attachment to the uniquely heightened endothelial cells of the post-capillary venules of lymph nodes. They then pass into and through, not between, the endothelial cells and transmigrate into the lymph node.[17] It was suggested early that lymphocytes have surface receptors that recognize the heightened endothelium of these specialized venules.[20,21] The small lymphocytes were shown to be able to bind to the heightened endothelium of even glutaraldehyde-fixed sections of lymph node.[22] In contrast, labeled thoracic duct large lymphocytes injected iv soon left the blood and localized mainly in the wall of the small intestine, where they took on the appearance of the plasma cell line.[17]

Recent research[22a] has revealed that a) both T- and B-lymphocytes are involved in the transendothelial homing into lymphoid organs, b) expression of lymphocyte homing receptors is developmentally regulated during early T- and B-cell development in the thymus or bone marrow, respectively, c) there are at least two independent lymphocyte homing receptors, one for peripheral lymph nodes and another for Peyer's Patches, and d) most antigen-activated lymphocytes transiently downregulate the expression of their organ specific endothelium homing receptors. The lymph node homing receptor is a branched-chain, ubiquitinated cell-surface glycoprotein,[22a] and the lymph node heightened endothelium receptor is a lectin, one of the sugars recognized being mannose-6-phosphate, present either as a single sugar or as part of a 6-phosphomannosyl-conjugated mannan.[22b]

Recent evidence suggests that specific homing of hemopoietic stem cells (HSC) is likewise the result of surface interactions between HSC and the capillary endothelium of hemopoietic tissues. A recognition mechanism, based on the interaction of membrane glycoproteins and lectin-like substances capable of specific interaction with sugar residues of glycoprotein, again appears to be involved.[23-28]

It has been suggested that homing receptor genes may be part of a multigene family involved in cell–cell interactions.[22a] Undoubtedly, many other receptor-mediated homing and cell–cell interaction pathways and mechanisms, involving the many developmental stages of the pluripotent hemopoietic stem cell and its multiple lines of differentiation, will be elucidated. The multiple endothelia and stromal cells of the various hemopoietic and lymphoid organs also will be elucidated.

Unexplained Failure of Marrow Isografts

In 1962, Fernbach and Trentin[29] reported the failure of isologous marrow from a well twin to take in his 3-yr-old identical twin with aplastic anemia that developed after numerous 7–10 d treatments with chloramphenicol during the preceeding 24 mo, plus a 1 wk course of chloramphenicol combined with "triple sulfa" approximately 1 mo prior to onset of severe purpura. Identity of the twins was confirmed by identity of 22 out of 22 blood groups tested and successful cross-transplantation of full thickness skin grafts of 9 mo duration. Yet, the marrow transplantation, done October 30, 1959, was ineffective, as was a second marrow graft from the well twin done December 22, 1959. In reporting the results, we stated "It is possible that in the present patient the bone marrow cavity has been rendered incapable of supporting marrow growth by the initial exposure to, persistence of, or reexposure to an unknown etiologic factor(s). Injury to some hypothetical 'proliferative' or 'homing' factor might be responsible for the persisting bone marrow hypoplasia in this identical twin even after isologous bone marrow transplantation."

Subsequently, purpura became a significant clinical problem and the child was placed on prednisone combined with testosterone enanthate at regular intervals. This therapy was continued for almost 1 yr, during which time the hemoglobin gradually returned to normal levels and transfusions were no longer necessary. The white blood count remained between 3,000 and 5,000, fluctuating frequently, but the platelet count remained 15,000. The medications were discontinued when the hemoglobin remained stable for several months. Thereafter, the boy was followed with regular counts, but the thrombocytopenia persisted. Early in 1964, E. Donnell Thomas of Seattle was consulted regarding what steps of the marrow transplants might have been at fault. He could find none and recommended trying a third marrow transplant from the well twin. Prior to the third try, the patient's hemoglobin was normal, but he was minimally leukopenic. His platelet count remained below 15,000 and he continued to have occasional petechiae and ecchymoses. At the time of the last transplant in June of 1964, his only hematological defect was thrombocytopenia. His bone marrow was moderately cellular with scattered, but decreased, numbers of megakaryocytes and a slight increase in fat content. The third marrow transplant also failed to improve the patient's hematological status. The sequential recovery during steroid therapy, first of his red cell production, then his white blood cell production, but not his platelet count, again suggested that the defect was not of the pluripotent hemopoietic stem cell, but of some hypothetical host factors controlling its differentiation into the erythroid, granulocytic, or megakaryocytic cell lines, or controlling proliferation within each of these cell lines.

In 1982, Nara et al.[30] reported that chloramphenicol (CP), added to in vitro cultures of human bone marrow, suppressed both stem cells, measured by CFU-C, and hemopoietic inductive microenvironments (HIM), measured by CFU-F. To more critically measure the in vivo effect of CP on HIM separately from its effect on CFU-S, they used the subcutaneous mouse femur transplant method of Hotta.[31] The marrow of the implanted femurs, with ends cut off, completely degenerates within 1 wk, but thereafter regenerates and is repopulated by host CFU-S as a function of HIM. Femurs from mice that received six daily injections of CP, and were transplanted into untreated isologous mice, yielded, after 5 wk, 70% as many nucleated cells and only 28% as many CFU-S as similarly transplanted femurs from sham-treated mice.

Spleen Colony Types

Decision

The demonstrated clonality of spleen colonies, in an organ normally highly lymphoid in nature, led us to seek spleen colonies of lymphocytes to test the clonal selection theory of antibody production.[32,33] To our disappointment, none of the spleen colonies were lymphoid in nature. They consisted instead of only four lines of hemopoietic differentiation: erythroid, neutrophilic granuloid, megakaryocytic, and eosinophilic granuloid[2,5,6,34-37] (*see* color Figs. 1–5 of ref. 2). The first report of spleen colonies dealt only with relatively large late colonies that were found to contain mixtures of hemopoietic cells.[13] Because of their evidence that spleen colonies were clonal in origin, but contained mixtures of different hemopoietic cell types and CFU-S in widely different proportions, and because factors controlling decision for differentiation were not known, Till et al.[38] proposed in 1964 a 'stochastic' model of CFU-S self-renewal (birth) or differentiation (death) based solely on numbers of CFU-S detected in 10-d-old and 12-d-old spleen colonies on retransplantation. The numbers of CFU-S per colony were very heterogeneous and fitted a 'gamma' distribution better than a Poisson distribution. They set up a Monte Carlo chance model with any given cell division of the original CFU-S and its self-renewed CFU-S progeny having an arbitrary 60% chance of self-renewal (producing two CFU-S) and a 40% chance of death (producing only terminally differentiated progeny). Two examples of pyramid diagrams were presented showing that, after six generations, one could have as few as two CFU-S, or as many as 10. They conclude that the data suggest a lax, rather than rigid, control of CFU-S self-renewal or differentiation, supporting a probabilistic control mechanism. They state that "If the probabilistic view is found to be correct, it will still be necessary to determine what kind of control mechanisms could act to alter the probabilities and to define their modes of action." Simultaneously, spleen colonies of earlier ages were found by several laboratories to consist usually of a single line of hemopoietic differentiation, with the percentage of mixed colonies increasing with colony age (Table 1).[5,34]

Four-d-old spleen colonies are not yet visible macroscopically, but subserial histological sections of the spleen revealed that 66% of the developing colonies showed only erythropoietic differentiation, 22% only neutrophilic granulopoietic differentiation and 12% were as yet undifferentiated (Table 2).[5] The *erythroid colonies* are the fastest growing and largest colonies and the first to appear grossly visible at 6 d. The slower growing *granulocytic colonies* do not begin to appear grossly visible until 8 d of age. Microscopic *megakaryocytic colonies* appear as separate colonies, at about 6 d, as a cluster of megakaryocytes. Such colonies constitute ± 15% of the total number of colonies. *Colonies of only eosinophilic granulopoiesis* are the rarest (1% or less) of the spleen colonies and, unlike neutrophilic colonies, rarely achieve gross visibility. Thus, unless one performs the laborious procedure of microscopic examination of serial or subserial sections of the entire spleen, one misses two of the four spleen colony types.[5]

At *8 d of colony age*, the percentage of spleen colonies that express erythroid, neutrophilic granuloid, megakaryocytic, or eosinophilic granuloid differentiation, approximates 60, 20, 15, and 1% respectively. For both the erythroid and neutrophilic colonies, immature cells were found more frequently in the periphery, forming a "shell" around the more differentiated central cells. After 8 d, foci of granulopoiesis appeared in the periphery of more and more of the large erythroid colonies, and they were then classified as mixed.[5] At *10 d of colony age*, erythroid colonies were found to have a mean cell number of 873,000, compared to only 298,000 for the neutrophilic granuloid colonies. At the same time, the fewer mixed colonies were the largest, with a mean of 2,120,000 cells, and the histologic appearance of large erythroid colonies that acquired peripheral areas of neutrophilic granulopoiesis, megakaryocytopoiesis, or both[5], which appearance was noted also in the original report of mixed spleen colonies by Till and McCulloch.[13] This was our first clue that the initial limitation of erythroid colonies to a single line of differentiation was more a function of size (distance from the center of origin to the peripheral area of secondary differentiation) than of time *per se*.

Table 1

Percentage of the Various Types of Spleen Colonies as Reported in the Literature[a]

Source of CFU	Identification Method	Colony age, d	Percent of Colony Types[b]					Reference
			Ery.	Gran.	Meg.	Un.	Mixed	
Transplanted Bone Marrow	Histological sections	9	42	21	21	NC[c]	16	Lewis and Trobaugh (1964)
		9	47	22	19	NC	12	Trobaugh and Lewis (1964)
		10	45	14	18	NC	23	Juraskova et al. (1964)
		10	50	20	0	NC	30	Mekori and Feldman (1965)
		10	35	15	6	16	28	Schooley (1964)
		8	68	25	NC	NC	7	Curry et al. (1964)
	Stained smears	10	62	17	0	NC	21	Juraskova et al (1964)
Endogenous	Histological sections	10	75	0	0	NC	25	Mekori and Feldman (1965)
Peripheral leukocytes	Histological sections	9	36	36	24	19	12	Trobaugh and Lewis (1964)

[a]After Curry, J. L. and Trentin, J. J. (1967) *Developmental Biology* 15, 395–413.
[b]Ery., erythoid: Gran., granulocytic; Meg., megakaryocyte; Un., undifferentiated.
[c]NC, colonies of this cell type not counted.

Table 2

Effect of Colony Age and Method of Identification on Number and Type of Spleen colonies Found[a]

Expt. No.	Method of study	Colony age, d	Number of spleens	Total colonies counted	Mean total colony count per spleen		Percent of colony types[c]				
					Gross	Microscopic	Ery.	Gran.	Meg.	Un.	Mixed
1	Gross counts only	4	6	0	0	ND[b]	ND	ND	ND	ND	ND
	Histological sections	4	6	49	5.1	8.2	66	22	0	12	0
2	Dissect out and imprint	6	10	51	8.4	ND	100	0	0	0	0
		9	12	101	8.9	ND	72	17	0	0	11
		12	11	98	8.9	ND	23	9	0	0	68
	Histological sections	6	11	129	4.9	11.7	59	23	1	7	10
		9	10	113	8.1	11.3	52	17	10	5	16
		12	12	145	9.3	12.1	31	10	12	0	47

[a] Each (C57 × Af) F_1 mouse received 850 R and 8×10^4 viable isogenic nucleated bone marrow cells. After Curry, J. L. and Trentin, J. J. (1967) *Developmental Biology* **15**, 395–413.

[b] ND, Not done.

[c] Ery., erythroid; Gran., granulocytic; Meg., megakaryocyte; Un., undifferentiated.

This repeatedly observed, strikingly different, but, consistent ratio of the four spleen colony types, each limited for a prolonged period and a size of over a million cells to only one line of hemopoietic differentiation, was so nonrandom that it raised questions about the pluripotency of CFU-S or the stochastic theory of pluripotent stem cell decision for differentiation, or both. We were forced to consider the possibility that each spleen colony was formed by a committed stem cell, and that the late appearance of mixing on the periphery of the largest colonies occurred by confluence or transmigration.

Spleen Colony Retransplantation

If CFU-S are monocommitted, then retransplantation of cells from individual early colonies of only erythropoietic or of granulopoietic differentiation, each into a secondary irradiated mouse, should lead to repopulation with only one line of hemopoietic differentiation. Lewis and Trobaugh transplanted half of each of nine erythroid spleen colonies, 10-d-old, into a single irradiated mouse. Nine days later, six of the nine secondary spleens were found to contain colonies of either erythroid, granuloid, or megakaryocytic type, or of mixtures thereof.[39] We transplanted larger numbers of erythroid and also granuloid spleen colonies, of different ages, each into an individual secondary irradiated recipient.[6] At 7 d of primary colony age, the granuloid colonies are not yet large enough to see and dissect out; the erythroid colonies are. All 12 of the retransplanted, 7-d-old erythroid colonies failed to give secondary spleen colonies (Table 3). At 9 and 10 d of primary colony age, some or all of both erythroid and granuloid retransplanted colonies yielded secondary colonies. Although the granuloid colonies contain only about one-third as many cells as the erythroid colonies, a higher percentage of the granuloid colonies of either age gave secondary colonies than did erythroid colonies of the

Table 3
Number and Types of Secondary Progeny Spleen Colonies
Formed by Transplantation of Individual Primary Spleen
Colonies of a Single Differentiation Line Into an
850 R-Irradiated Secondary Recipient[a]

Primary Spleen Colony Age, d	Primary Spleen Colony Type	No. of Primary Colonies Transplanted	% Giving Secondary Progeny Colonies	Overall Mean Progeny Colonies Per Primary Colony ± SEM	% of Progeny Colonies Predominantly Erythroid
7	Erythroid	12	0	0	
7	Granuloid	0[b]	–	–	
9	Erythroid	47	55	2.0 ± 0.37	79
9	Granuloid	13	69	4.7 ± 1.0	60
10	Erythroid	31	74	> 4.8[c]	76
10	Granuloid	19	100	>17.4[d]	63[e]

[a]After Curry, J. L., Trentin, J. J., and Wolf, N. (1967) *Jour. Exp. Med.* **125**, 703–720.

[b]Too small to dissect out.

[c]Two of 31 primary colonies yielded too many secondary colonies to count accurately (>20).

[d]Eleven of 19 primary colonies yielded too many secondary colonies to count accurately (>20).

[e]$p < .01$ for significance of difference in the percent erythroid progeny of erythroid vs granuloid primary colonies, by X^2 test.

same age, and the overall mean number of secondary spleen colonies was higher per granuloid than per erythoid primary colony! This indicated a higher level of CFU-S renewal in granuloid than in erythroid colony microenvironments. Both erythroid and granuloid primary colonies gave both erythroid and granuloid secondary colonies. Indeed, 60–63% of erythroid progeny colonies of granuloid primary colonies was the same as if normal marrow cells had been transfused. But 76–79% of erythroid progeny colonies of erythroid primary colonies was slightly, but significantly, increased ($p < .01$). We attributed this to the probability that "some colonies may be formed by cells already monocommitted to either the erythroid or granuloid cell line."[6]

This seemed confirmed by the facts that a) among spleen colonies formed by transplantation of spleen cell suspensions rather than marrow cell suspensions, there is a much higher ratio of erythroid to granuloid colonies (Table 4),[40, 41] b) the number of CFU-S required to reduce radiation mortality from 100 to 50% (therapeutic efficiency) of spleen-derived CFU-S is only half as much as bone marrow-derived CFU-S,[42] and c) marrow CFU-S are twice as effective as spleen-derived CFU-S in giving rise to daughter CFU-S.[43] Interestingly, the E:G colony ratio of spleen-derived hemopoietic colonies growing in bone marrow was as low as marrow-derived hematopoietic colonies (Table 5).[40]

Spleen cells injected into intermediate irradiated mice, then recovered within 2-1/2 h from the spleen and marrow, and injected into secondary irradiated mice, behaved as spleen CFU-S, i.e., gave a high proportion of erythroid colonies in the spleen and a low proportion of erythroid colonies in the marrow of the secondary mice, regardless of whether they were recovered from the intermediate host's spleen or marrow (Table 6).[40] These results indicate that the higher proportions of erythroid, rather than granuloid colonies given by CFU in the spleen, but not in the marrow of a primary irradiated recipient, is not a result of selective migration of erythroid-committed CFU-S to the spleen rather than the marrow. The erythroid-committed spleen CFU-S are not altered in their secondary

Table 4
Proportion of Erythropoietic and Granulopoietic Colonies
(E:G ratios) in Spleens of Irradiated (1100 R) Mice
Injected with Spleen or Bone Marrow Cells[a,b]

Expt. No.	Donor Cells[c]	No. Mice	No. Col.	Percent Ery.	Percent Gran.	E:G Ratio	E:G Ratio Diff.	Sig. Level
1	B.M.	7	91	45.1	26.4	1.7		
	Spleen	8	79	75.9	8.9	8.6	5.1	$p < .005$
2	B.M.	6	61	44.3	34.4	1.3		
	Spleen	6	52	75.0	13.4	5.6	4.3	$p < .005$
3	B.M.	6	69	59.4	21.7	2.7		
	Spleen	5	31	87.1	3.2	27.0	10.0	$p < .025$
4	B.M.	5	54	59.3	31.5	1.9		
	Spleen	6	28	78.6	7.1	11.0	5.8	$p < .05$
5	B.M.	6	59	62.7	13.0	4.6		
	Spleen	6	40	80.0	10.0	8.0	1.7	$p < .05$

[a]After Wolf, N. S., Jenkins, V. K., and Trentin, J. J. (1972) *Exper. Hematol.* 22, 37, 38.

[b]Donor and recipient mice were 3–4-mo-old (C57 BL6 × A)F$_1$ hybrids maintained in a specific pathogen-free colony. Spleens were removed for examination 8 d after irradiation and hemopoietic cell transplantation.

[c]5×10^4 bone marrow cells or 5×10^5 spleen cells were injected via the lateral tail vein.

colony types in spleen vs marrow by 2-1/2 h of residence in the marrow of an intermediate mouse, and the spleen stroma is more conducive to the growth of an erythroid-committed CFU-S into an erythroid hemopoietic colony than is the marrow stroma.

Unfortunately, this and other evidence that not all CFU-S are pluripotent was either unknown to or ignored by most investigators, who persisted in speaking of CFU-S as "the"

Table 5

Erythropoietic to Granulopoietic (E:G) Colony Ratios in Spleens
and Bone Marrow of Irradiated (1000–1100 R) Mice Injected
with Spleen or Bone Marrow Cells[a]

	Spleen			Bone Marrow		
Donor[b]	No. Mice	No. Colonies	E:G Ratios	No. Mice	No. Colonies	E:G Ratios
B. M.	11	134	2.2	10	33	0.6
Spleen	27	303	9.0	27	44	0.9

[a]Donor and recipient mice were 3- to 4-mo-old (C57 Bl6 × A)F$_1$ hybrid mice maintained in a specific pathogen-free or conventional colony. The colonies were counted 7–8 d after irradiation and hemopoietic cell injection. The data were combined from three experiments, only one of which contained bone marrow-injected mice. After Wolf, N. S., Jenkins, V. K., and Trentin J. J. (1972) *Exper. Hematol.* **22**, 37, 38.

[b]5×10^4 bone marrow cells or 5×10^5 spleen cells were injected via the lateral tail vein.

pluripotent hemopoietic stem cell, despite many occasions at national and international meetings when attention was called to their heterogeneity, ignored, that is, until the Magli, Iscove, Odartchenko publication[44] to be discussed later.

Effect of Erythropoietin Deprivation on Spleen Colony Types

At this point, we were confronted with a dilemma. The data on spleen colony types indicated that CFU-S were committed. The data on spleen colony retransplantation indicated that they were pluripotent. More questions needed to be asked of and answered by the spleen colonies.

If most CFU-S are indeed pluripotent stem cells, and the splenic environment is conducive to their commitment and ex-

Table 6

Erythropoietic to Granulopoietic (E:G) Colony Ratios in Spleens
and Bone Marrow of Irradiated (1000–1100 R) Mice Injected
with Hemopoietic Stem Cells from Intermediate Hosts[a]

Inter. Donor Cells[b]	Spleen			Bone Marrow		
	No. Mice	No. Colonies	E:G Ratio	No. Mice	No. Colonies	E:G Ratio
B.M.	6	10	10	6	5	1.0
Spleen	12	78	11.7	12	14	0.8

[a]Donor, intermediate hosts and final recipients were 3- to 4 mo–old (C57 Bl6 × A)F$_1$ hybrid mice. The final recipients were sacrificed 7 d after irradiation and hemopoietic cell injection, and the numbers and types of colonies determined. After Wolf, N. S., Jenkins, V. K. and Trentin, J. J. (1972) *Exper. Hematol.* **22**, 37, 38.

[b]The intermediate donors were irradiated and injected with 5×10^7 spleen cells, sacrificed within 2.5 h, and 0.4–0.8% of the total number of spleen cells or 0.8–1.6% of the total number of cells from both femurs were injected into each final recipient.

pression of four lines of hemopoietic differentiation, what would happen if erythropoiesis is blocked by erythropoietin-deprivation brought about by hypertransfusion-induced polycythemia before and during spleen colony growth? Presumably the 60% of the pluripotent CFU-S that ordinarily would become erythroid colonies, would now be free to become granuloid or megakaryocytic colonies.

Results from several laboratories were in agreement that polycythemia prevented the appearance of most or all spleen colonies and that exogenous erythropoietin (EPO) prevented this effect, permitting normal numbers, but not more, of erythroid colonies to develop.[6,34,45–49] Some early reports suggested a shunting of the polycythemia-suppressed erythroid spleen colonies to other types of differentiation.[45,47,50] Our own data showed only a slight increase in the number of granuloid colonies.[34,51] We wondered if this slight increase was real, or secondary to loss of erythropoiesis in what would otherwise have been classified as a mixed erythroid and granuloid colony. We undertook additional experiments.

Visualization of Erythropoietin-Sensitive Stem Cell Colonies

What had become of the missing erythroid colonies? Was it possible that careful histological examination of serial or subserial spleen sections would reveal small, undernourished erythroid colonies?

An experiment was set up with 20 normocythemic and 20 polycythemic irradiated recipient mice, the latter kept polycythemic by a third hypertransfusion 4 d postirradiation and marrow injection. At 8 d, the spleens were harvested and approximately 40 subserial longitudinal histological sections, at 50 μm intervals, were made through each of the 40 spleens. Careful microscopic examination did, indeed, reveal the missing colonies, but they were not erythroid. They were microscopic foci estimated to consist of only 100–200 undifferentiated cells (Fig. 1). The increase in the number of such undifferentiated colonies, vs the control group, matched the number of missing erythroid colonies, 189–187 (Table 7). The slight increase in the number of neutrophilic granuloid colonies in polycythemic mice was accounted for by the decrease in the number of mixed erythroid plus granuloid colonies, owing to the absence of erythropoiesis, causing them to be classified as granuloid only.[6] This gave the important answer that either the CFU-S of erythroid colonies were all precommitted, or that in an erythroid microenvironment of the spleen, the progeny of a pluripotent CFU-S, not called on by EPO to differentiate, could not divert to a different line of hemopoiesis, such as granulopoiesis or megakaryocytopoiesis even though other similar pluripotent CFU-S that had lodged only millimeters away in

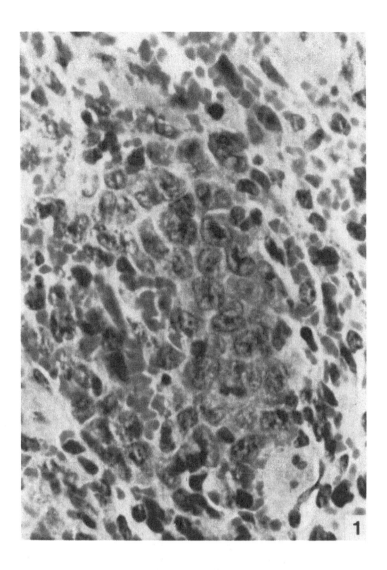

Fig. 1. Small, undifferentiated colony appearing as the predominant colony type in the spleens of polycythemic mice, 8 d postirradiation (900 R whole body) and isologous marrow injection (6×10^4 viable nucleated cells). Because of their small size and fairly nondescript characteristics, these colonies are difficult to find at low magnification. Cells are characterized by abundant, pale, reticulated cytoplasm, large nuclei with a peripheral chromatin distribution, and one or several very prominent nucleoli. Generally they fit description of the hemohistioblast traditionally believed to be the marrow "stem cell" (Hematoxylin and eosin, × 1975) (Curry, J. L., Trentin, J. J., and Wolf, N. (1967) *J. Exp. Med.* **125,** 703–720, courtesy of The Rockefeller University Press; and Gordon, A. (1970) *Regulation of Hematopoiesis*, courtesy of Appleton-Century-Crofts).

Table 7
Survey of All Types of Microscopically Identifiable 8-Day Colonies in the Spleens
of Control and Polycythemic Mice Receiving 900 R and 12×10^4 Isologous Marrow Cells[a]

Group	No. of spleens	Mean gross counts	Ery.[b]	Neut.[b]	Eos.[b]	Meg.[b]	Undiff.[b]	Mixed				Total
								Ery. + N	Ery. + M	N + M	Ery. + N + M	
Controls	20	11.5	193	74	1	51	18	23	9	6	3	378
Polycythemic	20	4.2	6	83	2	68	207	2	0	9	0	377

[a] After Curry, J. L., Trentin, J. J., and Wolf, N. (1967) J. Exp. Med. 125, 703–720.
[b] Ery. = Erythroid; neut. = N = neutrophilic; eos. = eosinophilic; meg. = M = megakaryocytic; and undiff. = undifferentiated.

the same spleen were developing into granuloid or megakaryocyte colonies!

In additional experiments in which erythropoietin was administered to polycythemic mice during only the last 4 d of colony growth, these tiny, undifferentiated colonies were converted into intermediate-sized pan-erythroid colonies containing up to 100,000 cells in all stages of erythropoiesis (*see* Fig. 4 of ref. 6). In contrast, if erythropoietin was given only during the first 4 d of colony growth, these tiny, undifferentiated colonies were converted to intermediate-sized undifferentiated colonies containing an estimated 5000–10,000 cells (Fig. 2). These experiments permitted visualization, for the first time, of colonies of the erythropoietin-sensitive stem cells, which cells, indirect evidence indicated must exist.[52-55] The colonies of Figs. 1 and 2 must be composed largely of both erythropoietin-sensitive and pluripotent stem cells.

Decision for Lineage-Specific Differentiation

These latter experiments would have an added great significance regarding decision for differentiation if some of the CFU-S were indeed pluripotent stem cells, since the CFU-S themselves were known not to be responsive to erythropoietin.[52-55] If the CFU-S of origin of an erythroid colony is pluripotent, then these experiments demonstrated that within the first few days of its residence in an erythroid microenvironment of the spleen, its few hundred progeny cells had acquired responsiveness to erythropoietin. This would indicate that decision for erythropoiesis in an erythroid microenvironment is not random or lax, but rigidly controlled by microenvironmental factors.

Because of the obvious importance of resolving the question of whether CFU-S were pluripotent or monocommitted,

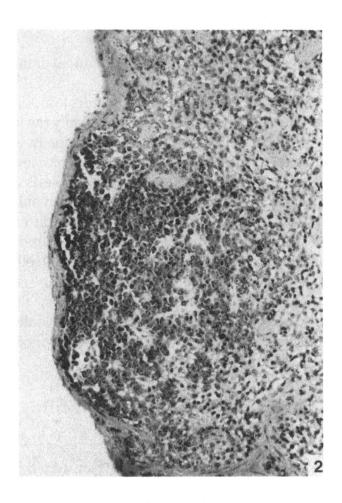

Fig. 2. Intermediate size undifferentiated colony; microphotograph of a polycythemic mouse spleen receiving 900 R whole body x-irradiation, daily injections of sheep erythropoietin (ESF) for first 4 d postirradiation, and a third hypertransfusion 4 d postirradiation; sacrificed after 8 d. This type of colony, characteristic of such a treatment schedule, is significantly larger than very small undifferentiated colony, yet shows no differentiated elements. It is postulated that the four doses of ESF caused both an increased rate of proliferation and waves of differentiation, but during the 4 d of polycythemia without ESF stimulation, differentiating elements completed the maturation process and entered the circulation, leaving only proliferating, undifferentiated, but ESF-sensitive cells in the colony (Hematoxylin and eosin, × 380) (Curry, J. L., Trentin, J. J., and Wolf, N. (1967) *J. Exp. Med.* **125**, 703–720, courtesy of The Rockefeller University Press; and Gordon, A. (1970) *Regulation of Hematopoiesis*, courtesy of Appleton-Century-Crofts).

we used T6 chromosome-marked bone marrow suspensions to determine directly whether the peripheral appearance of a second differentiation line within an enlarging spleen colony arose from within the clone, or from adjacent colonies of a different type, by transmigration of cells or fusion of colonies.

Endoclonal Origin of the Second Line of Differentiation

Irradiated mice were injected with a 50/50 mixture of bone marrow from mice with or without two T6 marker chromosomes, designated T6$^+$ and T6$^-$, respectively. Spleen colonies were harvested at d 7, 10, 11, and 12, and each colony was examined for the percentage of erythroid and granuloid cells in Giemsa-stained imprints, and karyotyped for the number of T6$^+$ and T6$^-$ mitotic cells.[56] All 49 of the 7-d-old colonies and all six of the 10-d-old colonies were a single line of hemopoietic differentiation. Of these 55 colonies, 53 were of single T6 karyotype, approximately half of them T6$^+$ and half T6$^-$. The remaining two colonies had only a minor component of mitotic cells bearing the second karyotype (1$^+$, 76$^-$ and 58$^+$, 2$^-$) (Table 8).

Results of the 11- and 12-d-old colonies were pooled. Of these, 45 still had a single line of differentiation and 48 were mixed erythroid and granuloid. The great majority of these late colonies of either single or mixed differentiation lines contained only a single T6 karyotype, roughly half of them T6$^+$ and half T6$^-$ (Table 9). Of the 48 colonies of mixed erythroid and granuloid cytology, if the second differentiation line had entered by fusion or migration from other colonies, it should have introduced the second karyotype in approximately half of the cases. Instead, 43 of 48 had only a single karyotype, with the second karyotype represented again by only 1–3 cells, except in one mixed colony with 11 of the 71 mitoses showing a second karyotype. In none of the 48 mixed colonies, in which the per-

Table 8

Relationship of Cytology to T6 Karyotype
of Spleen Colonies Arising in Irradiated Mice
Receiving a 50/50 mixture of T6$^+$ and T6$^-$ Bone Marrow Cells[a]

Colony age, d	No. of Colonies	Hematologic cell lines of differentiation	T6 karyotype, No. of colonies	
			Single	Mixed[b]
7	49	single	47	2(1+/76-, 58+/2-)
10	6	single	6	0
11–12	45	single	42	3(73+/1-, 1+/65-, 22+/1-)
11–12	48	mixed	43	5(72+/1-, 1+/45-, 3+/180-, 50+/1-, 60+/11-)

[a]After Trentin, J. J. (1971) *Am. J. Path.* **65**, 621–628.
[b]Numbers in parentheses are No. of cells in each mixed colony.

centage of erythroid and granuloid cells ranged widely from predominantly erythroid to predominantly granuloid, did the percentage of T6$^+$ and T6$^-$ cells resemble the percentage of erythroid or granuloid cells (Table 9). These data reaffirmed past evidence that spleen colonies are clonal in origin and clearly and directly indicated that the late appearing second differentiation line arose from within the clone of origin of the colony and the CFU-S of origin must, of necessity, have been pluripotent in at least most of the spleen colonies. The pluripotent CFU-S of origin must, of necessity, have undergone self-renewal as well as committing others of its progeny to the first line of differentiation, and most important, the differentiation of the CFU-S of origin and its pluripotent progeny is somehow limited initially to a single line of hemopoiesis, apparently by its initial microenvironment.

Chen and Schooley used marrow from irradiation chimeric mice bearing three kinds of chromosome-marked cells in their bone marrow and also obtained results reaffirming the clonal origin of spleen colonies. Unfortunately, they did not

Table 9
Comparison of the Percent of Erythroid and Granuloid Cells
in Spleen Colonies of "Mixed" Type with the Number
of T6[+] and T6[-] Cells in that Colony[a]

Differential, %		Karyotype, No. of Cells	
Erythroid	Granuloid	T6[+]	T6[-]
62	8	0	47
64	2	0	15
67	5	0	85
60	5	0	33
76	11	0	16
32	44	0	46
45	32	0	105
3	45	0	19
38	27	0	60
60	17	0	92
45	27	0	58
69	11	0	152
74	5	122	0
75	2	32	0
42	9	40	0
71	4	22	0
53	21	35	0
55	6	16	0
57	11	34	0
44	6	67	0
59	15	77	0
39	28	72	1
41	9	50	1
71	3	1	45
62	3	3	180
29	42	60	11

[a]Each of the 26 lines represents one 11- or 12-d-old spleen colony from the group of 48 mixed spleen colonies of Table 8. After Trentin, J. J. (1971) *Am. J. Path.* **65,** 621–628.

study the type or types of hemopoietic differentiation in the spleen colonies that they karyotyped.[58]

The Working Hypothesis

In 1964, on the basis of preliminary evidence, we reported to the old "Bone Marrow Transplantation Group" (the forerunner of the International Society for Experimental Hematology) that spleen "colony forming units (CFU's) are not all pluripotential stem cell, but rather that under these conditions most CFU's are committed to the erythroid series (or become quickly committed following lodgment in the spleen, perhaps as a result of microenvironmental influences), are nevertheless dependent on endogenous or exogenous erythropoietin to develop into a colony, and if prevented by hypertransfusion from developing into an erythroid colony, do not develop into colonies of other cell types." This appeared in a publication of the Biology Division of Oak Ridge National Laboratory called Experimental Hematology[34] the forerunner of the current journal of the same name that is the official publication of the International Society for Experimental Hematology.

In 1967, on the basis of further data, we proposed as a working hypothesis[6] that "most but perhaps not all spleen colony-forming units are pluripotent hemopoietic stem cells. It is further postulated that hemopoietic-inductive microenvironments (HIM) of different kinds exist in both the spleen and bone marrow, and that these determine the differentiation of pluripotent stem cells into each of the lines of hemopoietic differentiation. Erythropoietin therefore may 'induce' erythroid differentiation of only those stem cells under the influence of an erythroid HIM. Alternatively erythropoietin may act only as a growth and function stimulant of those stem cells that have been 'induced' by an erythroid HIM into a state of erythropoietin responsiveness. In the latter case morphological differentiation presumably results from the functional activity stimulated by ESF." In speculating on the nature of HIM, we stated that: "Hormones in general stimulate mitosis and/or secretion by target cells that have been 'induced' into a state of hormone responsiveness by a prior local induction phenomenon classically involving specific mesenchyme as the inducer."[6] In today's state of knowledge, acquistion of responsiveness to a hormone or growth factor is synonymous with acquisition of receptors for the hormone or growth factor.

Tests of the Working Hypothesis

Bone Marrow Colonies and Characteristics

About this time, we wondered whether repopulation of the marrow was similarly colonial, and, if so, what types of colonies appeared in the marrow and in what proportion. Since the marrow was known to be more granulopoietic than erythropoietic, would there be relatively more granuloid colonies? Because marrow regeneration could not be seen as grossly visible or easily dissectible colonies, such as those occurring in the spleen, we undertook the laborious task of fixing, decalcifying, and subserial sectioning four long bones (femurs and tibias) and the sternum of each mouse used in spleen colony studies. Discrete foci of hemopoietic repopulation (bone marrow 'colonies') were found in the marrow, just as in the spleen. Their numbers were, like spleen colonies, also directly proportional to the number of marrow cells injected intravenously, and so were presumably also clonal in origin.[37] Like spleen colonies, they were again of a single differentiation type and the same four types as in the spleen (*see* Figs. 6–10 of ref. 2). But one major difference was immediately apparent. Instead of erythroid colonies outnumbering granuloid colonies by approximately 3 to 1, granuloid colonies outnumbered erythroid colonies by a factor of about 2 to 1. For uniformity of expression, we began using the term E to G colony ratio, i.e., the E:G ratio of spleen colonies is approximately 3 and of marrow colonies, it is approximately 0.5.[2,37]

Ever wary about the question of pluripotency vs mono-commitment of CFU, we wondered if CFU-BM might be comprised of a high percentage of granuloid-committed colony precursors that 'home' to the bone marrow to account for the lower E:G colony ratio among marrow colonies. Therefore, we reharvested the marrow cells that had 'homed' to the bone marrow 18–24 h after iv injection into primary irradiated recipients and retransplanted them intravenously into secondary irradiated recipients. They again 'homed' to both the spleen and marrow, giving E:G ratios in each characteristic of the organ, just as if normal marrow cells had been injected for the first time. The results did not indicate a selective homing of pre-committed cells, but rather a difference in the organ stromal influence on pluripotent stem cell differentation.[2,37]

Hemopoietic Colony Characteristics in Transplanted Spleen or Bone Marrow Stroma

Whole Spleen Transplantation

Groups of mice were transplanted subcutaneously (sc) with 4, 8, or 16 isologous whole adult spleens and allowed 60 d to revascularize and repair the ischemic damage that ensued. The mice were then lethally irradiated and injected iv with 6×10^4 isologous marrow cells. The transplanted spleens developed spleen colonies with the same ratio of erythroid colonies to granuloid colonies as the spleen *in situ*, i.e., 3.5, whereas the E:G ratio of the colonies that developed in the bone marrow *in situ* in these same mice was 0.7. Although each transplanted spleen before irradiation was only 1/5 the size and weight of a normal spleen, in those mice with 16 subcutaneous spleens, the aggregate number of colonies therein was slightly more than twice the number of colonies in the spleen *in situ*. The individual colonies in the transplanted spleens were, however, smaller than those in the spleen *in situ*.[37] The average number of colonies per mouse in both spleen *in situ* and marrow of the five bones of the four groups of this experiment with 0, 4, 8, or 16 (sc) transplanted spleens was fairly uniform, i.e., 11.9, 10.7, 12.6, and 10.4, respectively. The average number of additional colonies per mouse in the 4, 8, or 16 transplanted spleens of the last three groups was 5.6, 6.4, and 17.6. This indicates that the more hemopoietic organ stroma available, the more of the injected CFU's find "fertile soil" and express themselves as hemopoietic colonies. It further suggests that there may not be continuous recirculation until most or all injected CFU's find a home, in which case one would have expected to find progressively fewer colonies in the spleen *in situ*, plus the marrow, as the number of transplanted spleens competing for circulating CFU's increased.[37]

These experiments demonstrated that the capacity of the spleen stroma to 'trap' circulating CFU-S and promote hemopoietic colony growth survived surgical transplantation, without benefit of vascular anastamosis. Tavassoli et al.[59,60] reported that subcutaneously transplanted pieces of rat or mouse spleen were reconstituted from a thin peripheral strip of surviving splenic tissue. Wolf later studied the effect of ligation of the vascular stalk of the spleen *in situ*. He documented the ischemic degeneration that resulted, followed by regeneration of the characteristic spleen stroma, starting from the spleen capsule and proceeding centrally to architectural completion within 40 d. Extramedullary hematopoiesis returned as soon as stromal reconstruction was complete, always found just behind the leading edge of the new stromal ingrowth, and seemed always to precede restoration of the lymphoid components.[61] Tavassoli et al.[62] reported that following in vitro irradiation of pieces of rat spleen with 500, 1000, or 1500 rad, the percentage that regenerated following subcutaneously autoimplantation was 100, 70, and 0, respectively.

Wolf[63] studied the limits of regeneration of mouse spleen hemopoietic microenvironmental functions following either irradiation or ligation of the blood supply, or a combination of both. Spleen colony number, size, type, ^{59}Fe uptake, and microscopic study of splenic structure were used as means of assessment. The most severe or least repaired damage was induced by high dose irradiation (4000 rads), by 1000 rads followed immediately by splenic ligation, and by two successive splenic ligations separated by a 30-d recovery period. It was seen that reduction of CFU-S lodgment, as measured by f factor, played a very major role in the lesser number of spleen colonies formed after either kind of damage. Following the several treatments, the numbers of spleen colonies formed, their size and typing as erythrocytic or granulocytic, varied independently of each other, suggesting that these functions of the microenvironment and the cell types responsible for them, are independent of each other. The exhaustion of regenerative capacity, displayed by repeatedly ligated spleens, suggested a maximal limit for stromal cell replications commensurate with Hayflick's hypothesis.

Intact Marrow Stroma Transplantation

Primary recipient mice, irradiated by 1000 R, were given 2.5×10^6 to 3×10^7 isologous marrow cells iv and sacrificed 18–24 h later. A femur was cracked open and pieces, as much as possible, of a single femoral marrow stroma (usually 1/4–1/2) was implanted by trocar into the spleens of 1000 R irradiated isologous secondary recipients. Marrow cells, flushed from the opposite femur of the primary recipient, were injected iv into another irradiated secondary recipient. The marrow fragments, being in a highly vascular site, sustained hemopoietic colony growth and, as hoped, some of their CFU-S also migrated into the spleen stroma (Fig. 3) (*see* also Fig. 11 of ref. 2). In three pooled experiments, those that grew primarily in the implanted marrow stroma gave a preponderance of granuloid colonies (E:G colony ratio of 0.1) as did those that migrated to the bones of the secondary host (E:G colony ratio = 0.3). Those that grew in the spleen gave a preponderance of erythroid colonies (E:G colony ratio of 2.4). In another set of experiments, the protocol was such that CFU'S were required to migrate from the spleen into the implanted irradiated pieces of marrow stroma, with similar results. In both sets of experiments, the most revealing result related to the 19 mixed colonies that straddled the border, growing partly in marrow stroma and partly in spleen stroma. In every case, that portion of the colony proliferating in the spleen stroma was erythropoietic and the portion in the marrow stroma was granulopoietic! (Fig. 4) (*see* also Figs. 5 and 7 of ref. 37, and Fig. 12 of ref. 2). This permitted direct visualization of what the earlier experiments had indicated, i.e., the important influence of hemopoietic organ stromal microenvironments on the type of hemopoiesis within a pluripotent hemopoietic stem cell clone.

Whole Spleen Stroma Transplant 'Cure' of Sl/Sl^d Anemia

At the UTMD Anderson Symposium in 1967, James Till spoke of the genetically determined macrocytic anemia of Sl/Sl^d mutant mice that have normal CFU-S and elevated erythropoietin, but cannot support normal erythropoiesis.[64] At the same symposium and later on, I postulated that their anemia might result from a deficit of the erythroid HIM.[65,2] Both Seldon Bernstein[66] and I[56] tested this by transplantation of whole spleens from +/+ or Sl/+ nonanemic littermates into Sl/Sl^d anemic mice. Whereas normal marrow or spleen cell suspensions from such donors, injected intravenously into Sl/Sl^d

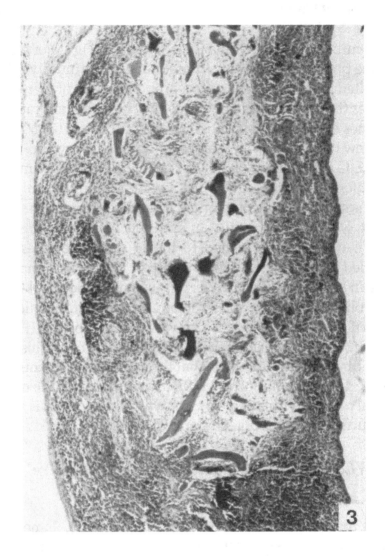

Fig. 3. Spleen containing a trocar implant of bone marrow stroma. Limits of the marrow stromal graft are evident from the bone spicules and less dense stroma of the marrow graft. The marrow stromal graft was obtained 18–24 h after 1000 R whole body irradiation followed by iv injection of a bone marrow cell suspension. It was then trocar-implanted directly into the spleen of a 1000 R-irradiated secondary recipient. The spleen was harvested 7 d later. The only source of CFU's in the secondary recipient of this experiment is the bone marrow stromal implant. Hemopoietic colonies are developing both in the marrow implant and the adjacent spleen. Some colonies straddle the border between marrow implant and spleen (Hematoxylin and eosin, × 92) (Wolf, N. S. and Trentin, J. J. (1968) *J. Exp. Med.* **127,** 205–214, courtesy of The Rockefeller University Press).

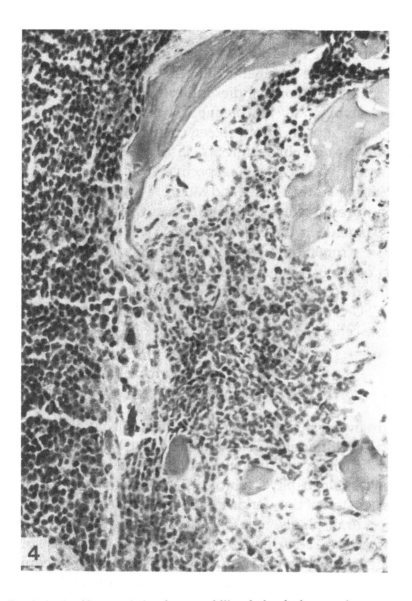

Fig. 4. A mixed hemopoietic colony straddling the border between bone marrow stromal implant and adjacent spleen. In this experiment, 1000 R-irradiated bone marrow stroma, plus a 1 mm piece of unirradiated spleen, were trocar-implanted into the spleen of a 1000 R-irradiated recipient. The only source of CFU's was the 1 mm unirradiated spleen graft. Note that the portion of the colony in the spleen stroma (left and upper) is erythropoietic, whereas the portion in the marrow stroma (right and lower) is granulopoietic (Hematoxylin and eosin, × 375) (Wolf, N. S. and Trentin, J. J. (1968) *J. Exp. Med.* **127**, 205–214, courtesy of The Rockefeller University Press).

mice, does not cure their anemia, transplantation of intact spleens from the nonanemic littermates did 'cure' their anemia.[56,66] Spleen colony studies indicated that irradiated Sl/Sl[d] mice receiving 1×10^5 nonanemic Sl/+ marrow cells did indeed have a deficit of erythroid spleen colonies, compared to their similarly treated nonanemic Sl/+ littermates, 1 erythroid colony/spleen vs 5.9/spleen, respectively.[56]

Subsequently, Dexter and Moore,[57] using long-term marrow cultures in which CFU-S self-renewal and differentiation is dependent on an interaction with an adherent layer of marrow stromal cells, were able to duplicate the stromal cell defect of the Sl/Sl[d] mouse and the stem cell defect of W/W[v] mice, and "cure" each in terms of total nonadherent cells and total CFU-C produced per culture over 6 wk by adding Sl/Sl[d] marrow cells to W/W[v] adherent cells.

Effect of Mouse Hemopoietic Microenvironments on Rat CFU-S

In several studies performed in rats, spleen colonies were reported to differentiate only along the erythroid line or remain partly or wholly undifferentiated.[67] Could it be that the rat spleen contained only erythroid HIM? We envisioned a possible severe test of the working hypothesis based on xenogeneic marrow transplants, mouse to rat and rat to mouse. Using Lewis rats, we confirmed the fact that their isologous spleen colonies exhibited only erythroid differentiation and required 11–12 d to grow to grossly visible size, rather than 8 d for the mouse to mouse spleen colonies. Increasing numbers of Lewis rat marrow cells, between 10^5 and 10^6, injected into irradiated mice gave increasing numbers of spleen colonies in mouse strains A, Balb/c, DBA, C3H, and CBA, but none in the C57 BL/6 strain or the (C57 × A)F$_1$ hybrid![68] In the latter two strains, when the rat marrow cell dose was increased to 10^7, it would confluently repopulate the marrow at 8 d and ensure 30-d survival in the absence of spleen colonies or spleen repopulation at 8 d, but with confluent spleen repopulation at 30 d! When the rat marrow cell dose was increased to 2.6×10^7, the spleens of the $(C57 \times A)F_1$ mice still remained resistant to 8 d spleen colonies or repopulation, but at the next higher dose of 3.7×10^7 cells, the spleens were confluently repopulated at 8 d without ever, at any marrow cell dose, developing discrete spleen "colonies."

Several common characteristics were found to exist between this atypical "xenogeneic resistance" of some mouse strains to rat marrow transplants[68] and atypical "allogeneic resistance" to some allogeneic marrow transplants[69] and to F_1 "hybrid resistance" to some parental strain marrow transplants,[69] the latter sometimes encountered unrecognized and named "CFU repression"[70] and "poor growth phenomenon."[71] Because of the genetic specificity of the donor-recipient combinations, in which hybrid, allogeneic, and xenogeneic resistance occurred,[68,72] they were grouped under the name of "genetic resistance" to bone marrow transplantation.[73] They were subsequently found to be NK cell mediated[74,75] and "hybrid resistance" to be related to genetic resistance to lymphoma–leukemia.[76] In our attempts to study mouse marrow cell-derived spleen colonies in the rat, no spleen colonies were ever observed with cell doses of 10^6 to 3.15×10^8 of either $(C57 \times A)F_1$ or C3H marrow in Lewis rats in four separate trials.[77] Therefore, we tested the HIM hypothesis with Lewis rat marrow in three mouse strains, C3H, A, and Balb/c. Of 643 isologous Lewis rat spleen colonies, 490 were erythroid and 153 were undifferentiated. No granuloid, megakaryocytic, or mixed colonies were observed at 11 or 12 d. The E:G colony ratio, therefore, was an extreme 490:0.

In contrast, Lewis rat marrow, growing in C3H, A, and Balb/c mice, gave 162 erythroid, 55 granuloid, 82 mixed, 5 undifferentiated, and no megakaryocytic colonies, for an E:G colony ratio of 3:1, typical of mouse spleen colonies.[77] Karyotype analysis confirmed that the colonies were composed of rat cells. The mouse spleen hemopoietic microenvironments not only elicited granulopoietic colonies of rat CFU-S, with the same E:G colony ratio as if they were mouse CFU-S, but also caused the colonies to reach macroscopically visible size in 8 d, rather than 12 d required in the rat. Although rat megakaryocytic colonies were not observed in either the rat or mouse spleens, they were observed in the mouse marrow. Again the existence of functional stromal hemopoietic microenvironments was reaffirmed. In addition, these experiments gave the important information that one cannot assume that the types and ratios of hemopoietic microenvironments found in the spleen of one species will necessarily pertain to another.

Microenvironmental Control of Eosinophilic Granulocyte Response to Tetanus Toxoid

Sensitization of mice to tetanus toxoid produces a great eosinophilic granulocytosis and peritoneal eosinophil exudation.[78,79] Because the percentage of eosinophilic spleen colonies is normally very low and of eosinophilic marrow colonies only slightly higher, we studied the spleen and marrow eosinophil colonies and eosinophil cell numbers in irradiated, marrow cell-injected mice. It was found that tetanus toxoid antigen did increase the number of eosinophilic granuloid colonies. Attempts were made to determine whether the antigen produces its effect by an action on the colony-forming stem cells of the marrow donor, or on the host stromal microenvironments for eosinophilic granulopoiesis.

Antigen treatment of the marrow cell donors did not consistently increase the number of spleen and bone marrow colonies in recipient animals or change the percentage of eosinophil or other hemopoietic colony types. Antigen pretreatment of the irradiated recipients increased the percentage of eosinophil-containing colonies in the spleen and femoral bone marrow, without significantly changing the total number of either spleen or marrow colonies. Antigen treatment of both the bone marrow cell donor and recipient produced a further increase in the percentage of eosinophil-containing colonies in the marrow cavity, but not the spleen. Antigen treatment of the irradiated recipient increased the number of eosinophilic cells (but not the total number of cells) in both the peritoneal exudate and bone marrow. Antigen treatment of both the marrow donor and recipient produced a further increase in the number of eosinophilic cells in the peritoneal cavity, but not in a single femur. Since antigen treatment of the marrow recipient, or recipient and donor, but not the marrow donor alone, results in increased eosinophilic cell and colony numbers, the effect of antigen appears to be mediated through some host factor(s), perhaps the eosinophilic hemopoietic microenvironment, rather than directly on the hemopoietic stem cells.[80]

Microenvironmental Control of Mast Cell Differentiation

Until the late 1970's, and despite their many similarities, basophilic granulocytes and tissue mast cells were thought to be independent cell lineages, the former of marrow origin and the latter of connective tissue origin.[81] In a series of very fine publications, Kitamura and associates, using C57 BL-Bgj/Bgj mice whose mast cells have distinctively large granules, demonstrated that marrow-donor type mast cells appeared in irradiated recipient caecum and glandular stomach by 42 d, forestomach by 63 d, mesentery by 96 d, and skin by 152 d, indicating that differentiation from marrow precursors is locally controlled.[82] Mast cell precursors are derived from hematopoietic tissues rather than lymphopoietic ones, and differentiation is not thymic dependent.[83] Both W/W^v and Sl/Sl^d mice have less than 1% of the number of tissue mast cells found in congenic +/+ mice. The mast cell defect of W/W^v mice is a stem cell defect, that of Sl/Sl^d mice is not, but appears to be owing to a defect localized in the peripheral tissues where they differentiate.[84,85] Mast cell colonies in the mesentery of W/W^v mice 15 wk after injection of a 50/50 mixture of marrow cells from beige and normal C57 BL6 mice were clonal in nature.[86] Development of skin mast cells from bone marrow-derived precursors was under local control, as revealed by skin painting with methylcholanthrene.[87] These studies reveal the existence of HIM in surprising new locations.

Dissecting the Hemopoietic Microenvironment

In a series of investigations on this subject, Norman Wolf reported that *lodgment* of CFU-S in spleen, measured by f factor, was the same in Sl/Sl^d and +/+ mice and that *commitment*, although characteristically different for spleen compared to bone marrow, was subnormal in Sl/Sl^d spleens. The *stimulus to proliferate*, as measured by spleen colony size and cell type content, was even more reduced.[88] An additional defect was a mean daily loss of 2.5 to 3% of its total blood volume via the intestinal tract.[89]

When half an Sl/Sl^d spleen was grafted to half an *in situ* spleen of an irradiated, congenic +/+ mouse, or vice versa, the "chimeric" spleen supported erythropoiesis in the +/+ region, not in the Sl/Sl^d region, regardless of which genotype was the irradiated, marrow-injected host mouse. Implants of normal bone marrow stroma within the spleens of irradiated Sl/Sl^d mice also supported normal proportions of erythrocytic and granulocytic hemopoiesis. Implants of normal +/+ spleen stroma, particularly capsular portions, into unirradiated Sl/Sl^d host mouse spleens supported erythropoiesis by Sl/Sl^d stem cells within and in the immediate vicinity of the implant. The evidence indicated that the stromal defect of the Sl/Sl^d spleen involved an erythropoietic stimulatory factor lacking in the Sl/Sl^d mouse.[90]

Other Evidence of the Roles of Marrow, Spleen, and Thymus Organ Stroma in Hemopoiesis and Lymphopoiesis

These include:

1. The secondary and permanent late aplasia of those areas of bone marrow and spleen receiving very high doses of local irradiation.[91,92]
2. The delay of return of hemopoietic stem cells and hemopoiesis to transplanted regenerating pieces of bone marrow or curetted aplastic areas of bone marrow until the late stages of regeneration of the characteristic organ stroma.[93-95] In these studies, the sequential stages of regeneration were carefully documented histologically and hemopoiesis did not resume until full architectural restoration of the stromal and vascular elements occurred.
3. The impairment of the ability of spleen or marrow stroma to support hemopoiesis following graft vs host injury to these organs.[96-98]
4. During regeneration of the thymus, after sublethal irradiation, the thymic stromal architecture is restored before the expression of cell surface-associated reticular MHC staining patterns. The observed sequential changes in the thymic microenvironment are related to the lymphoid repopulation of the thymus.[99]

Hemopoiesis on Intraperitoneal Cellulose Acetate Membranes

Seki[100] introduced cellulose acetate membranes intraperitoneally in mice. Over a period of days, they acquired an adherent layer of peritoneal cells; on injection of bone marrow cells intraperitoneally, small granulopoietic colonies developed on the coated membranes.

Knospe modified the technique by spreading pastes of gently homogenized spleen, marrow, bone, or regenerating endosteal tissue onto the membranes, folding them into rolls, and implanting them intraperitoneally. Over a period of weeks and months, they acquired trilineal hematopoiesis with resemblance to normal marrow.[101–103]

CFU-S Heterogeneity

In 1982, Magli et al.[104] reported that, by comparison of autopsy spleen colonies in Balb/c mice with an earlier spleen inspection by laparotomy, some early spleen colonies were transient in nature and disappeared, whereas others did not appear until later. A higher proportion of 9–12 d colonies than 7–8 d colonies were found to have primitive precursor cells identified by erythroid or mononuclear/granulocyte colonies in vitro. This was interpreted as new evidence challenging the pluripotentiality of CFU-S. In fact, it is not discordant with earlier reports that some spleen colonies may be formed by erythroid-committed progenitors,[6,40] that granuloid colonies appear later than erythroid colonies,[5] that the numbers of detectable CFU-S in spleen colonies increases with colony age and is greater in granuloid than erythroid colonies of the same age,[6] that some individual CFU-S can give rise to two, three, or four colonies,[105] that CFU-S can be physically separated into fractions with greater or lesser capacity for self-renewal,[106] that myelotoxic drugs can alter the self-renewal capacity of surviving CFU-S,[107–109] and that CFU-S subpopulations can be demonstrated to differ in self-renewal capacity associated with antigenic differences.[110, 110a]

Novel in the Magli publication were the reported proportions of the numbers of colonies disappearing early and appearing late and the conclusions. Of 101 colonies present on d 7–8, most were erythroblastic. Only 50 persisted to d 10, but were supplemented by 97 other colonies not present on d 7–8, but making a delayed appearance by d 10. The authors concluded that most 7–8 d colonies contain no primitive precursor cells and soon vanish by terminal differentiation, whereas 2/3 of the colonies appearing by d 10 had no visible antecedents on d 7 or 8, contained more primitive precursor cells, arose from slower growing pluripotent CFU-S, and that the spleen colony method provides a measure of pluripotential cells capable of extensive proliferation only where macroscopic colonies are scored at 11 d or later, contrary to usage in almost the entire literature on the subject. These conclusions are discordant with the data of Table 3[6] wherein, depending on colony type and age, 55–100% of d 9 and 10 erythroid or granuloid spleen colonies were demonstrably pluripotent, each giving rise to both erythroid and granuloid spleen colonies in secondary irradiated host mice, at an age when such colonies were demonstrably monoclonal by chromosome markers (Table 8).[56]

The great advantage of the provocative Magli publication[104] was that it got the attention of the hemopoietic research community in a way that the earlier data never did, regarding the fact that not all CFU-S are pluripotent. There are now a great number of desirable investigations into the heterogeneity of CFU-S[111–117] with particular reference to the ability to give rise to "early" (8 d) and "late" (12–14 d) spleen colonies. Unfortunately, the pendulum seemed to have swung too far in the opposite direction, such that all 8 d spleen colonies became suspect in most circles of being formed by nonpluripotent stem cells.

In order to more frequently examine and quantitate the appearance and disappearance of spleen colonies, Priestley and Wolf[118] developed an ingenious "spleen window," a subcutaneous chamber filled with balanced saline and a removable cover to examine, photograph, and plot colonies of the subcutaneously exteriorized spleen daily. They reported that spleen colonies were both appearing and disappearing each day between d 8 and 12, but reported that, in AB_6F_1 and $B_6D_2F_1$ mice, 60 and 58%, respectively of 8 d colonies persisted until d 12. In the AB_6F_1 mice, 22 colonies that disappeared were replaced by 27 new ones. In the $B_6D_2F_1$ mice, 21 colonies that disappeared were replaced by 35 new ones, but in Bouin's fixed spleens, as normally used for colony counts, the 8 and 12 d $B_6D_2F_1$ spleen colony counts did not differ, suggesting that some of the small colonies escape detection in d 8 visual counts on fresh spleens and the need to increase colony visibility in unfixed viable spleens.

In a more extensive study, Wolf and Priestly[119] recently reported that in groups of Balb/c and $B_6D_2F_1$ mice killed on d 7–12, the daily mean spleen colony numbers did not vary significantly over this time period. Daughter CFU-S content of spleen colonies on retransplantation was found to be proportional to colony size and age; even early-appearing colonies contained daughter CFU-S, although their presence was masked by low early colony cell numbers and seeding efficiency (f factor). Half of the "early" 8 d colonies produced one or more 11 d daughter colonies in secondary recipients. By the 11–12th d, the persisting early (8 and 9 d) spleen colonies contained as many "early" and "late" daughter CFU-S as late (10–12 d) appearing colonies. The intercolonial spleen tissue was found to contain CFU-S in increasing numbers between d 7 and 12, but by chromosome marker studies, these were not found to contaminate 12 d spleen colonies, but did contaminate some 14 d colonies. Reirradiation of the exteriorized spleen on d 3 revealed that approximately half of 12 d spleen colonies arise from CFU-S migrating to the spleen after 3 d! Indirect evidence indicated that these migrated from the repopulating marrow, in agreement with Van Zant's evidence that the great increase in late 8–14 d spleen colonies derived from 5 FU-treated marrow donors[108,109] comes from the marrow, since it does not occur in ^{89}Sr-pretreated recipient mice.[120]

Taken together, the data of Wolf[119] and Van Zant[120] that many normal and most 5-FU-marrow-derived late spleen colonies, respectively, arrive by secondary migration of CFU-S from the regenerating marrow, indicate that a) such "late" spleen colonies are not old, slow-growing, permanently resident spleen colonies, but rather are new immigrant, fast-growing colonies that are $3 + x$ days younger in the spleen than had been assumed, and b) CFU-S are apparently being renewed faster and in larger (exportable) numbers in regenerating marrow than in regenerating spleen. The reason for the latter may relate to the data of Table 3 herein, indicating that a higher percentage of retransplanted 9- and 10-d-old granuloid spleen colonies produce secondary spleen colonies, of both erythroid and granuloid types, and in larger numbers, than do the 3 times larger erythroid colonies of the same age. As indicated earlier, the ratio of granuloid to erythroid colonies is much greater in the marrow than in the spleen.[37] It is also possible that there are still better microenvironments for pluripotent CFU-S renewal in the marrow than in granuloid spleen colonies.

Granting that some spleen cell-derived and some marrow cell-derived CFU-S may be erythroid committed progenitor cells as suggested earlier, it does not necessarily follow that all such cells could give rise to a grossly visible 7 or 8 d spleen colony before it disappeared. Some may terminally differentiate and disappear while still only microscopic "colonies." Nor does it follow that colonies formed by a pluripotent CFU-S cannot appear and disappear early. A pluripotent CFU-S trans-

planted iv might, on reaching the spleen, encounter a microenvironment conducive for commitment before it encountered
one for self-renewal. Such a colony might thereafter behave as
one formed initially by a committed CFU-S.

Molineau et al.,[121] using a low marrow cell dose to give
only one d 8 spleen colony, and an occlusive ligature around
the middle of d 8 spleens containing only one colony, were able
to document the subsequent appearance of new colonies on
one or both sides of the ligature by autopsy on d 11, but were
unable, by the direct method, to document the persistence of d
8 colonies to d 11. However, in an informative study of the relationship between early and late spleen colony ratio and self-
renewal capacity in selected CFU-S populations, they verified
that spleen cell-derived CFU-S give a low ratio of d 11 to d 8
spleen colonies, and a low mean CFU per d 11 colony, compared to marrow-derived CFU-S. They also found that after
cytotoxic treatment of mice with cyclophosphamide, busulfan,
or BCNU, a high d 11 to d 8 spleen colony ratio is not necessarily
correlated with a high self-renewal capacity of the CFU-S population that forms the d 11 colonies.

Reversible Effect of Marrow and Spleen Microenvironments on Thymic Progenitor Cell Differentiation and Proliferation

In 1976, Duplan's laboratory[122] reported that marrow-
derived cells competitively repopulate the thymus of irradiated mice more rapidly than spleen-derived cells injected into
the same mouse, even when the number of injected spleen
CFU-S was twice the number of marrow CFU-S. The difference
in growth rates of the two populations subsided within 20 d
after injection into the new hosts. They hypothesized that the
microenvironment of the spleen inhibits the development of
one or more stem cell subpopulations with greatest capacity for

proliferation and production of thymic precursors, and transplanted spleen CFU-S that relocate in the marrow recover, after some time, the proliferative and thymic repopulating capacity of marrow stem cells. To test this hypothesis, they transplanted approximately equal numbers of either marrow or spleen CFU-S into lethally irradiated primary recipient mice and recovered them from both marrow and spleen of the primary recipient after 7, 9, 14, and 21 d.[123] At each interval, they tested the four groups of recovered cells in secondary irradiated recipients, as well as normal marrow and spleen cells in two groups of primary irradiated recipients, for rapidity of repopulation of the thymus. They measured this by the percentage of donor karyotypes in the six groups of recipients sacrificed at 14, 20, 25, and 30 d. By 30 d, donor type repopulation had reached virtually 100% in all groups.

The superiority of normal marrow over normal spleen cells for rapidity of thymic repopulation in the control groups was most evident at 20 d, at which time 72 and 43%, respectively of the thymic karyotypes were of donor origin. In this respect, cells of original marrow or spleen origin, after recovery from either the orthotopic (same) or heterotopic organ (marrow cells from spleen or spleen cells from marrow) still behaved as normal marrow or spleen after 9 and 14 d in the orthotopic site and after 7 or 9 d in the heterotopic site. But by 14 d (and 21 d) of residence in the heterotopic organ, cells of marrow origin now acted as normal spleen cells (24% of thymic karyotypes of donor origin at 20 d) and cells of spleen origin acted as normal marrow cells (70% of thymic karyotypes of donor origin at 20 d). They point out that marrow contains a T-precursor cell population with the enzyme terminal deoxyribonucleotidyl transferase, whereas in the spleen precursor pool this enzyme is absent,[124] confirming that the spleen contains T-cell progenitors, but not precursors. They conclude that "bone marrow and spleen microenvironments act differently on the differentiation process of T-progenitors and precursors. In addition, when marrow or spleen CFU-S are transferred into a new environment, the production of T-progenitors and precursors proceeds 7–9 days according to the pattern imprinted by the original micro-environment."[123] They point out that 9 d corresponds roughly to the time necessary for reconstitution of the stem cell pool.[125]

Reversible Predisposition of CFU-S
for Direction of Differentiation

In 1978, Wolf[126] reported that, just as observed earlier[40] for CFU-S of spleen origin (Table 4), early (13–14 d) fetal liver CFU-S gave a higher E:G spleen colony ratio than marrow-derived CFU-S, but even more so: E:G spleen colony ratio for marrow CFU-S = 2.6, spleen CFU-S = 8.6, and fetal liver CFU-S = 49.7! Again, as for the earlier experiments (Table 5), the E:G hemopoietic colony ratio in the marrow of these same recipient mice was only slightly increased for spleen-derived CFU-S and only slightly more for fetal liver CFU-S: E:G marrow colony ratio for marrow CFU-S = 0.47, spleen CFU-S = 0.85, and fetal liver CFU-S = 2.01.[126]

In the earlier experiments comparing spleen-derived with marrow-derived CFU-S, marrow or spleen CFU-S recovered from primary irradiated recipients marrow or spleen within 2-1/2 h, and injected into a secondary recipient, gave E:G colony ratios in the spleen and marrow characteristic of the original organ source (spleen or marrow), regardless of whether they were recovered from marrow or spleen of the primary recipient (Table 6). When the same comparison was made of fetal liver vs marrow CFU-S recovered 2–5 h from the primary recipient's marrow or spleen, again the E:G colony ratio in the marrow and spleen of the secondary recipient was characteristic of the original donor organ source of the CFU-S (fetal liver or marrow) regardless of whether recovered from the primary recipient's marrow or spleen.[126] In the earlier experiments, [40] since the therapeutic efficiency of spleen CFU-S is low, we had interpreted the higher E:G ratio of spleen CFU-S-derived spleen colonies to be owing to an excess of terminally committed erythroid CFU-S in spleen that can be expressed in the spleen, but not in the marrow stroma of the primary recipient. However, the therapeutic efficiency of fetal liver CFU-S is even higher than that of marrow CFU-S, and they produce rapidly, growing very large erythroid colonies that develop mixed hemopoiesis. Approximately 10 fetal liver CFU-S gives the same therapeutic efficiency as 20 bone marrow, or 40 spleen CFU-S.[42] Moreover, the ratio of total colonies formed in the spleens, relative to the total number formed in the five bones examined per mouse in the primary and secondary recipients, was essentially the same regardless of the original cell source (FL or BM) or intermediate organ of lodgment.

Wolf interprets these data as not compatible with either selective lodgment by precommitted CFU, nonexpression of erythroid-committed CFU in marrow, or granuloid-committed CFU in spleen. Instead, he concludes that CFU derived from fetal liver or adult spleen, compared to bone marrow, appear to carry with them a strong, but not irreversible predisposition to form erythrocytic colonies on lodgment in spleen. However, if they lodge in the predominantly granulocytic microenvironment of marrow, many of them will lose their "predisposition" and become granuloid colonies.[126] As a possible explanation, he envisions the concept of numerous specific receptor sites in the wall of the pluripotent stem cell and separate specific messenger molecules directing activity toward each line of differentiation.[127]

These interesting new data[126] present an alternate explanation for the high E:G colony ratios of spleen colonies formed by spleen cells rather than marrow cells being due to an excess of erythroid "mono" committed CFU-S that form only small, early-disappearing spleen colonies. This original explanation is not applicable to the even higher E:G colony ratios of spleen colonies formed by highly proliferative pluripotent fetal liver CFU-S. Instead, they suggest that the high E:G colony ratios produced by spleen and fetal liver CFU-S may be a reversible predisposition "imprinted" by the organ stromal microenvironment of their origin, possibly related to growth factor receptor numbers or activity. Whether differences of CFU-S from fetal liver, marrow, or spleen, with respect to capacity for self-renewal vs differentiation, is likewise a function of the microenvironment of "birth," or of CFU-S generation "aging" in the progression from fetal liver to marrow to spleen, remained to be determined.

Hemopoietic Hormone (Growth Factor) Receptors

When, on the basis of in vivo hemopoietic colony studies, we first proposed the concept of hemopoietic "microenvironmental influences"[34] and the working hypothesis of "hemopoietic inductive microenvironments (HIM) of different kinds,"[5] erythropoietin was already an accepted hormone and there were suggestive indications of the existence of granulopoietins and lymphopoietins. Available data indicated that the CFU-S of origin of spleen colonies was pluripotent and not itself responsive to erythropoietin,[52-55] but gave rise to the erythropoietin-sensitive stem cell. Within 4 d after the pluripotent CFU-S lodged in an erythroid HIM, its progeny cells of the tiny, undifferentiated, presumptive erythroid colonies were demonstrably sensitive to erythropoietin.[6] This suggested that the function of the erythroid HIM included or consisted of induction of responsiveness to erythropoietin.[6] To date, the technology for demonstrating specific receptors for erythropoietin is just maturing. But thanks to the purification of the four granulocyte–macrophage-mixed colony stimulating factors (CSF's), and gene cloning for both GM-CSF and multi-CSF, much is already known about their receptors.[128,129,129a] Each CSF receptor appears to bind to only a single species of CSF. Since most granulocytes and macrophages are able to respond to more than one CSF, these cells simultaneously exhibit more than one type of CSF receptor. It remains uncertain how many cells exhibit only a single species of receptor. Stimulation of granulocytes and macrophages, by a combination of two different CSF's, enhances the resulting proliferation, but exposure of cells to one CSF can down regulate other CSF receptors![128] Receptors for GM-CSF, G-CSF, and multi-CSF are very low in number (100–500/cell), whereas those for M-CSF are somewhat higher (3000–16,000/cell). Degradation of M-CSF receptor complexes is very rapid, but G-CSF receptor complexes are degraded much more slowly.[129]

Pluripotency of Hemopoietic CFU-S for Lymphoid Differentiation

By chromosome marker methods, it was recognized early that not only the hemopoietic, but also the lymphoid system of lethally irradiated mice, protected with bone marrow cells, was repopulated from cells of donor marrow origin and that there was traffic of stem cells between the bone marrow and the lymphoid organs.[130] Cells of the same karyotypically distinct marrow donor clone could be found in reconstituted irradiated normal or unirradiated stem cell defective anemic W/W^v mice in both the lymphoid and hemopoietic tissues, including spleen colonies.[131-133] This did not distinguish, however, whether the hemopoietically pluripotent spleen colony forming CFU-S could itself give rise also to lymphoid progeny or was descended from an even more pluripotent stem cell that could give rise to hemopoietic and lymphoid stem cells. This was resolved by the demonstration that either a single spleen colony[32] or a few spleen colonies[33] could reconstitute the hemopoietic and the lymphoid systems of irradiated mice, verified by chromosome marker. Moreover, mice so reconstituted with one or a few clones of cells derived from such hemopoietically and lymphopoietically pluripotent CFU-S, and immunized with defined Salmonella antigens, bovine serum albumin, and sheep red blood cells, produced an antibody to each antigen. This further indicated that any clonal restriction to antigen recognition and antibody production must occur downstream of the pluripotent CFU-S.[33]

Lymphoid-Inductive Microenvironments

When it became apparent that none of the spleen colonies were composed of lymphocytes, but only four different lines of hemopoiesis, and that lymphoid repopulation of the spleen occurred only secondarily, starting at about 14 d if a large enough marrow cell dose is administered to insure survival, it was suggested[2] that "These cells presumably differentiated from pluripotent CFU elsewhere, probably in central lymphoid organs such as the thymus, recapitulating ontogeny." It was further suggested that "Since thymic lymphocytes are more involved in delayed hypersensitivity reactions, and bursal or gut-derived lymphocytes are involved with antibody production, it seems probable that there may be at least two kinds of LIM, just as there are at least four kinds of HIM."

Since that time, it has been demonstrated that not only does T-cell differentiation occur by interaction of marrow-derived prethymic precursor cells with thymic stromal epithelial cells, which occur throughout the thymus, but that there may exist microenvironmental differences between the cortical vs medullary thymic epithelial cells, with respect to their influence on T-lymphocyte differentiation and proliferation.[134,135] Wekerle et al. have described a large thymic epithelial cell that engulfs many thymocytes into a large lymphoepithelial cell complex.[136]

It has also been shown that postnatally in mammals the bone marrow is the central lymphoid organ for the differentiation and proliferation of B-lymphocytes.[135] In mice and other rodents, small lymphocytes comprise approximately 1/4 of all nucleated cells of the bone marrow. The origin of most marrow lymphocytes has been shown to be from dividing precursor cells within the marrow itself. Some regional concentrations of surface IgM-bearing cells are apparent, suggesting that "the basal level of marrow B-cell genesis is determined by short-range microenviromental factors and inductive interaction with local stromal cells."[137]

Spangrude, Heimfeld, and Weissman have more recently given great impetus to the isolation, characterization, and demonstration of the in vivo differentiation sites of the mouse pluripotent hemopoietic stem cell (PHSC).[137a] By a combination of negative and positive immunoselection and sorting procedures, they have purified, isolated and identified as the PHSC, a minor population of mouse bone marrow cells that are Thy-1 low, lineage antigen negative and stem cell antigen-1 positive. They present evidence that these Thy-1^{lo} Lin$^-$ Sca-1^+ cells can proliferate and differentiate with approximately unit efficiency, into myelomonocytic cells, B cells, or T cells. Only 30 such cells injected intravenously saved 50% of lethally irradiated mice and reconstituted all blood cell types of the survivors. In the spleen they formed erythroid, myeloid and mixed colonies, but not lymphoid colonies. When injected directly into the thymus of 700 rad-irradiated mice they formed T cell colonies, with close to unit efficiency, but no myeloerythroid colonies. These findings are in accord with the important role of the hemopoietic organ stromal cells on the differentiation of the PHSC.

Metcalf and Johnson[138] reported the presence of in vitro B-lymphocyte colony forming cells (BL-CFC) in 7- to 13-d-old erythroid, granuloid, or mixed spleen colonies derived from bone marrow or 12 d fetal liver, i.e., before the fetal liver itself contains BL-CFC. Lala and Johnson, using T6 chromosome marked fetal liver or bone marrow, determined that the BL-CFC arose monoclonally from within the spleen colony, derived from the initiating CFU-S.[139] BL-CFC were found in 42% of 437 individual spleen colonies assayed between 6 and 13 d post-irradiation and marrow injection. They were found in 72% of 65 mainly erythroid spleen colonies, and 65% of 17 mainly granulocytic spleen colonies. The total number per spleen colony was from less than 200 to more than 4×10^3 BL-CFC, but 53% of 182 positive colonies contained less than 200 BL-CFC. The total number of BL-CFC per colony was inversely related to the total spleen colony cell count, being highest (515 BL-CFC/10^5 spleen colony cells) in colonies with less than 200,000 total cells. This, together with the fact that 24% of 75 d 8 spleen colonies contained BL-CFC, that are relatively mature B-cell progenitors, indicates that generation of BL-CFC from the CFU-S of origin was a relatively early event. It further indicates that conditions for generation and propagation of BL-CFC in erythroid and granuloid spleen colonies are suboptimal compared to those for generation of committed erythropoietic or granulopoietic progenitor cells by the pluripotent CFU-S of origin, which latter cells and their progeny progressively outnumbered the BL-CFC.

It is unresolved whether the origin of the BL-CFC from the pluripotent CFU-S was a random or directed event. It could have conceivably occurred by a spleen colony outgrowing its original microenvironment and encompassing a B-cell microenvironment, just as large erythroid colonies develop areas of granulopoiesis in their peripheral cuff of less differentiated cells as they outgrow their original microenvironment. Indeed, if a sparse number of B-cell "inductive" stromal microenvironments exist in spleen, in addition to the known "B- and T-cell areas" (functional microenvironments) of the spleen, that provide homes for the proliferation and function of immigrant T- and B-lymphocytes produced elsewhere, it seems highly probable that the marrow stroma is much richer in such B-cell inductive microenvironments, in light of its dominant role in the "central" generation of B-lymphocytes in adult rodents.[135]

In Vitro Bone Marrow Cultures

Early Methods

The advent of in vitro clonal cultures of hemopoietic cells in semisolid medium[140,141] gave great impetus to the discovery and study of the many colony stimulating factors necessary for in vitro growth of the many differentiated hemopoietic cell lines.[128,142] The short life-span of such cultures made it apparent that these were terminally differentiating colonies formed by committed progenitor cells, with no evidence of the important stromal microenvironmental influences on early commitment and differentiation and CFU-S self-renewal, that spleen colony and other studies had revealed in vivo.[2] At the Second International Workshop on Hemopoiesis in Culture, at which Arthur Axelrad reported his new BFU-E colony method, this discussant called attention to the stromal cell microenvironmental influences that occur in vivo, and asked "Are the several in vitro marrow culture methods dependent on such interactions in vivo, or limited by their absence in vitro? Or do such interactions occur in vitro? It might be profitable to look for them in vitro, in particular in connection with Dr. Axelrad's burst of colonies."[143]

The Dexter Method

In 1971, Chang and Anderson[144] reported that in relatively short-term liquid cultures of mouse bone marrow cells, there developed adherent foci of "natural feeder cells," upon which granulocytic colonies formed, and that "it seemed likely that the feeder cell was actually contributing some factor which was required for the formation and development of the colony." In 1973, Dexter and Lajtha reported a truly major advance in hemopoietic cell culture.[145] They described a liquid coculture system of mouse thymus and bone marrow cells in which an adherent layer of cells formed, in some of which granulopoiesis continued for many weeks and CFU-S were shown to actually proliferate and, after 7–9 wk in culture, to protect lethally irradiated mice. For the first time, it was possible not just to maintain, but proliferate the pluripotent CFU-S in culture! They soon modified the technique to achieve similar results with liquid cultures of bone marrow alone. However, this required recharging the cultures with fresh isologous bone marrow after 3 wk when an adherent layer of at least three stromal cell types had formed.[146,147] CFU-S replication and granulopoiesis occurred in close association with certain areas of adherent cells. The authors conclude that "as the composite layer of 'giant,' 'epithelial' and phagocytic mononuclear cells is necessary for extended stem cell proliferation and granulopoiesis, these areas may be supplying a necessary microenvironment for their proliferation and differentiation. This in vitro system may provide useful means to investigate some of the factors (cellular and humoral) controlling haemopoietic processes."[147] At last, the in vitro hemopoietic culture systems revealed the necessity of stromal cell–CFU-S interactions so evident earlier in vivo for CFU-S proliferation and differentiation![2]

The Greenberger Modification

An initial impediment to the widespread use of this valuable new method was the esoteric and baffling serum requirement. Of several types of sera from many sources, only certain horse sera were effective in supporting long-term proliferation of CFU-S. Only some batches obtained from Flow Laboratories in Scotland were effective, although all the batches tested stimulated CFU-C. None of the horse sera tested from Gibco were effective, nor were several batches of fetal calf sera obtained from either Flow or Gibco.[146] It remained for Joel Greenberger, in a brilliant piece of deductive reasoning and research, to demonstrate, with the aid of a horse serum batch reported by Dexter to induce lipid accumulation in marrow cells in vitro, that mouse marrow preadipocytes are insulin-resistant, but corticosteroid responsive, with respect to lipogenesis, and that corticosteroids, but not other steroid hormones, when added to a 'negative' horse serum, would cause it to stimulate both lipogenesis and long-term CFU-S replication in culture.[148] It soon became apparent that virtually any batch of horse, fetal calf, or goat serum, supplemented with hydrocortisone, would promote rapid development of an adherent layer of bone marrow cells necessary for long-term proliferation of CFU-S and continuing granulopoiesis.[149] "Recharge" of cultures with fresh, isologous marrow after 3 wk became unnecessary, and longevity of the cultures was improved such that granulocytes, GM-CFU, and CFU-S were produced for over 1 yr in vitro, depending on the mouse strain.[149-151]

The stromal cells composing the adherent layer have been described as endothelial cells, reticulum cells, fibroblasts, adipocytes, macrophages, and "blanket" cells.[150,152,153] "Cobblestone" areas are regions of active granulopoiesis composed of macrophage-associated granulocytes beneath a blanket cell layer.[150] Tavassoli and Takahashi[152] noted that "Granulopoiesis was observed in the culture system in the absence of colony-stimulating activity in the supernatant, suggesting direct cellular interaction or short-range factors in the induction of granulopoiesis. Widespread cellular interactions were noted between macrophages and epithelioid cells, the latter often completely embracing the former and both extending cytoplasmic processes toward each other. This is reminiscent of the cooperative interaction of endoderm and mesoderm in chick embryo hemopoiesis and may be necessary for the maintenance of stem cells in these cultures."

Cell–cell interactions are clearly important because if the stem cells are separated from the stromal cells by a thin agar layer[154] or a diffusion chamber membrane,[155] they die rapidly and hemopoiesis declines. In reference to these, and extracellular matrix, and other stromal cell "domains" in vitro, Dexter et al.[150] point out that regulatory molecules such as GM-CSF, which need not be added to such cultures and are not readily detected therein,[152] may be produced by the stromal cells and presented directly to the developing hemopoietic cells. They state[150] that "regulation of hemopoiesis as a whole should be seen in the context of interacting cell populations producing local islands of the appropriate regulatory molecules, i.e., a series of stromal cell domains that influence stem cell proliferation and progenitor cell development,[156,157] similar to the model proposed many years ago by Trentin.[2]" In response to questions regarding whether the in vitro microenvironments he described are inductive or permissive, Dexter answered that they are "determinative environments," and that "the whole system is very rigidly controlled, presumably by the kinds of cell interactions we have been discussing."[150]

B-Lymphocyte Cultures

In vitro studies in long-term, marrow-derived B-lymphocyte cultures have also given considerable support for local microenvironmental marrow-derived stromal accessory cell interactions to facilitate the transition from pre-B to B-cells,[158] and to sustain B-cell presursors long-term.[159] In the latter study, it was suggested that the precursor of the long-term in vitro B-cell may be either a pluripotent hemopoietic stem cell, or lymphoid stem cell.

For the long-term success of the Whitlock-Witte B-lymphocyte cultures,[160] an adherent multilayer of several stromal cell types is needed, just as in the predominantly myelopoietic long-term Dexter marrow cultures.[161] These may include fibroblasts, macrophages, adipocytes, epithelioid cells, and reticular cells in a three-dimensional framework mimicking marrow stroma in vivo.[162] In both of these long-term marrow culture systems, lymphocytopoiesis or myelopoiesis occurs within the adherent cell layers, providing an excellent opportunity for studying close range interactions of stem cells with stromal cells to determine which stromal cells are responsible for what, and whether by direct cell–cell contact or very short-range mediators. In the long-term B-lymphocyte cultures, Dorshkind et al.[163] have described a large epithelial nurse cell whose numerous membrane infoldings completely engulf as many as 14 B-lymphocytes, with striking morphological similarity to the thymic nurse cells described by Wekerle et al. that similary engulf many thymocytes in the thymus.[136] In the B-cell cultures, these large epithelial cells appeared to be the key B-cell interactive component of the stromal cell layer.

Distinctive Stromal Cells of Erythroid and Granuloid Spleen Colonies

Erythroid Colonies

In 1971, LaPushin and de Harven reported finding distinctive dendritic dark reticular cells in intimate association with clusters of glucocorticosteriod-sensitive thymocytes.[164] In 1977,

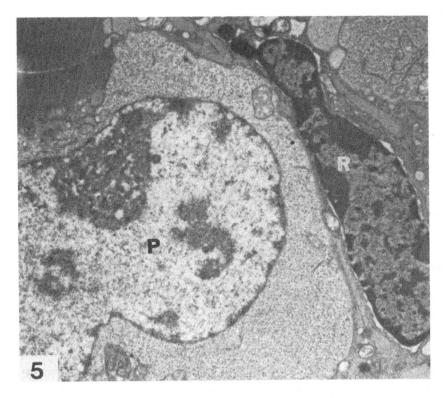

Fig. 5. Electron micrograph of a proerythroblast from a splenic erythroid colony, d 7. Note the typical proerythroblast (P), characterized by numerous cytoplasmic polyribosomes and a prominent nucleus with a well-defined nucleolus and extensive euchromatin, in close contact with other cellular elements, especially the fusiform reticular cell (R) (×8400) (LaPushin, R. W., and Trentin, J. J. (1977) *Exp. Hematol.* **5**, 505–522, courtesy of Munksgaard, Copenhagen).

LaPushin and Trentin reported a study of erythroid and granuloid spleen colonies for possible distinctive stromal cell types. Light and electron microscopy of 7 d erythroid spleen colonies revealed distinctive highly dendritic reticular cells, often in aggregates, indigenous to these early erythroid colonies (Figs. 5 and 6). They were not observed outside the erythroid colonies or in granuloid colonies, or within the spleens of control irradiated mice not injected with bone marrow. The dendritic form of these cells, therefore, was a result of their interaction

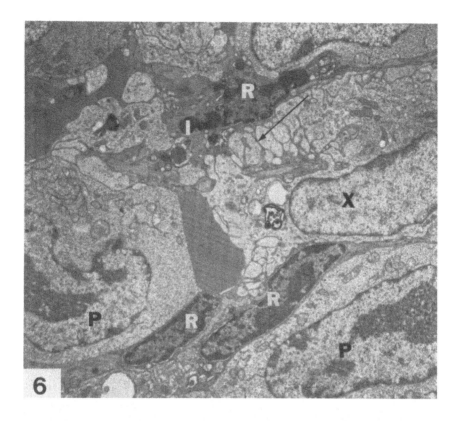

Fig. 6. Electron micrograph showing two oblate reticular cells (R) between a group of proerythroblasts (P) with no demonstrable extracellular spaces surrounding them. A third reticular cell containing lysosomes (l) and manifold cytoplasmic processes (←) is shown interdigitating with the cytoplasm of a proerythroblast, or perhaps a cell slightly earlier in differentiation (x) (×5600). (LaPushin, R. W., and Trentin, J. J. (1977) *Exp. Hematol.* 5, 505–522, courtesy of Munksgaard, Copenhagen).

with the surrounding proerythroblasts that they completely encircled and enveloped.[165] The cytoplasm of the reticular cells was electron dense and contained isolated ribosomes, contrasting sharply with the less dense cytoplasm and polyribosomes of the proerythroblasts. This permitted observation of very complex interdigitation areas of the dendritic processes of stromal reticular cells into blunt processes of proerythroblasts, providing an opportunity for the exchange of materials between them (Figs. 6 and 7). From d 7 to 8, there was a marked

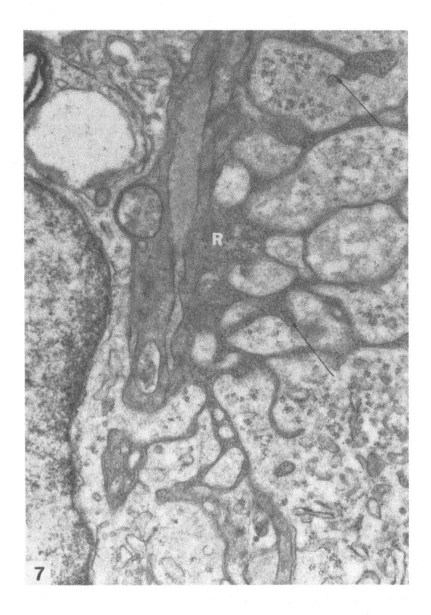

Fig. 7. Higher power micrograph of interdigitation areas in Fig. 6. The reticular cell processes (R) are dense, with numerous isolated ribosomes setting them apart from the cytoplasm of the erythroblast whose cytoplasm is less intensely stained and whose ribosomes are in the polyribosomal configuration. The complexity of the interdigitations provides for areas of possible exchange of material as indicated ($\leftarrow$) ($\times$ 31,000), (LaPushin, R. W., and Trentin, J. J. (1977) *Exp. Hematol.* **5**, 505–522, courtesy of Munksgaard, Copenhagen).

shift in the cytology of the erythroid colonies. On d 7, approximately 75% of the erythroid cells were proerythroblasts. By d 8, approximately 60% of the cells were basophilic, polychromatophilic, and orthochromatophilic erythroblasts.

Paralleling the shift to more mature cells, the dendritic reticular cells were seen less frequently, but were still primarily associated with clusters of proerythroblasts. It is possible that these dendritic reticular cells correspond to the phagocytic reticular cells of erythroblastic islets in human and mouse bone marrow[166,167] since Ben-Ishay and Yoffey[168,169] have described phagocytic reticular cells of erythroblastic islands of rat marrow that have cytoplasmic fine processes in close association with developing erythroblasts during primary hypoxia, but which become smaller and retract their processes posthypoxia as the erythroblasts disappeared. Chen and Weiss[170] showed that reticular cells with long processes, in human fetal bone marrow, appeared to form an association with hematopoietic cells. They interpreted their observations as being in accord with the concept of hemopoietic inductive microenvironments. Macario et al.[171] have isolated "erythroblastic nests" from highly erythropoietic mouse spleens by density gradient separation. These consist of a corona of proerythroblasts and erythroblasts around a central cell, characterized as usually a macrophage, less often a monocyte. It seems probable that these cells, intimately associated with the early stages of intense erythropoiesis and variously observed and described as phagocytic reticular cells, dendritic reticular cells, phagocytic reticular cells with fine processes, reticular cells, and on isolation in vitro, as macrophages or monocytes, may all be different functional and/or developmental stages of the same or of two closely related cell types.

In view of the now abundant evidence for production of a variety of interleukins and hemopoietic growth regulatory factors by cells of the T lymphocyte lineage, as well as by cells of the monocyte-macrophage lineage, it seems quite probable that the tissue phase of these and possibly other "blood" cells, may be involved, directly or indirectly, in some of the hemopoietic organ "stromal" microenvironment functions.

Granuloid Colonies

Because granuloid spleen colonies are less numerous, slower growing, and smaller than erythroid colonies, hypertransfusion-induced polycythemia was used to suppress erythroid colony formation, and granuloid colonies were dissected out at d 10.[165] These colonies consisted primarily of myeloblasts, with occasional metamyelocytes. Distinctive fibroblast-like stromal cells were pleiomorphic, exhibiting fusiform, spindle, or stellate configurations. None of the stromal cells formed aggregates as in erythroid colonies. Neither did they stain with the acidified Giemsa differential stain that stained distinctive dendritic reticular cells of the early erythroid colonies. The cytoplasm of the fusiform- and spindle-shaped stromal cells was characteristic of cells engaged in protein synthesis; the cisternae of the endoplasmic reticulum were often distended with secretory material.

The stellate stromal cells possessed abundant cytoplasm with extensive Golgi regions and numerous electron-dense bodies (Fig. 8). Their processes were not as complex as the erythroid colony stromal cells and, although they made contact with adjacent myeloblasts, they did not exhibit the complex interdigitations with the cytoplasm of the myeloblasts as the erythroid colony stromal cells did with proerythroblasts. A consistent finding was the appearance in these granuloid colonies of a cell closely resembling a conventional macrophage, round to ovoid in shape, containing densely staining coarse cytoplasmic inclusions that were highly irregular in contour (Fig. 9). Although such macrophages were found in lethally

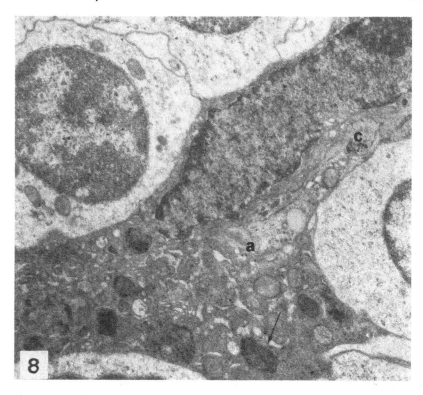

Fig. 8. An electron micrograph of the stellate stromal cell of the granuloid colony. Note numerous dense bodies (←), amorphous ground substance (a) and possible modest collagen deposition (c) (× 12,500), (LaPushin, R. W. and Trentin, J. J. (1977) *Exp. Hematol.* **5,** 505–522, courtesy of Munksgaard, Copenhagen).

irradiated control spleens without marrow cell injection, they were absent from erythroid colonies.[165] Whether any of these macrophages could also represent the macrophages of granulocyte–macrophage colonies in vitro is uncertain.

Other Candidate In Vivo Hemopoietic Microenvironment Stromal Cells

More recently, Westen and Bainton[172] have described, in mouse and rat bone marrow a) a fibroblast-type of reticulum cell characterized by having alkaline phosphatase associated

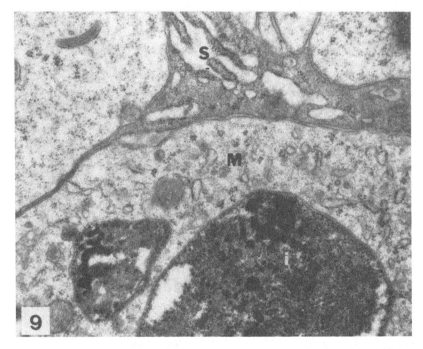

Fig. 9. Ultrastructure of a portion of the cytoplasm of a macrophage (M) from a granuloid colony. Note inclusions (i) within macrophage. Compare cytoplasm of macrophage and adjacent stromal cell (S) (7,500×). (LaPushin, R. W. and Trentin, J. J. (1977) *Exp. Hematol.* **5**, 505–522, courtesy of Munksgaard, Copenhagen).

with its plasma membrane (Al-RC), closely associated with granulocytic precursors, particularly myeloblasts and neutrophilic promyelocytes; b) a macrophage type of reticulum cell characterized by its abundance of lysosomal acid phosphatase, mainly associated with erythroid precursors. In a developmental study of the association of hemopoiesis with Al-RC,[173] it was found that at 9 d of gestational age, no Al-RC were found in blood islands of the yolk sac (the erythropoiesis site) or in the fetal liver. By 16 d, the fetal liver contained Al-RC interspersed with hematopoietic cells, as well as alkaline phosphatase in bile canaliculi. In addition to immature erythroid cells, there were immature and mature granulocytes and megakaryocytes. In the 18 d fetal femur, Al-RC were identified in the extravascular spaces by their positive reaction and processes. These spaces also contained many mature granulocytes. Distinct from these cells, alkaline phosphatase was also present extracellularly in the areas of calcifying cartilage.

In 1974, Friedenstein et al.[174] reported that slow growing, relatively radioresistant, extremely adhesive clonogenic fibroblast cultures of repeatedly passaged bone marrow or spleen cells of guinea pigs or rabbits, when transplanted under the kidney capsule of the autologous host of origin, resulted in the formation of primitive hemopoietic tissue. If the fibroblasts originated from bone marrow cultures, the regenerated tissue contained bone and was populated with myeloid cells. When the fibroblasts originated from spleen cultures, the regenerated tissue contained no bone or myeloid cells, but was populated with lymphoid cells. Their interpretation was that regenerated stromal tissue was of donor origin, representing the cells responsible for transferring the microenvironment of the hemopoietic tissue of origin, i.e., marrow or spleen, respectively. However, ectopic bone formation with hemopoiesis can be induced by implantation of demineralized (acid insoluble), allogeneic bone powder in a variety of tissues,[175–177] or implantation of urinary bladder transitional epithelium.[178,179] In any event, whether the regenerated stroma is of donor or recipient origin, if indeed fibroblasts from spleen vs bone marrow induce a different type of regenerated tissue specific of the organ of origin (lymphopoiesis vs hemopoiesis), this would be a highly significant observation.

A large number of hemopoietic stromal cell types and lines have been or are being isolated and cloned by cell cultures in many laboratories. Some appear to have little or no effect on hemopoiesis. Others have been shown to produce one or another of the hemopoietic colony stimulating factors, including multi-CSF (IL-3), a 41,000 mol wt glycoprotein fraction of

WEHI-3 cell conditioned medium.[179a] It is well established that murine multipotential and committed progenitor cell lines require the presence of IL-3 for in vitro proliferation and differentiation.[179b] A number of adherent cell lines, including a cloned bone marrow cell line, stimulate multipotential eythroid and other hemopoietic progenitor cells by close cell–cell contact in the absence of detectable IL-3.[179b] Cell types such as these are excellent candidates for the hemopoietic stromal microenvironmental influences earlier observed in vivo.

Hemopoiesis

Random or Controlled?

As mentioned earlier, Till et al.[38] first proposed a "stochastic" model of CFU-S self-renewal (birth) or differentiation (death) based on CFU-S numbers found in 10- and 12-d-old spleen colonies. In 1973, Korn et al.[180] fitted mathematical formulas of stochastic models to some published data on spleen colonies of different ages, based on their estimates of the contents of erythroid and granuloid differentiated cells only. They state "The stochastic model assumes that the decision of the pluripotent stem cell (S) to self-renew, differentiate to the precursor of the erythroid line (E) or differentiate to the precursor of the granulocytic line (G) is a random event determined by the three probabilities P_S, P_E, P_G respectively." Two sets of parameters for the stochastic model were chosen to give good agreement with the available experimental data. One set had equal probability of differentiation into erythroid or granuloid lines ($P_E = P_G$). The other set had more than a 10 times greater probability of differentiation into granuloid than erythroid.

On the basis of additional comparisons of experimental and calculated scatter plots, they chose, as the best match, the set with 10 times greater probability of differentiation into the granuloid rather than the erythroid line. They state that the model "accounts for the heterogeneity in cell numbers of different types in macroscopic spleen colonies. It agrees with the observed trend that colonies are predominantly of one type early, heterogeneous later. Moreover, it fixes the as yet unmeasured generation time of the cell in the granulocytic line at 12 ± 1 h and predicts that despite the fact that at late times erythroid cells are in the vast majority in the colonies, the decision to differentiate to the granulocytic line is favored over the erythroid line by a factor of 10." The authors point out "one serious flaw" of fixed generation times, and that the model ignored all secondary controls, such as feedback from increasing cell populations or the action of erythropoietin. Not mentioned was lack of consideration of the evidence of in vivo stromal microenvironmental influences on early differentiation into E vs G colonies or secondary cell lines. This includes different geographic points of origin of these two colony types in the spleen; delayed, yet endoclonal occurrence of granulopoiesis in the peripheral area of less differentiated cells of the largest erythroid colonies; failure of undifferentiated erythroid colonies to develop granulopoiesis in a polycythemic host, whereas the expected numbers of granulopoietic colonies are developing normally in the same spleen; markedly different ratios of erythroid to granuloid colonies developing in the marrow, compared to the spleen of the same animal; and the abrupt line of transition between erythropoiesis and granulopoiesis within a single colony (clone) as it grows from spleen stroma to marrow stroma implanted in the spleen, or vice versa.[37] Nor was mention made of the evidence of greater self-renewal of CFU-S in granulopoietic than erythropoietic spleen colonies (Table 3).[6]

On the other hand, given the existence of hemopoietic stromal microenvironmental influences, it must be conceded that random events must also exist in the process, such as the possibility of a given intravenously injected CFU being circulated first to the spleen rather than marrow, or vice versa; the possibility within each organ of making first contact by chance with one stromal cell type vs other types; or the possibility of a hemopoietic progenitor cell with multiple hormone receptors, as for the four known granulocyte–macrophage, multipotential colony stimulating factors,[129] being pre-empted first by one vs another colony stimulating factor, possibly by chance proximity to a stromal cell producing one CSF vs another.

In vitro, in the absence of stromal influences, the existence of apparently random events of differentiation and proliferation of multilineage hemopoietic blast cells and their progeny has been directly demonstrated by the still more recent elegant work of Ogawa and his associates. In 1982, Nakahata and Ogawa reported late appearing, small undifferentiated, slow growing "stem cell colonies" arising from bone marrow or spleen cells in methylcellulose cultures with pokeweed mitogen-stimulated spleen cell-conditioned medium (PWM-SCM) and erythropoietin.[181] Replating revealed self-renewal capacity and extensive ability to generate secondary colonies, some colonies having 100% replating efficiencies. Individual primary blast cell colonies had concurrent and high incidences of d 9 spleen colony forming units, and multilineal CFU-GEMM. Replating comparisons revealed the progenitors of blast cell colonies to be more primitive stem cells than CFU-GEMM. Of 68 blast cell colonies replated, 35 contained progenitors of blast cell colonies and 67 contained CFU-GEMM, the distribution of each in individual colonies being extremely heterogeneous.

In the absence of PWM-SCM or IL-3, no blast cell colony growth was observed. Delayed addition resulted in a reduction of blast cell colonies that became multilineage colonies, but did not alter the proliferative characteristics of late emerging blast cell colonies.[182] Using blast cell colonies derived from spleen cells of 5-FU-treated mice and micromanipulator techniques, they studied the differentiation of single progenitor cells and paired daughter cells through several single cell transfer passages. Some first generation colonies contained blast cells and all six differentiated cell lines in roughly the following order of frequency: monocyte–macrophage, neutrophil, mast cells, megakaryocytes, erythrocytic, blast, and eosinophilic. Others showed no progeny or only a single differentiated cell line, usually monocyte–macrophage or neutrophil. Others showed two or more of the differentiated cell lines in a suprisingly large number of combinations and relative frequencies. Paired daughter cells, placed in separate culture dishes, might give rise to similar or dissimilar differentiated cell types.[183,184] IL-3, in place of PWM-SCM, resulted in greater neutrophil and eosinophil expression and gave lineage combinations not seen with PWM-SCM.[182] With PWM-SCM, there was progressive and random loss of one or more differentiated progeny types from one generation to the next. This could go directly from six to one type in one generation, or less abruptly. The monocyte–macrophage and neutrophil cell lines were the last to be lost, in contrast to the obligatory erythrocytic differentiation data of Johnson.[185] In no case was there reacquisition of lost differentiation potential.

They concluded that self-renewal and commitment to differentiation of the primitive hemopoietic stem cells appear to be governed by a stochastic rule, although the distribution parameter (p) may be under regulation of humoral factors and that the current model supports a more complex and multistep process of differentiation of multipotential to monopotential progenitors, i.e., progressive and stochastic loss of potencies.[186] No mention was made of receptors for CSF's.

Although these results are extremely interesting and informative, it should be noted that the frequencies and order of appearance of differentiated cell types are markedly different than those in spleen colonies developing in vivo. Of great significance is that, during the first 16 d in primary culture of normal spleen cells, the undifferentiated cells of these blast cell colonies multiplied slowly and remained undifferentiated, whereas other cells were undergoing rapid multiplication and multilineage differentiation into large colonies, as if the more primitive blast cell colonies lacked receptors present on the less primitive colony-formers, receptors for the multiple colony stimulating factors present in PWM-SCM, receptors probably acquired in vivo. Indeed, most of the small blast cell colonies were not originally discovered until most of the large colonies degenerated. The sequence of events was clarified by primary cultures of spleen cells from 5-FU-treated mice, in which the more mature progenitors and their fast growing early differentiating colonies were eliminated. Small slow-growing, undifferentiated colonies made their first appearance every day from d 3 through 16 in the following numbers: 4, 2, 3, 7, 7, 14, 2,5, 3, 2, 3, 1, 2, 2.[187] These numbers plot as a sigmoid-type curve, typical of the dose-response curve for CSF concentration and the number of GM colonies developing in a culture dish, that is thought to relate to the 10-fold variation in GM-CSF receptor numbers observed on individual normal progenitor cells.[129] At 16 d, these 57 colonies consisted of 22 GEMM, 12 large GM (pure macrophage), 8 GMM, 8 megakaryocyte, 6 blast, and 1 GEM colony. Emerging blast cell colonies matured to GEMM colonies at a relatively constant number of days after first appearance, regardless of that time. In general, the appearance sequence of differentiated cells was megakaryocytic, granulocytic, and erythrocytic.

It would appear from these results that at least low levels of receptors for various CSF's are being acquired or increased in numbers or activity in vitro in the absence of direct stem cell–stromal cell contact. This could result from a genetically preprogrammed maturational event, possibly set in motion by the displacement of pluripotent stem cells from their G_o niches (microenvironment) in vivo. On the other hand, in embryo-genesis and organogenesis, there are examples of dependence on mesenchymal cell interaction with either endoderm or ecto-derm, involving the acquisition of hormone responsiveness, as in the case of the ingrowth of mammary buds. Early data in-dicated that CFU-S are not responsive to erythropoietin (EPO), but give rise to EPO-responsive stem cells.[52-55] Early spleen colony studies demonstrated that soon after CFU-S lodgment in an erythropoietic microenvironment of the spleen, it and/or its undifferentiated progeny acquired responsiveness to EPO, presumably by influence of the stromal cells of that microenvi-ronment, resulting in rapid proliferation and erythroid differ-entiation.[6] This suggests that the local stem cell–stromal cell interactions in hemopoietic microenvironments are mediated by local production and transfer of appropriate regulatory molecules for induction of the expression of receptors on stem cells for one or more CSF's.

Alternatively, if the appearance of low levels of receptors to multiple CSF's is genetically preprogrammed, the role of microenvironmental stromal cells may be to selectively in-crease or activate one or another type of receptor and/or to pro-duce one or another CSF for local use. Multi-CSF (IL-3), with stimulation properties for granulocytes, macrophages, erythroid cells, eosinophils, megakaryocytes, mast cells, and stem cells, is not normally detectable in circulation and is presumed to be produced and act short range upon local target cells, possibly by cell–cell contact.[129] Since responsiveness to CSF's of these multiple cell lines appears to develop concurrently in the blast cell colonies, the survival, growth, and differentiation of which are IL-3 dependent, IL-3 may be involved in the activation and/or utilization of receptors to multiple CSF's. The abun-dant evidence for a controlling influence of local microenviron-mental stromal cells on hemopoietic stem cell self-renewal and differentiation in vivo, and in the Dexter-type long-term marrow cultures in vitro, cannot be ignored. As mentioned earlier, regarding long-term liquid cultures of bone marrow in which CFU-S proliferation does occur, but only in cell–cell contact with an obligatory stromal cell layer, Dexter describes the system as very rigidly controlled, presumably by cell–cell interactions.[150] Nor can the evidence of additional random stochastic events in vivo, as mentioned above, and in vitro, in the absence of stromal cell interactions, be ignored.

How then can these seemingly conflicting observations be rationalized? It is suggested that PHSC's have the genetic potential for expression of receptors for the many CSF's of each of its many possible lines of differentiation. However, while still in resting reserve in G_o niches of the marrow stroma, these receptors may be either not expressed or some or all may be expressed at very low levels. But on appropriate regulatory signals, one or more or a combination of receptors may be either expressed or upregulated or both. Release of PHSC from the G_o stromal niches appears to be triggered by remote (humoral) signal(s) since subtotal irradiation of mice is reported to result in an increase in circulating CFU-S, presumably from the unirradiated marrow. Expression or upregulation of receptors for some CSF's of some lines of differentiation appears to be locally controlled, since the PHSC acquires responsiveness to EPO shortly after lodgment in an erythroid stromal microenvironment of the spleen.[6] It seems logical that not all stem cells or progenitors of other lines of differentiation should be highly responsive to EPO, lest a hypoxic condition needlessly drain cell lines other than erythropoietic. The same should apply to responsiveness to CSF's of other lines of differentiation. The different hemopoietic and lymphopoietic stromal microenvironments may thus serve to allocate subsets of PHSC for responsiveness to CSF's of one or another line of differentiation as needed.

It is apparent that some hemopoietic progenitor stem cells of freshly collected bone marrow or spleen cell suspensions have already acquired responsiveness (upregulated receptors) for CSF's of one or another line of differentiation, as a result of prior in vivo interactions, as in the acquisition of responsiveness to EPO in an erythroid stromal microenvironment. Such cells should behave accordingly when transplanted in vivo, or cultured in vitro. In methyl cellulose cultures, they presumably account for the early developing and rapidly differentiating colonies of single lineage, dependent on appropriate cultural conditions and CSF's for that line of differentiation.

Other PHSC of freshly collected marrow, perhaps just released from their resting state in G_0 niches of the marrow stroma, may not yet have acquired such responsiveness to a single line of differentiation. These may account for the blast cells of the late developing "stem cell" colonies in methylcellulose cultures. It is suggested that in the absence of the strong in vivo stromal microenvironmental influences on these processes, the blast cells of the methylcellulose "stem cell" colonies slowly acquire low levels of receptors for one or more of the different CSF's, either genetically preprogrammed or under the influence of added IL-3, or of IL-1, IL-3, or related factors, known or unknown, alone or in combination, in the polk weed mitogen-spleen conditioned medium. Those stem cells with newly acquired or activated receptors are then susceptible to competitive preemption by any one of the corresponding colony stimulating factors in the culture medium, in a seemingly random manner.

It is further suggested that in vivo, as a rapidly expanding pluripotent but initially erythropoietic spleen colony grows outward from its original erythropoietic microenvironment, and self-renewing PHSC in its peripheral zone of morphologically less differentiated cells[5] encounter granulopoietic or mega-karyocytic stromal microenvironments and develop endoclonal foci of these differentiation lines,[56] it may also occupy some areas lacking strong stromal CSF influences, such that some of its progenitor cells, with receptors recently appeared but not yet preempted by CSF's may, on transfer to in vitro culture, be detected as a progenitor stem cell of one or another line of differentiation.[187a,187b]

It is further suggested that in vitro, in the absence of continued reinforcement, as receptors for different CSF's are degraded and lost,[129] the differentiation capacity for that cell line is lost, accounting for the "progressive and stochastic loss of potencies" observed by Ogawa et al.[186] Depending on differences in starting cells and cultural conditions, this would also account for the differences in the last line of (obligatory) differentiation seen by Johnson[185] and Ogawa et al.[186] Competition for preemption of pluripotent stem cells with multiple receptors, by one or another humoral factor, is in accord also with the competition observed by Van Zant and Goldwasser[188] between erythropoietin and GM-CSF for target cells in mouse bone marrow.

It is further suggested that the degradation of receptors initially induced or selectively increased by the dominant receptor-inducing or reinforcing microenvironments of the spleen, marrow, or fetal liver, and the reacquisition of a new set of receptors, after transplantation, in the dominant receptor-inducing or reinforcing microenvironment of one of the other organs, could account for the reversal of Duplan's "reversible imprint" of marrow or spleen stem cells for competitive repopulation of the thymus, after 9 d residence in the other organ.[122,123] It could also account for Wolf's[126] "reversible predisposition" for direction of differentiation by fetal liver cells depending on whether they form hemopoietic colonies in the spleen (E:G colony ratio of 50) or marrow (E:G colony ratio of 2). This assumes that CFU from fetal liver have hormone receptors for both EPO and G-M CSF's, but that the dominant spleen microenvironments selectively reinforce the erythropoietin receptors and/ or are much more highly competitive for preemption, via the EPO receptors, for expression of erythroid differentiation, whereas the reverse is true of the dominant marrow microenvironments. The "adaptive differentiation" of Natural killer (NK) large granular lymphocytes and T-lymphocytes, and their "plasticity" in vitro has been reviewed by Grossman and Herberman.[189]

Projections

The "G-M people" have made a good start at CSF receptor research.[129] The same is sorely needed for erythropoietin receptors. The perfection of the multiple hemopoietic and lymphopoietic hormone receptor technologies and their application, both in vitro and in vivo, will resolve many of the remaining puzzles regarding which stromal cells do what, to which stem cells, and when, where, and how, with reference to self-renewal, differentiation, proliferation, and terminal maturation. Among these are the questions of how many stromal cells, and in what arrangement, constitute a given hemopoietic or lymphoid microenvironment; which cells act by inducing or enhancing the expression of a receptor; which cells produce CSF's that act short range; which cells act by direct cell to cell contact; what are the regulatory molecules involved, and their mechanisms of action; and are there such things as malignancy-inducing microenvironments?

Malignancy-Inducing Microenvironments?

If stromal cell–stem cell microenvironmental interactions can so importantly control the self-renewal and differentiation of the pluripotent bone marrow stem cell and its progeny in more than a dozen different normal myeloid and lymphoid cell lines, is it possible that an aberrant stromal cell regulatory message may result in malignant myeloid or lymphoid cells? Thymic lymphoma–leukemia occurs spontaneously in some strains of mice. It originates in the thymus, spreads to other organs, and has a terminal leukemic phase. In other strains, it can be readily induced by irradiation, chemicals, estrogen, or viruses.[190–192] Most, if not all, strains of mice have vertically transmitted leukemia-like retroviruses that can be found in the thymus. Spontaneous murine lymphoma–leukemia can be transmitted by retrovirus. Irradiation-induced murine leukemia is indirectly mediated and transmissible by endogenous retrovirus (Rad LV).[190,192] Thymectomy of young adult mice prevents or virtually eliminates T-cell lymphoma–leukemia, whether spontaneously occurring or caused by irradiation, chemicals, estrogen, or virus, even though such mice still have extrathymic T-cells and virus.[193,194] The murine thymus, probably because of its primary role in T-cell differentiation, and retrovirus activity, indeed appears to contain malignancy-inducing microenvironments.

Acknowledgments

The author gratefully acknowledges the valuable consultation of Norman Wolf, Mehdi Tavassoli, and Dennis Osmond in the preparation of this manuscript. The author's investigations presented herein were supported by USPHS grants K06-CA-14219, CA-03367, CA-05021, CA-12093, and AM-30857.

References

[1]Tavassoli, M. (1980) *Blood, Pure and Eloquent* (Wintrobe, M. M., ed.), McGraw Hill, New York, pp. 57–79.

[2]Trentin, J. J. (1970) *Regulation of Hematopoiesis* (Gordon, A., ed.), Appleton Century-Crofts, New York, pp. 161–186.

[3]Tavassoli, M. (1975) *Exp. Hematol.* **3,** 213–226.

[4]Tavassoli, M. and Friedenstein, A. (1983) *Am. J. Hematol.* **15,** 195–203.

[5]Curry, J. L. and Trentin, J. J. (1967) *Developmental Biology* **15,** 395–413.

[6]Curry, J. L., Trentin, J. J., and Wolf, N. (1967) *J. Exp. Med.* **125,** 703–720.

[7]Jacobson, L. O., Marks, E. K., Gaston, E. O., Robson, M. J., and Zirkel, R. E. (1949) *Proc. Soc. Exp. Biol. Med.* **70,** 740–742.

[8]Jacobson, L. O., Simmons, E. L., Marks, E. K., and Eldridge, J. (1951) *Science* **113,** 510, 511.

[9]Lorenz, E., Uphoff, D., Reid, T. R., and Shelton, M. (1951) *J. Natl. Cancer Inst.* **12,** 197–201.

[10]Trentin, J. J. (1956) *Proc. Soc. Exp. Biol. Med.* **92,** 688–693.

[11]Trentin, J. J. (1957) *Proc. Soc. Exp. Biol. Med.* **96,** 139–144.

[12]Ford, C. E., Micklem, H. S., and Gray, S. M. (1959) *Br. J. Radiol.* **32,** 280 (abstract).

[13]Till, J. E. and McCulloch, E. A. (1961) *Rad. Res.* **14,** 213–222.

[14]Becker, A. J., McCulloch, E. A., and Till, J. E. (1963) *Nature* (London) **197,** 452–454.

[15]Ford, C. E., Ilbery, P. L. T., and Loutit, J. F. (1957) *J. Cell. Comp. Physiol.* **50,** 109–121.

[16]Everett, N. B., Riche, W. O., and Caffrey, R. W. (1964) *The Thymus in Immunobiology* (Good, R. A. and Gabrielsen, A. E., eds.), Hoeber Medical Books, New York, pp. 291–297.

[17]Gowans, J. L. (1964) *The Thymus in Immunobiology* (Good, R. A. and Gabrielsen, A. E., eds.), Hoeber Medical Books, New York, pp. 255–273.

[18]Ford, C. E. (1966) *Ciba Foundation Symposium: The Thymus: Experimental and Clinical Studies* (Wolstenbolme, G. E. W., ed.), Little, Brown, Boston, pp. 131–152.

[19]Barnes, D. W. H. and Loutit, J. F. (1967) *Lancet* **2,** 1138–1141.

[20]Gesner, B. M. and Ginsburg, V. (1964) *Proc. Natl. Acad. Sci. USA* **52,** 750–755.

[21]Woodruff, J. and Gesner, B. M. (1968) *Science* **161,** 176–178.

[22]Stamper, H. B., Jr. and Woodruff, J. J. (1976) *J. Exp. Med.* **144,** 828–833.

[22a]Gallatin, M., St. John, T. P., Siegelman, M., Reichert, R., Butcher, E. C., and Weissman, I. L. (1986) *Cell* **44,** 673–680.

[22b]Stoolman, L. M., Tenforde, T. S., and Rosen, S. D. (1984) *J. Cell Biol.* **99,** 1535–1540.

[23]Tavassoli, M., Kishimoto, T., Harjes, K., and Collier, B. (1985) *Exp. Hematol.* **13,** 968–973.

[24]Kataoka, M. and Tavassoli, M. (1985) *Blood* **65,** 1163–1171.

[25]Soda, R. and Tavassoli, M. (1983) *J. Ultrastruct. Res.* **84,** 299–310.

[26]Soda, R. and Tavassoli, M. (1984) *J. Ultrastruct. Res.* **87,** 242–251.

[27]Pino, R.M. (1984) *Am. J. Anat.* **169,** 259–272.

[28]Hardy, C. L., Kishimoto, T., Harjes, K., Tavassoli, M., and Greenberger, J. (1986) *Exp. Hematol.* **14,** 636–642.

[29]Fernbach, D. J. and Trentin, J. J. (1962) *Proceeding of the VIIIth International Congress of Hematology,* vol. 1, Pan-Pacific, Tokyo, pp. 150–155.

[30]Nara, N., Bessho, M., Hirashima, K., and Momoi, H. (1982) *Exp. Hematol.* **10,** 20–25.

[31]Hotta, T. (1980) *Acta Haematol. Jap.* **43,** 649–660.

[32]Trentin, J. J. and Fahlberg, W. J. (1963) *Conceptual Advances in Immunology and Oncology,* Harper and Row, Hoeber Medical Division, New York, pp. 66–74.

[33]Trentin, J. J., Wolf, N., Cheng, V., Fahlberg, W., Weiss, D., and Bonhag, R. (1967) *J. Immunol.* **98,** 1326–1337.

[34]Curry, J. L., Trentin, J. J., and Wolf, N. S. (1964) ORNL *Exp. Hematol.* **7,** 80.

[35]Curry, J. L., Trentin, J. J., and Cheng, V. (1967) *J. Immunol.* **99,** 907–916.

[36]Curry, J. L. and Trentin, J. J. (1967) *J. Exp. Med.* **126,** 819–832.

[37]Wolf, N. S. and Trentin, J. J. (1968) *J. Exp. Med.* **127,** 205–214.

[38]Till, J. E., McCulloch, E. A., and Siminovitch, L. (1964) *Proc. Natl. Acad. Sci. USA* **51,** 29–36.

[39]Lewis, J. P. and Trobaugh, F. E., Jr. (1964) *Nature* **204,** 589, 590.

[40]Wolf, N. S., Jenkins, V. K., and Trentin, J. J. (1972) *Exp. Hematol.* **22,** 37, 38.

[41]Wolf, N. S. (1974) *Cell Tissue Kinet.* **7,** 89–98.

[42]Duplan, J. F., Legrand, E., Castaignos, C., and de Calignon, E. (1979) *Int. J. Radiat. Biol.* **36,** 595–600.

[43]Lahiri, S. K. and Van Putten, L. M. (1969) *Cell Tissue Kinet.* **2,** 21–28.

[44]Magli, M. C., Iscove, N. N., and Odartchenko, N. (1982) *Nature* **295,** 527–529.

[45]Schooley, J. C. (1964) *Exp. Hematol.* **7,** 79.

[46]Lirion, M. and Feldman, M. (1965) *Israel J. Med. Sci.* **1,** 86–88.

[47]Bleiberg, I., Lirion, M., and Feldman, M. (1965) *Transplantation* **3,** 706–710.

[48]O'Grady, L. F., Lewis, J. P., Lange, R., and Trobaugh, F. E. (1966) *Exp. Hematol.* **9,** 77–80.

[49]Marsh, J. C., Boggs, D. R., Chervenick, P. A., Cartwright, G. E., and Wintrobe, M. M. (1968) *J. Cell. Physiol.* **71,** 65–76.

[50]Bleiberg, I., Lirion, M., and Feldman, M. (1967) *Blood* **29,** 469–480.

[51]Trentin, J. J., Curry, J. L., Wolf, N., and Cheng, V. (1968) *The Proliferation and Spread of Neoplastic Cells,* Williams and Wilkins, Baltimore, pp. 713–731.

[52]Bruce, W. R. and McCulloch, E. A. (1964) *Blood* **23,** 216–232.

[53]Fried, W., Martinson, D., Weisman, M., and Gurney, C. W. (1966) *Exp. Hematol.* **10,** 22.

⁵⁴Schooley, J. C. (1966) *J. Cell Physiol.* **68**, 249–262.
⁵⁵Till, J. E., Siminovitch, L., and McCulloch, E. A. (1966) *Exp. Hematol.* **9**, 59.
⁵⁶Trentin, J. J. (1971) *Amer. J. Path.* **65**, 621–628.
⁵⁷Dexter, T. M. and Moore, M. A. S. (1977) *Nature* **269**, 412–414.
⁵⁸Chen, M. G. and Schooley, J. C. (1968) *Transplantation* **6**, 121–126.
⁵⁹Tavassoli, M., Ratzan, R. J., and Crosby, W. H. (1973) *Blood* **41**, 701–709.
⁶⁰Tavassoli, M., Ratzan, R. J., Maniatis, A., and Crosby, W. H. (1973) *J. Reticuloendothel. Soc.* **13**, 518–526.
⁶¹Wolf, N. S. (1982) *Exp. Hematol.* **10**, 98–107.
⁶²Tavassoli, M., Sacks, P. V., and Crosby, W. H. (1975) *Proc. Soc. Exp. Biol. Med.* **148**, 780–783.
⁶³Wolf, N. S. (1982) *Exp. Hematol.* **10**, 108–118.
⁶⁴Till, J. E., McCulloch, E. A., Phillips, R. A., and Siminovitch, L. (1968) *The Proliferation and Spread of Neoplastic Cells*, Williams and Wilkins, Baltimore, pp. 235–245.
⁶⁵Trentin, J. J., Curry, J. L., Wolf, N. S., and Cheng, V. (1968) *The Proliferation and Spread of Neoplastic Cells*, Williams and Wilkins, Baltimore, pp. 713–731.
⁶⁶Bernstein, S. E. (1970) *Am. J. Surgery* **119**, 448–451.
⁶⁷Dunn, C. D. R. and Elson, L. A. (1970) *Br. J. Haematol.* **19**, 755–764.
⁶⁸Rauchwerger, J. M., Gallagher, M. T., and Trentin, J. J. (1973) *Proc. Soc. Exp. Biol. Med.* **143**, 145,146.
⁶⁹Cudkowicz, G. and Bennett, J. (1971) *J. Exp. Med.* **134**, 83–102.
⁷⁰McCulloch, E. A. and Till, J. E. (1963) *J. Cell. Comp. Physiol.* **61**, 301–308.
⁷¹Goodman, J. W. and Wheeler, H. B. (1968) *Transplantation* **6**, 173–186.
⁷²Lotzova, E., Dicke, K. S., Trentin, J. J., and Gallagher, M. T. (1977) *Transpl. Proc.* **9**, 289–292.
⁷³Trentin, J. J., Rauchwerger, J. M., and Gallagher, M. T. (1973) *Biomedicine* **18**, 86–88.
⁷⁴Trentin, J. J., Kiessling, R., Wigzell, H., Gallagher, M. T., Datta, S. K., and Kulkarni, S. S. (1977) *Experimental Hematology Today* (Baum, S. J. and Ledney, G. D., eds.), Springer-Verlag, New York, pp. 179–183.
⁷⁵Datta, S. K., Gallagher, M. T., Trentin, J. J., Kiessling, R., and Wigzell, H. (1979) *Biomedicine* **31**, 62–66.
⁷⁶Trentin, J. J., Gallagher, M. T., and Lotzova, E. (1976) *Transpl. Proc.* **8**, 463–468.
⁷⁷Rauchwerger, J. M., Gallagher, M. T., and Trentin, J. J. (1973) *Transplantation* **15**, 610–613.
⁷⁸Speirs, R. S. and Speirs, E. E. (1964) *J. Immunol.* **92**, 540–549.
⁷⁹Speirs, R. S. and Turner, M. X. (1969) *Blood* **34**, 320–330.
⁸⁰Jenkins, V. K., Trentin, J. J., Speirs, R. S., and McGarry, M. P. (1972) *J. Cellu-*

lar Physiology **79**, 413–422.

81Block, M. H. (1976) *Text-Atlas of Hematology,* Lea and Febiger, Philadelphia, Plates XXXIX–XL, pp. 39, 40.

82Kitamura, Y., Shimada, M., Hatanaka, K., and Miyano, Y. (1977) *Nature* **268**, 442, 443.

83Kitamura, Y., Shimada, M., Go, S., Matsuda, H., Hatanaka, K., and Seki, M. (1979) *J. Exp. Med.* **150**, 482–490.

84Kitamura, Y., Go, S., and Hatanaka, K. (1978) *Blood* **52**, 447–452.

85Kitamura, Y. and Go, S. (1979) *Blood* **53**, 492–497.

86Kitamura, Y., Matsuda, H., and Hatanaka, K. (1979) *Nature* **281**, 154, 155.

87Hatanaka, K., Kitamura, Y., and Nishiomune, Y. (1979) *Blood* **53**, 142–147.

88Wolf, N. S. (1974) *Cell Tissue Kinet.* **7**, 89–98.

89Wolf, N. S. (1978) *Cell Tissue Kinet.* **11**, 325–334.

90Wolf, N. S. (1978) *Cell Tissue Kinet.* **11**, 335–345.

91Knospe, W. H., Blom, J., and Crosby, W. H. (1966) *Blood* **28**, 398–415.

92Jenkins, V. K., Trentin, J. J. , and Wolf, N. S. (1970) *Radiat. Res.* **43**, 212.

93Tavassoli, M. and Crosby, W. H. (1968) *Science* **161**, 54–56.

94Knospe, W. H., Blom, J., and Crosby, W. H. (1968) *Blood* **31**, 400–405.

95Knospe, W. H., Gregory, S. A., Husseini, S. G., Fried, W., and Trobaugh, F. E., Jr. (1972) *Blood* **39**, 331–340.

96Kitamura, Y., Kawata, T., Suda, O., and Ezumi, K. (1970) *Transplantation* **10**, 455–462.

97Knospe, W. H., Blom, J., Goldstein, H. B., and Crosby, W. H. (1971) *Radiat. Res.* **47**, 199–212.

98Kitamura, Y., Kawata, T., Kanamaru, A., and Seki, M. (1973) *Exp. Hematol.* **1**, 350–361.

99Huiskamp, R., van Vliet, E., and Van Ewijk, W. J. (1985) *Immunol.* **134**, 2170–2178.

100Seki, M. (1973) *Transplantation* **16**, 544–549.

101Knospe, W. H., Mortenson, R., Husseini, S., and Trobaugh, F. E., Jr. (1978) *Exp. Hematol.* **6**, 233–245.

102Knospe, W. H., Husseini, S., and Trobaugh, F. E., Jr. (1978) *Exp. Hematol.* **6**, 601–612.

103Knospe, W. H., Husseini, S., and Adler, S. S. (1983) *Exp. Hematol.* **11**, 512–521.

104Magli, M. C., Iscove, N. N., and Odartchenko, N. (1982) *Nature* **295**, 527–529.

105Barnes, D. W. H., Evans, E. P., Ford, C. E., and West, B. J. (1968) *Nature* **219**, 518–520.

106Worton, R. G., McCulloch, E. A., and Till, J. E. (1969) *J. Exp. Med.* **130**, 91–103.

107Schofield, R. and Lajtha, G. (1973) *Br. J. Haematol.* **25**, 195–202.

[108]Hodgson, G. S. and Bradley, T. R. (1979) *Nature* **281**, 381, 382.

[109]Hodgson, G. S., Bradley, T. R., and Radley, J. M. (1982) *Exp. Hematol.* **10**, 26–35.

[110]Monette, F. C. and Stockel, J. B. (1981) *Stem Cells* **1**, 38–52.

[110a]Muller-Sieburg, C. E., Whitlock, C. A., and Weissman, I. L. (1986) *Cell* **44**, 653–662.

[111]Baines, P. and Visser, J. W. M. (1983) *Exp. Hematol.* **11**, 701–708.

[112]Porcellini, A., Manna, A., Talevi, N., Sparoventi, G., Marchetti-Rossi, M. T., Baronciani, D., and De Biagi, M. (1984) *Exp. Hematol.* **12**, 863–866.

[113]Harris, R. A., Hogarth, P. M., Wadeson, L. J., Collins, P., McKenzie, I. F. C., and Pennington, D. G. (1984) *Nature* **307**, 638–641.

[114]Visser, J. W. M., Bauman, J. G. J., Mulder, A. H., Eliason, J. F., and De Leeuw, A. M. (1984) *J. Exp. Med.* **159**, 1576–1590.

[115]Mulder, A. H., Visser, J. W. M., and van den Engh, G. J. (1985) *Exp. Hematol.* **13**, 768–775.

[116]Peterson, H. P., Von Wangenheim, K. H., and Feinendegen, L. E. (1986) *Exp. Hematol.* **14**, 776–781.

[117]Martens, A. C. M., van Bekkum, D. W., and Hagenbeek, A. (1986) *Exp. Hematol.* **14**, 714–718.

[118]Priestley, G. V. and Wolf, N. S. (1985) *Exp. Hematol.* **12**, 733–735.

[119]Wolf, N. S. and Priestley, G. V. (1986) *Exp. Hematol.* **14**, 676–682.

[120]van Zant, G. (1984) *J. Exp. Med.* **159**, 679–690.

[121]Molineau, G., Schofield, R., and Testa, N. G. (1986) *Exp. Hematol.* **14**, 710–713.

[122]Muramatsu, S., Monnot, P., and Duplan, J. F. (1976) *Exp. Hematol.* **4**, 188–200.

[123]Legrand, E., Daculsi, R., and Duplan, J. F. (1979) *Leuk. Res.* **3**, 253–259.

[124]Basch, R. S., Kadish, J. L., and Goldstein, G. (1978) *J. Exp. Med.* **147**, 1843–1848.

[125]Schofield, R. and Lajtha, L. G. (1969) *Cell Tiss. Kinet.* **2**, 147–155.

[126]Wolf, N. S. (1978) *Blood Cells* **4**, 37–51.

[127]Wolf, N. S. (1983) *Frontiers in Experimental Hematology* (Torelli, U., Bagnaro, G. P., Brunelli, M. A., Custaldini, C., and DiPrisco, A. U. , eds.), Serono Symposia, Rome, pp. 233–251.

[128]Metcalf, D. (1984) *The Hemopoietic Colony Stimulating Factors*, Elsevier, Amsterdam, p. 493.

[129]Metcalf, D. (1985) *Science* **229**, 16–22.

[129a]Clark, S. C. and Kamen, R. (1987) *Science* **236**, 1229–1237.

[130]Harris, J. E., Ford, C. E., Barnes, D. W. H., and Evans, E. P. (1964) *Nature* **201**, 884–887.

[131]Barnes, D. W. H., Ford, C. E., Gray, S. M., and Loutit, J. F. (1959) *Progress in Nuclear Energy*, Series VI (2) (Bugher, J. C., Coursaget, J., and Loutit,

J. F., eds.), Pergammon, London, pp. 1–10.

[132]Ford, C. E. and Clarke, C. M. (1963) *Proc. Fifth Canadian Consec. Conf.,* National Cancer Institute of Canada, Academic, New York, pp. 129–146.

[133]Wu, A. M., Till, J. E., Siminovitch, L., and McCulloch, E. A. (1968) *J. Exp. Med.* **127,** 455–464.

[134]Ewijk, W. V. (1984) *Am. J. Anat.* **170,** 311–330.

[135]Osmond, D. G. (1985) *J. Inv. Derm.* **85,** Suppl. 1, 2s–9s.

[136]Wekerle, H., Ketelsen, V. P., and Ernst, M. (1980) *J. Exp. Med.* **151,** 925–944.

[137]Osmond, D. G. and Batten, S. J. (1984) *Am. J. Anat.* **170,** 349–365.

[137a]Spangrude, G. J., Heimfeld, S., and Weissman, T. L. (1988) *Science* **241,** 58–62.

[138]Metcalf, D. and Johnson, G. R. (1976) *Immuno-aspects of the Spleen* (Batisto, J. R. and Streilein, J. W., eds.), Elsevier, Amsterdam, pp. 27–36.

[139]Lala, P. K. and Johnson, G. R. (1978) *J. Exp. Med.* **148,** 1468–1477.

[140]Bradley, T. R. and Metcalf, D. (1966) *Aust. J. Exp. Biol. Med. Sci.* **44,** 287–300.

[141]Ichikawa, Y., Pluznik, D. H., and Sachs, L. (1966) *Proc. Natl. Acad. Sci. USA* **56,** 488–495.

[142]McCulloch, E. A., ed. (1984) *Clinics in Hematology* **13,** 2, Saunders, London.

[143]Robinson, W. A., ed. (1973) *Hemopoiesis in Culture,* Second International Workshop, May 23–26, D. H. E. W. Publication No. (NIH) 74-205, US Government Printing Office, Washington, DC, pp. 277, 278.

[144]Chang, Y. T. and Andersen, R. N. (1971) *J. Reticuloendothel. Soc.* **9,** 568–579.

[145]Dexter, T. M. and Lajtha, L. G. (1973) *Br. J. Hematol.* **28,** 525–530.

[146]Dexter, T. M. and Testa, N. G. (1976) *Differentiation and Proliferation of Hemopoietic Cells in Culture in Methods in Cell Biology,* vol. XIV (Prescott, D. M., ed.), Academic, New York, pp. 387–405.

[147]Allen, T. D. and Dexter T. M. (1976) *Differentiation* **6,** 191–194.

[148]Greenberger, J. S. (1978) *Nature* **275,** 752–754.

[149]Greenberger, J. S. (1984) *Methods in Hematology: Hematopoiesis* (Golde, D. W., ed.), Churchill Livingstone, New York, pp. 203–242.

[150]Dexter, T. M., Spooncer, E., Simmons, P., and Allen, T. D. (1984) *Long-Term Bone Marrow Culture* (Wright, D. G. and Greenberger, J. S., eds.), Liss, New York, pp. 57–96.

[151]Greenberger, J. S. (1984) *Long-Term Bone Marrow Culture* (Wright, D. G. and Greenberger, J. S., eds.), Liss, New York, pp. 119–131.

[152]Tavassoli, M. and Takahashi, K. (1982) *Am. J. Anat.* **164,** 91–111.

[153]Allen, T. D. (1980) *Microenvironments in Haemopoietic and Lymphoid Differentiation* (Porter, R. and Whelan, J., eds.), Pitman, London, pp. 38–67.

[154]Dexter, T. M., Heyworth, C. M., and Spooncer, E. (1985) *Mediators of Immune Regulation and Immunotherapy* (Singhal, S. K. and Delovitch, T. L., eds.), Elsevier, New York, pp. 101–111.

[155]Bentley, S. A. (1981) *Exp. Hematol.* **9**, 308–312.

[156]Dexter, T. M., Spooncer, E., Varga, G., Allen, T. D., and Lanotte, M. (1983) *Haemopoietic Stem Cells*, Alfred Benzon Symposium No. 18 (Killman S. V. -A. A., Cronkite, E. P., and Muler-Berat, C. N., eds.), Munksguard, Copenhagen, pp. 303–322.

[157]Dexter, T. M., Simmons, P. Purnell, R. A., Spooncer, E., and Schofield, R. (1984) *Aplastic Anemia: Stem Cell Biology and Advances in Treatment* (Young, N. S., Levine, A. S., and Humphries, A. K., eds.), Liss, New York, pp. 13–33.

[158]Kincade, P. W., Lee, G., Paige, G. J., and Scheid, M. P. (1981) *J. Immunol.* **127**, 255–260.

[159]Dorshkind, K. and Phillips, R.A. (1983) *J. Immunol.* **131**, 2240–2245.

[160]Whitlock, S. A. and Witte, O. N. (1982) *Natl. Acad. Sci. USA* **79**, 3608–3612.

[161]Dexter, T. M. (1976) *Differentiation* **6**, 191–194.

[162]Weiss, L. (1976) *Anat. Rec.* **186**, 161–184.

[163]Dorshkind, K., Schouest, L., and Fletcher, W. H. (1985) *Cell Tissue Res.* **239**, 375–382.

[164]La Pushin, R. W. and de Harven, E. (1971) *J. Cell Biol.* **50**, 583–597.

[165]La Pushin, R. W. and Trentin, J. J. (1977) *Exp. Hematol.* **5**, 505–522.

[166]Bessis, M. C. and Breton-Gorius, J. (1962) *Blood* **19**, 635–663.

[167]Berman, I. (1967) *J. Ultrastruct. Res.* **17**, 291–313.

[168]Ben-Ishay, Z. and Yoffey, J. M. (1971) *J. Reticuloendoth. Soc.* **10**, 482–500.

[169]Ben-Ishay, Z. and Yoffey, J. M. (1972) *Lab. Invest.* **26**, 637–647.

[170]Chen, L. T. and Weiss, L. (1975) *Blood* **46**, 389–408.

[171]Macario, A. J. L., de Macario, E. C., and Dugan, C. B. (1983) *Cell Separation Methods and Selected Applications*, Academic, New York, pp. 273–316.

[172]Westen, H. and Bainton, D. F. (1979) *J. Exp. Med.* **150**, 919–937.

[173]Ahmad, L. A. and Bainton, D. F. (1986) *Exp. Hematol.* **14**, 705–709.

[174]Friedenstein, A. J., Chailakhyan, R. K., Latsinik, N. V., Panasyuk, A. F., and Keiliss-Borok, I. V. (1974) *Transplantation* **17**, 331–340.

[175]Urist, M. R. (1965) *Science* **150**, 893–899.

[176]Reddi, A. H. and Anderson, W. A. (1976) *J. Cell Biol.* **69**, 557–572.

[177]Brockbank, K. G. M., Ogawa, M., and Spector, M. (1980) *Exp. Hematol.* **8**, 763–769.

[178]Huggins, C., McCarroll, H., and Blocksom, B. (1936) *Arch. Surg.* **32**, 915–931.

[179]Friedenstein, A. Y. (1968) *Clinical Orthopaedics and Related Research* **59**, 21–37.

[179a]Greenberger, J. S., Humphries, K., Eckner, R. J., and Sakakeeny, M. A. (1983) *Normal and Neoplastic Hematopoieses*, Liss, New York, pp. 157–178.

[179b]Li, C. L. and Johnson, G. R. (1985) *Nature* **316**, 633–636.

[180]Korn, A. P., Henkelman, R. M., Ottensmeyer, F. P., and Till, J. E. (1973) *Exp. Hematol.* **1**, 362–375.

[181]Nakahata, T. and Ogawa, M. (1982) *Proc. Natl. Acad. Sci. USA* **79**, 3843–3847.

[182]Ogawa, M., Pharr, P. N., and Suda, T. (1985) *Hematopoietic Stem Cell Physiology*, Liss, New York, pp. 11–19.

[183]Suda, T., Suda, J., and Ogawa, M. (1984) *Proc. Natl. Acad. Sci. USA* **81**, 2520–2524.

[184]Suda, J., Suda, T., and Ogawa, M. (1984) *Blood* **64**, 393–399.

[185]Johnson, G. R. (1981) *Experimental Hematology Today* (Baum, S. J., Ledney G. D., and Khan, A., eds.), Karger, Basel, pp. 13–20.

[186]Ogawa, M., Porter, P. N., and Nakahata, T. (1983) *Blood* **61**, 823–829.

[187]Suda, T., Suda, J., and Ogawa, M. (1983) *J. Cell Physiol.* **117**, 308–318.

[187a]Gregory, C. J., McCulloch, E. A., and Till, J. E. (1972) *Transplantation* **13**, 138–141.

[187b]Gregory, C. J. (1976) *J. Cellular Physiol.* **89**, 289–301.

[188]van Zant, G. and Goldwasser, E. (1979) *Blood* **53**, 946–965.

[189]Grossman, Z. and Herberman, R. B. (1986) *Cancer Res.* **46**, 2651–2658.

[190]Kaplan, H. S. (1967) *Cancer Res.* **27**, 1325–1340.

[191]Gardner, W. U., Pfeiffer, C. A., and Trentin, J. J. (1959) *The Physiopathology of Cancer*, 2nd ed. (Homburger, F., ed.), Hoeber-Harper, New York, pp. 152–237.

[192]Gross, L. (1951) *Proc. Soc. Exp. Biol. and Med.* **78**, 342–348.

[193]McEndy, D. P., Boon, M. C., and Furth, J. (1944) *Cancer Res.* **4**, 377–390.

[194]Trentin, J. J. (1964) *The Thymus in Immunobiology* (Good, R. A. and Gabrielsen, A. E. eds.), Hoeber and Row, New York, pp. 753–762.

Chapter 2

Molecular and Cellular Traffic Across the Marrow Sinuses

Marshall A. Lichtman,
Charles H. Packman,
and Louis S. Constine

Introduction

In those species in which hemopoiesis is confined to the extravascular compartment of marrow, the marrow sinus wall separates the hemopoietic cells from the circulation. This vascular barrier regulates the traffic of cells and macromolecules that move from blood to marrow or marrow to blood. In this chapter, we review the current state of knowledge regarding the transfer of cells and molecules across the marrow sinus wall.

Marrow Structure

Extensive studies of marrow have been performed on animals, principally rodents.[1-36] Certain animals like the mouse, provide advantages to the anatomist. The mouse has active hemopoiesis in its femoral marrow, and its central femur contains no trabecular bone or fat cells. Thus, for transmission electron microscopy, the femur can be excised rapidly and fixed by immersion, or it can be perfused *in situ* with fixative, removed, and decorticated prior to preparation for examination. Decalcification and sectioning through bone is avoided, and excellent specimens can be prepared for examination. The femurs fixed by perfusion are good specimens for study by scanning electron microscopy since their vascular sinuses are cleared of blood, permitting visualization of the luminal surface. Much of what we know of the structure of the marrow derives from studies of the mouse and the rat, both of which have femurs with active hemopoiesis and without trabecular bone, although the rat femur, unlike that of the mouse, contains a small proportion of fat cells.

Arterial and Venous Circulation

The arterial blood supply of marrow comes from two major sources.[15] The nutrient artery, the principal source, penetrates the cortex through the nutrient canal. In the marrow cavity, it bifurcates into ascending and descending medullary arteries from which radial branches travel to the inner face of the cortex. After penetrating the endosteum, the radial vessels diminish in caliber to structures of capillary size that course within the canalicular system of the cortex. Here arterial blood from the nutrient artery can mix with arterial blood that enters the cortical capillary system from the periosteal capillaries. The latter, a second major source of arterial blood, are derived from muscular arteries. Derivatives of radial arteries in the marrow have also been found to communicate directly with the marrow sinus system.[1,23,37] The direct anastomosis of radial artery with marrow sinuses is quantitatively less important than the blood flow that enters the sinus from cortical capillaries. Thus, most arterial blood enters the cortical canalicular system prior to entering the marrow sinuses.

Specialized, thin-walled arterial segments that abruptly arise as continuations of arteries with walls of normal thickness, can be found in marrow.[33,34] These vessels give off nearly perpendicular branches analogous to arterial branching observed in the spleen and kidney. The functional significance of these unusual vascular structures is not known. They may serve to permit volume compensation for changes in intramedullary pressure.

It is not known what selective pressures led to the evolution of the medullary cavity of bone becoming the principal hemopoietic organ in mammals. The circulatory links between cortex and marrow may provide a clue to the possible dependence of marrow on contiguous components of bone. For example, a drop in pO_2 in the blood reaching marrow after traversing cortical capillaries may contribute to the optimal conditions for hemopoiesis. In vitro blood cell growth is facilitated at lower oxygen tensions.[38] Also, there may be a transfer of chemicals or cells from cortex to marrow in order to provide optimal conditions for hemopoiesis. With marrow injury, restitution of hemopoiesis may depend on the movement of cells, from the cortex to marrow,[39,40] that could occur because of the communication of cortical capillaries with marrow sinuses.

The cortical blood enters the marrow cavity at the endosteal surface. A highly branching network of medullary sinuses provides the channels whereby blood flows through the marrow. The marrow sinuses course through the medullary cavity and collect into a larger central sinus from which the blood enters the systemic venous circulation through emissary veins.

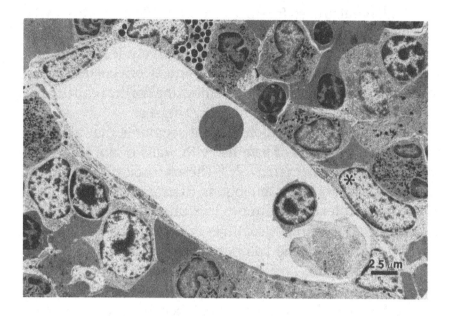

Fig. 1. TEM of a marrow sinus and neighboring hemopoietic tissue from the femur of a rat. An erythrocyte, a lymphocyte, and a large fragment of megakaryocyte cytoplasm are in the sinus lumen. Two endothelial cell nuclei are present at each end of the long axis of the sinus. The lumen of the sinus is covered by endothelial cell cytoplasm. An adventitial reticular cell is present on the abluminal surface of the sinus wall (asterisk).

Marrow Sinuses

In mammals, hemopoiesis takes place in the extravascular spaces between marrow sinuses. Thus, developing blood cells have a close relationship to the sinuses and must traverse the sinus wall to enter the circulation. The diameter of marrow sinuses in the mouse varies from 5 to 30 μm. The sinus wall is composed of a luminal layer of endothelial cells that form a complete inner lining and an abluminal coat of adventitial reticular cells that form an incomplete outer coat (Fig. 1). A thin, interrupted basement lamina is present between these cell layers.

Endothelial Cells

Endothelial cells form a complete covering for the inner surface of the sinus.[2,4-9,17,23,35,36] The endothelial cells are broad and flat. *En face*, the irregular edges of their cytoplasm often have overlapping unions. Their nuclei may protrude away from the sinus lumen or form a fusiform protrusion into the lumen. In cross section, the cell junctions are distinct and often are overlapping or interdigitating. The junctions are not tight ones, and this is thought to be a specialization of endothelial cells in marrow.[32] A very fine basement lamina underlies the endothelial cell layer. This complex layer composed of amorphous and fibrillar structures may be synthesized by the endothelial cells.[41] Its development in marrow sinus walls is less complete than in other vascular sites.

Holes in endothelium (0.1–3.0 µm diameter) are frequent in scanning micrographs of the luminal surface of sinus walls and can be seen also in transmission micrographs. Most holes are probably artifacts induced during the preparation of the marrow for microscopy. In some cases, they may be sites where cells in passage were lost during the rigors of preparation.[27] Marked attenuation of endothelial cell cytoplasm, short of discontinuity, may be seen in transmission micrographs. At these sites, endothelial cell cytoplasm has thinned to a diameter that approaches a double plasma membrane in thickness (fenestra with a diaphragm).[21] These attenuated areas may provide a *locus minoris resistentiae* for cell penetration, or may represent areas of early repair following migration of cells through the sinus wall. Studies have not established that such thinning is an absolute prerequisite to egress. Cells often can be seen in transit across the endothelium at sites that are not unduly thin, although it is possible that a short fenestra was the original site of penetration. Egress of marrow cells into the circulation requires the formation of a migration pore through the cytoplasm of endothelial cells. These pores are formed during cell migration and often appear close to an endothelial cell junction.[7,8,17,23,27] Parallel arrays of microfilaments have been found in endothelial cells, sometimes adjacent to migration pores.[17,18]

In contrast to the endothelial cells lining vessels in other tissues, the endothelium of marrow and liver sinusoids is actively endocytic.[42] Because they are the only marrow cells in direct contact with the circulation, sinus endothelial cells form the major barrier and control system for molecules and particles entering and leaving the hemopoietic spaces. Anatomic features related to these endocytic and transport functions[21,43] include clathrin-coated pits,[44] clathrin-coated vesicles, lysosomes, phagosomes, transfer tubules, and diaphragmed fenestrae[45] (Figs. 2 and 3).

ENDOCYTOSIS OF PARTICLES. Particles such as carbon, ferritin, and albumin-coated colloidal gold are endocytosed by endothelial cells primarily through clathrin-coated pits.[10,21,43,46] These pits, ranging in diameter from 100 to 210 nm, are considerably larger than those found in other fenestrated endothelium. They are normally present on the luminal surface of sinus endothelium and their numbers increase in the presence of intravascular particles.[21,46] Particles less frequently bind to smooth areas of membrane[21,43] and are not internalized at these sites.[43] Coated pits containing bound particles invaginate and detach from the plasma membrane to become clathrin-coated vesicles.[21,43] These coated vesicles may then fuse with one another, losing their coating in the process to become smooth vacuoles, prelysosomal compartments termed "phagosomes,"[21] "endosomes,"[47] or "receptosomes."[48] Carbon particles tend to remain sequestered in phagosomes,[21] whereas large clathrin-coated vesicles containing albumin-coated colloidal gold[43] or ferritin[21] fuse with smooth membraned "transfer tubules" or "pleomorphic vacuoles." Transfer tubules and pleomorphic vacuoles ultimately fuse with or become "dense bodies" that are lysosomes as judged by the presence of acid phosphatase.[21]

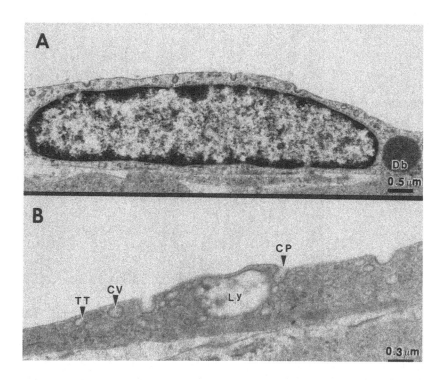

Fig. 2 (A) Perinuclear region of a sinus endothelial cell. Multiple coated pits and coated vesicles are seen at the luminal surface. A dense body (DB) is shown. (B) Portion of endothelial cell cytoplasm showing coated pits (CP), coated vesicles (CV), tubular structures (TT), and a lysosome (LY).

This process occurs very rapidly: within 20 s postinjection, 42% of endothelial-associated gold particles are internalized, and by 1 min 83% of particles are internalized, with a few already seen in dense bodies.[43] Gold particles are still detectable in dense bodies 1 wk postinjection.[43]

Clathrin-coated pits are sites for receptor-mediated endocytosis. It is difficult to conceive of a receptor-mediated process to explain the uptake of such diverse particles as ferritin, carbon and albumin-coated colloidal gold, and other mechanisms for uptake such as fluid phase pinocytosis or nonspecific ad-

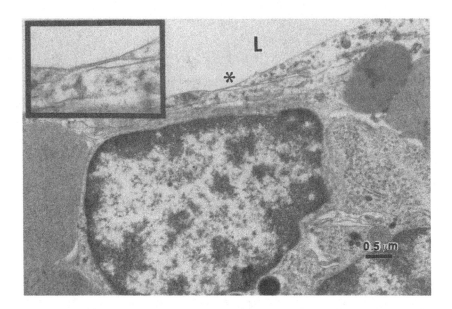

Fig. 3. TEM of a marrow sinus segment from the femur of a rat. The lumen is indicated by an "L." Endothelial cell cytoplasm lines the sinus wall and just below the asterisk, the endothelium thins to form a fenestra with a diaphragm. The inset shows the diaphragm at about three times the magnification of the figure. The highly endocytotic character of marrow sinus endothelium is evident. Adventitial cell cytoplasm is evident on the abluminal side of the endothelial cytoplasm and it is interrupted at the sites where reticulocytes abut the abluminal surface of the endothelium.

sorptive affinity have been considered. Yet, the site of uptake of these particles seems to be principally through coated pits.[21,43] Albumin that has been conformationally altered is endocytosed by a receptor-mediated process.[49,50] Recently, endogenous albumin has been recognized in clathrin-coated vesicles of marrow sinus endothelium.[42] These observations support the possibility that uptake of particles could be receptor-mediated as well, resulting from binding of plasma albumin to particle surfaces.[42,43]

TRANSCELLULAR PASSAGE OF PARTICLES. Although the sinusoidal lining of marrow is anatomically continuous, there are areas of the sinus wall that are markedly attenuated and have the appearance of a diaphragm. These fenestrae and channels with diaphragms, allow direct transcellular passage of carbon particles from the circulation to hemopoietic spaces.[45] Particles do not pass between endothelial cells.[45] Diaphragmed fenestrae allow carbon to enter the extravascular space within 3 min after injection. Within 15 min, particles may be found within the cytoplasm of parenchymal macrophages.[10]

Occasionally, clathrin-coated vesicles containing carbon[45] or colloidal gold[46] are seen at the abluminal side of endothelial cells. It is not known whether these vesicles have transported the carbon from the luminal surface in order to deposit it in the hemopoietic space or whether the carbon was endocytosed from the hemopoietic space by clathrin-coated pits on the abluminal surface of the sinus endothelium. However, coated pits are thought to be responsible for the transfer of iron transferrin-coated colloidal gold particles from the circulation to the hemopoietic space when the complexes are bound to and internalized by marrow erythroblasts.[51] This observation suggests that some transcellular passage may occur via coated pits.

SURFACE MOLECULES OF SINUS ENDOTHELIUM IN ENDOCYTOSIS AND TRANSCELLULAR PASSAGE. At the molecular level, marrow sinus endothelium exhibits several features that may be important in the regulation of cellular and molecular traffic. The charge distribution and sialic acid composition of the luminal surface of marrow sinus endothelium is discontinuous and not random.[30,52,53] Sialic acid groups are detectable along the luminal surface by means of the cationic markers, native ferritin, polycationic ferritin, and colloidal iron, but these groups are markedly less dense at sites of clathrin-coated pits,[30] diaphragmed fenestrae,[52] and near cells in transit.[53] There are also anionic charge groups that are insensitive to neuraminidase, present along the entire luminal surface, and that are increased at diaphragmed fenestrae and coated pits.[30,52,53] Since these structures have in common their association with endocytosis[21,43] and transendothelial passage of particles[45] and cells,[17,24,54] it has been postulated that regions of the membrane devoid of sialic acid containing moieties have an altered stability that permits passage to occur.[52,53] Supporting this idea are experiments that demonstrated increased phagocytosis by neuraminidase-treated monocytes.[55]

Molecular features of the marrow sinus endothelial surface have also been studied using lectins. Lectins are proteins or glycoproteins that bind to specific oligosaccharide structures and either agglutinate cells or precipitate glycoconjugates.[56,57] As determined by lectin binding, the luminal surface of marrow sinus endothelium contains α-D-mannosyl, β-D-galactosyl, N-acetylgalactosaminyl, N-acetyglucosaminyl and sialyl groups.[58,59] Lectin binding is sparse on the abluminal surface.[59] Fucosyl groups are conspicuous by their absence,[58,59] a property shared by liver sinus endothelium but not endothelium from other organs.[60] The saccharide groups identified by lectin binding are denser over the perinuclear plasma membrane, less dense over the tapered regions of the cell, and almost absent from regions of clathrin-coated vesicles and diaphragmed fenestrae.[58] This nonrandom distribution of saccharide groups with regard to known sites of molecular and cellular traffic implies an important role for these groups in endothelial membrane function. Under conditions of stimulated erythropoiesis, there is a marked decrease in sialyl groups without a change in other saccharide groups, further suggesting a possible role for sialic acid in regulating membrane stability and cell egress.[61]

The luminal surface of marrow sinus endothelium also contains a lectin-like substance that recognizes galactosyl residues and specifically mediates the removal of colloidal gold coated with galactosyl–bovine serum albumin, fluid phase galactosyl–bovine serum albumin, and asialotransferrin.[46,62]

Uptake of the galactosylated colloidal gold was most prominent at clathrin-coated pits.[46] Native bovine serum albumin
and mannosylated and fucosylated albumins were not removed in any specific fashion.[46] The biological significance of
this galactosyl receptor is unknown, but the receptor may play
a role in the recognition and removal of cells and molecules
with terminal galactosyl residues.

Endothelial cells from umbilical cords are known to be a
source of granulocyte–monocyte growth factor,[63] and if this
property is shared by endothelial cells of marrow sinuses, they
could contribute to hemopoietic cell growth.

Adventitial Reticular Cells

The abluminal or adventitial surface of the vascular sinus
is composed of reticular cells. These cells relate anatomically to
the sinus wall on their luminal side and to the hemopoietic cells
on their abluminal side.[3,5] The reticular cell bodies are contiguous with the sinus forming a part of its adventitial coat
(Fig. 1). Their extensive cytoplasmic processes envelop the
outer wall of the sinus to form an adventitial sheath.[2–7,14,17,19,22,35–37]
The proximal portion of their cytoplasmic processes are broad,
but branching. The adventitial sheath is heavily interrupted
and has been estimated to cover about 65% of the abluminal
surface of sinuses in the unperturbed mouse.[14,19] The reticular
cell cytoplasm is capable of major changes in its volume.
Several types of stress (e.g., endotoxemia and hypererythro-
poietinemia) have been shown to lead to a marked reduction in
the area of the outer surface of the sinus that is covered with
reticular cell processes.[14,19] This alteration is thought to favor
cell egress since reticular cell processes provide an impediment
to the transmural migration of mature cells.

The reticular cells are neither highly phagocytic[11] nor capable of developing into hemopoietic cells.[40] They synthesize
reticular (argentiphilic) fibers that, along with their cytoplas-

mic processes, provide much if not all of the physical support for hemopoietic cells. There is little information about the function of these cells. They undergo little if any proliferation unless marrow is damaged.[40] It is probable that they are vital to sustain the normal physiology of marrow since restoration of the marrow sinus network and the reticular cells precede the development of hemopoiesis in bones experimentally denuded of marrow[64] or in transplanted bone.[65] The intimate physical association of reticular cell processes with developing hemopoietic cells has suggested that they participate in cell–cell interactions that are inductive and regulatory in hemopoiesis.[37]

The cytoplasmic processes of reticular cells extend into the hemopoietic compartment as well as over the outer surface of the sinus wall. These processes are continuous with the reticular fiber network that stretches between sinuses and forms a meshwork on which hemopoietic cells rest. The cell bodies, and their broad processes and fibers, constitute the reticulum of marrow. Reticular cell processes and fibers often partially wrap around, or otherwise contact, hemopoietic cells. Other, more cylindrical, blunt processes terminate against hemopoietic cells. Histochemical studies of marrow show that adventitial reticular cells have a high concentration of alkaline phosphatase in their membrane compatible with being a type of fibroblast.[66]

Ultrastructural studies in the mouse suggest that the sinus adventitial reticular cell may be the principal fibroblast-like cell in the marrow, other than fibroblasts or fibroblast-related cells associated with the larger blood vessels, nerve trunks, and, bone. Thus, there may be few, if any, free fibroblasts in the hemopoietic spaces unassociated with vascular channels.[4,7,9,11,37] There are several implications of these considerations. When fibroblast cultures are established from marrow, the cells could be derived from blood vessels, marrow sinus reticular cells, or fibroblasts in hemopoietic spaces. The latter cells are rare in mouse marrow. If fibrosis in pathological states is a result of increased fiber synthesis and depositions by (and proliferation of) adventitial reticular cells, this may be a manifestation of vascular sinus proliferation. Thus, the increased blood flow through bones seen in myelofibrosis may reflect an increase in the number or size of vascular sinuses with a concomitant increase in adventitial reticular cells and fibers.[67]

Fat Cells

Adipocytes in marrow develop by lipogenesis in cells that are closely related to fibroblasts. In the mouse, the adventitial reticular cell is a preadipocyte[37] that can be converted to fat cells in vivo under certain experimental conditions.[35,36] Fat cells are absent from mouse femur, but are present in small numbers in rat femoral marrow. Nonhemopoietic cells in mouse[68–71] and human marrow[72–74] can undergo transformation to fat cells in vitro. This in vitro transformation may represent the transformation of reticular cells (or another fibroblast-like cell) to fat cells. Moreover, marrow fat cells have been found to transform into fibroblasts in culture by a process of lipolysis.[72,74] Adipocytes are often parasinal, which would be consistent with their origin in adventitial reticular cells, whose cell bodies are closely applied to the sinus wall (Fig. 4).

The regulation of the transformation of adventitial cells to adipocytes as well as their function is not known, but may relate to a "cushioning effect" within the medullary cavity. This could occur to a greater or lesser extent depending on the degree of ongoing hemopoiesis and, thus, the spatial requirements of the stimulated, quiescent, or retreating marrow.

Marrow Nerves

Arterial vessels can be identified in the hemopoietic spaces by electron microscopy. Nerves accompany the vessels. Mye-

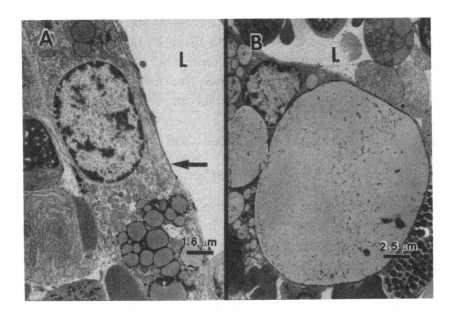

Fig. 4 (A) TEM of a marrow sinus segment from the femur of a rat. The lumen (L) of the sinus is lined by a very thin layer of endothelial cell cytoplasm (arrow). The adventitial reticular cell cytoplasm just beneath the endothelium (asterisk) shows early lipogenesis (area of multilocular fat droplets). (B) TEM of a segment of a marrow sinus from the femur of a rat. The lumen is shown by an L. The nucleus of a reticular cell is compressed by two large fat droplets. The lipogenesis in this adventitial reticular cell is more advanced than in (A) and could eventuate in a unilocular fat cell.

linated and nonmyelinated fibers are present in marrow.[13,75–77] The prevailing view is that the nerves function to regulate arterial vessel tone. Some investigators have suggested that nonmyelinated fibers may terminate in the hemopoietic spaces, implying that neurohumors elaborated from free-nerve terminals may affect hemopoiesis (Fig. 5).

Evidence for Discrimination in the Release of Marrow Cells

The quantitative evaluation of discriminatory release of blood cells begins with a consideration of the number of

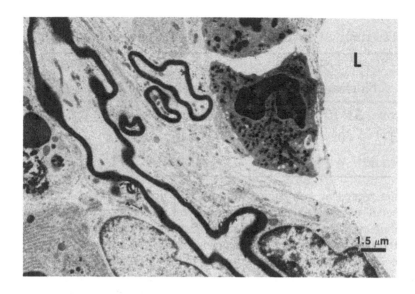

Fig. 5. TEM of a marrow sinus segment from the femur of a rat. The lumen of the sinus is indicated by an L. A granulocyte is separated from the lumen by an attenuated region of endothelium. Myelinated nerve fibers are evident in the hemopoietic space. Schwann cells also are present in association with the nerve fiber.

marrow cells and circulating blood cells of the same morphologic age. For example, the ratio of marrow myeloblasts to blood myeloblasts is very high compared to the ratio of marrow neutrophils to blood neutrophils. The more mature cells exhibit a lower marrow-to-blood ratio that is compatible with the proposal that mature cells are released more readily from marrow.

Table 1 shows the marrow-to-blood (M/B) ratios that can be derived from the prevalence of hemopoietic cells in marrow and blood.[78–80] Reticulocytes have a low M/B ratio (2/1) compared to nucleated red cells (M/B ratio ∞). Mature granulocytes exhibit a lower ratio (<10/1) than immature granulocytes (M/B ratio >10,000/1). Megakaryocytes can be found in the right heart blood in low concentrations in subjects without hemopoietic disease, but they have a very low extramedullary

Table 1
Distribution of Hemopoietic Cells in Marrow and Blood[a]

| | Red cells | | Granulocytes | | Megakaryo- |
	Nucleated	Reticulocyte	Immature	Mature	cytes
Marrow	3×10^9	6×10^9	5×10^9	6×10^9	6×10^6
Blood	0	3×10^9	$<5 \times 10^5$	0.6×10^9	2×10^2
M/B ratio	∞	2/1	>10,000/1	10/1	30,000/1

[a]Data represent number of cells per kilogram of body weight. The number of marrow red cells and granulocytes was taken from the studies of Donohue et al.,[78] the number of marrow megakaryocytes from Harker,[79] and the number of blood megakaryocytes from Kaufman et al.[80] The marrow/blood ratio does not consider the pool of extravascular neutrophils in the tissues. This pool, estimated by some to represent as much as 100-fold the blood neutrophil pool, would reduce further the marrow-to-extramedullary ratio of mature granulocytes.

prevalence compared to their numbers in marrow (M/B ratio > 30,000/1). The marrow-to-blood ratio of platelets cannot be calculated since there are no data regarding the number of free platelets in the hemopoietic spaces. It is probable that few, if any, detached platelets are normally present in the hemopoietic compartment, making such considerations meaningless.

The numerator and denominator of the M/B ratio may be influenced by factors that make interpretation difficult. For example, selective differences in circulation time, sequestration by the spleen, or death in the circulation could bias the denominator of the ratio. Also, the prevalence of immature cells outside the marrow is difficult to ascertain. The quantity of cells in or entering the tissues influences the interpretation. The marrow-to-blood ratio of neutrophils is a falsely high estimate since the tissue neutrophils are neglected. In most cases, the factors noted act to minimize the differences between the higher marrow-to-blood ratio of immature cells and the lower marrow-to-blood ratio of mature cells.

These ratios, despite the limitations that should be placed on the inferences drawn from them, provide strong support for the discriminatory release of differentiated, functional cells and the retention in marrow of incompletely differentiated cells.

Factors Governing Release of Hemopoietic Cells

The complex process of marrow cell egress is influenced by several factors.[26,81] Hemopoietic cells are in the extravascular spaces of marrow, which makes it necessary for them to penetrate the wall of the marrow sinus to enter the venous circulation. The proximity of certain cells to the marrow sinus (e.g., megakaryocytes and reticulocytes) may permit egress of platelets and red cells, respectively. The developmental change that occurs in the nucleus and cytoplasm of maturing cells allows translocation of terminally differentiated cells from the hemopoietic compartment to the marrow sinus. Cell-releasing substances, putative chemicals that facilitate the rate of release of specific morphologic cell types, may be responsible for the selective acceleration of the release of reticulocytes, neutrophils, and platelets depending on bodily needs. There is limited knowledge of the functional importance of nerve fibers in the marrow. Also, the precise regulation of blood flow in the marrow has resisted detailed study. In a global sense, the flow of blood through marrow vascular channels could influence the total delivery of new cells. The regulation of flow may be mediated by vasoactive compounds, nerves, or other factors that may influence the blood supply at the arteriolar level or the patency of smaller presinus or postsinus vessels. Neurogenic influences may exist independent of vasoregulatory fibers since some myelinated and nonmyelinated nerves course through marrow unassociated with the adventitia of arteries, and there may be a regulatory role for free, nonsynaptic nerve endings.

Biophysical Properties of Developing Hemopoietic Cells

During maturation of blood cells in the marrow, well-known and striking morphologic changes occur that coincide with the achievement of functional capability. The erythroid cell begins as a poorly differentiated blast cell and eventually becomes an anucleated diskoid sack of hemoglobin. The granulocytic cell, also a poorly differentiated blast cell initially, becomes a cell engorged with primary and specific granules with a segmented nucleus. The megakaryocyte begins as a blast cell and by endomitosis, becomes a multinucleate giant cell rich in cytoplasm and capable of producing platelets by cytoplasmic fragmentation and shedding.

In addition to these changes, evident by light microscopy, the cell changes in its ability to deform, move, and sustain directed movement (chemotaxis). The development of deformability, motility, and chemotaxis may be essential for normal and regulated marrow egress of cells. The structural changes that underlie the development of motility in hemopoietic cells during their maturation cannot be seen with the light microscope, but can be appreciated by physiologic studies of developing hemopoietic cells.

Cell Motility

Since egress of cells across the marrow sinus wall involves translocation in spatial terms, motility of the cell is required. Rapid, active motility, as judged by in vitro studies, is not a feature of immature hemopoietic cells. This limited rate of motility may contribute to their retention in marrow since some probing by pseudopods is probably required to initiate penetration of the sinus wall. A marked increase in the rate of motility occurs with maturation of the granulocyte, in particular. These cells become actively ameboid at the later stages of their development and this could contribute to their ability to search out the sinus wall and penetrate it.[82–84]

The reticulocyte displays some cell movement.[85] Its peripheral movements are desultory and not ameboid. Since the physical process of egress may initially involve probes (pseudopods) of reticulocyte cytoplasm,[17] it is possible that the movement of reticulocytes is an important feature for their exit from the marrow.[85] Reticulocytes are wedged between reticular fibers and may be jarred free by their vibratory motions.

The megakaryocyte also develops the ability to form pseudopods from its peripheral cytoplasm.[86] A megakaryocyte positioned next to the sinus wall can thrust out a projection of peripheral cytoplasm in a manner analogous to a granulocyte. Anatomically, this projection appears to be a pseudopod.[87–89]

The factors that underlie pseudopod formation have been the subject of intensive study.[90] The mechanism of cell movement involves contractile proteins analogous to muscle actin and myosin.[91] These proteins have been identified in granulocytes, monocytes, erythrocytes, and megakaryocytes.[92] The differences in the character of the movement of reticulocytes, granulocytes, and megakaryocytes are probably a function of the amount, type, and organization of contractile proteins in these cell types.

Cell Deformability

The ability of nucleated cells to deform is related to their ability to move. Highly ameboid cells are more easily deformable under in vitro conditions. Deformability of granulocytic, lymphoid, and erythroid cells of different stages of maturation has been examined by their ability to be filtered through micropore membranes,[93,94] penetrate micropore membranes actively,[82,94] and aspirated into glass microcapillary tubes.[83,84,93,95–97] Granulocytes and erythrocytes become more deformable as they mature. The erythroblast displays a marked increase in its ability to enter small diameter pores following enucleation. The mature granulocyte is able to enter 3-μm-pore-diameter capillary tubes and can penetrate a 1 to 3-μm Millipore filter during chemokinetic or chemotactic movement, whereas immature granulocytes cannot penetrate these size channels in vitro during 1–3 h of observation. The increased deformability of maturing cells may play a role in marrow egress since most cells are under marked deformation during migration through the marrow sinus wall.

Cell Chemotaxis

Chemotaxis of granulocytes is a feature of mature, rather than immature cells.[82] Chemotaxis may underlie the ability of mature marrow cells to accelerate their release in response to increased demand for cells. This aspect of cell release may be most important for granulocytes and monocytes, highly motile cells capable of increased directed movement in a chemotactic gradient. Whether marrow reticulocytes can respond to a chemoattractant is unknown. Platelet release may be accelerated by the more rapid penetration of megakaryocyte pseudopods through the sinus wall, a reaction that could be facilitated by a chemoattractant that interacts with megakaryocyte peripheral cytoplasm.

Cell Surface

The interaction of hemopoietic cells with stromal cells, processes, or fibers could be an important determinant of cell egress. Cell–cell interactions involving surface structures on immature hemopoietic cells could anchor these cells within the marrow spaces. During maturation, surface glycoproteins on hemopoietic cells could be altered resulting in detachment from stroma, making it possible to migrate or translocate toward the sinus wall. Changes on the cell surface of mature marrow cells may also play a role in penetrating the sinus wall.[98]

Cell Releasing Factors

Chemical releasing factors can accelerate the release of marrow cells.[99–102] Accelerated cell release could enhance blood counts in two ways. First, a rapid release of reticulocytes and neutrophils from the marrow could increase their circulating pools rapidly since two-thirds of the reticulocytes are in the marrow and 90% of the segmented neutrophils outside the tissues are in the marrow. There may be a small proportion of free platelets in the marrow.[103,104] Megakaryocyte cytoplasm is, in effect, a platelet pool and thus, blood platelet counts could be increased rapidly without the production of new cells.

Second, the later stages of the marrow transit time can be shortened by delivering newly produced cells into the circulation without a stay in a marrow storage pool. Accelerated release has a short period of effect unless increased production of cells ensues. This is particularly important in the case of cells with a short circulation of tissue survival time. Most physiologic studies have been directed at understanding the response of marrow granulocytes during periods of increased need. Less is known about the role of releasing factors in the delivery of red cells and platelets.

Candidate Factors

Evidence for a releasing factor for granulocytes has been obtained in studies of rats perfused with neutropenic plasma and in neutropenic dogs. The neutrophilia-inducing activity was not endotoxin and the neutrophilia was not caused by demargination of neutrophils, but was the result of a release of new cells from marrow.[105-107]

The C3e component of plasma complement is one identified factor capable of accelerating granulocyte release.[108-110] Complement could act to maintain the steady-state blood concentration of neutrophils, or to perturb the steady state and thus contribute to neutrophilia. Complement factors are known to be chemoattractants for mature, but not immature, granulocytes[82] and thus could call forth mature cells selectively. Glucocorticoid hormones and androgenic steroids can also induce release of mature granulocytes from marrow.[111-113] Their physiologic role is unclear.

Endotoxin also facilitates granulocyte egress,[14,114] possibly by activation of complement. Endotoxin may also effect accelerated granulocyte release by reducing adventitial cell cover on the abluminal surface of the sinus wall.[14] Purified leukocyte endogenous mediator, one of a triad of monokines that includes endogenous pyrogen and interleukin-1, has neutrophil-releasing activity.[115-117]

Erythropoietin has been implicated as a releasing factor for reticulocytes, in addition to its established role in stimulating proliferation of erythroid cells.[19,20,118,119] Thus, in the case of erythroid cells, the same chemical may be able to induce proliferation and accelerated release. The effect of erythropoietin on red cell release has not been fully elucidated. The hormone reduces the adventitial cell cover of the sinus wall and may facilitate access of the reticulocyte to the endothelial cell. The reduction of adventitial reticular cell cover does not explain selectivity of release since such a change should facilitate egress of any cell type.

Physiologic Studies

Accelerated release of marrow neutrophils in vivo occurs in response to neutropenia.[105,120,121] Plasma from animals with decreased granulocyte counts can increase the release of marrow cells as judged by the elution of cells from isolated perfused femurs.[100,106,107,122–125] The release of marrow neutrophils, in response to neutropenia, is mediated by a chemical releasing factor that is distinctive from endotoxin. Each cell type—reticulocytes, eosinophils, neutrophils, basophils, monocytes, and platelets—should have a factor that can specifically accelerate its release. The releasing factor for granulocytes is chemically distinct from the factors that increase proliferation and maturation.[126–128] Some overlap in the effect of releasing factors may occur. Neutrophilia and reticulocytosis or neutrophilia and thrombocytosis occur in reactive processes, such as hemolytic anemia or inflammation. The releasing factor may work nonspecifically, for instance, by decreasing the barrier presented by the marrow sinus wall. This would favor release of any cell type. Alternatively, several specific releasing factors could play a role in these occurrences. The site of elaboration of releasing factors, the physiologic systems that control their concentrations in the marrow, and the specific nature of their interaction with cells have not been defined.

Cell releasing factors could affect egress rate in several ways. They could function as specific chemoattractants, accelerating movement of differentiated cells into the marrow sinus. Porcine leukocytes release chemorecruitment molecules referred to as "leukorecruitins."[129,130] These chemicals could also act on the sinus wall or other stromal structures to reduce the impediment to egress. For example, a reduction in adventitial cell covering on the abluminal surface of the sinus may facilitate penetration of the endothelial cell by mature cells.[14,19] They could also act on the endothelial cell to reduce the thickness of its cytoplasm; cells are often seen migrating through these attenuated areas in endothelium. Alternatively, a releasing factor could provide a molecular bridge to attach the migrating cell to the abluminal surface of the sinus endothelial cell, initiating development of a migration channel.

Control of Blood Flow in Marrow

Several laboratories have examined the physiologic control of blood flow to bone.[131-133] Autonomic and autoregulatory mechanisms control blood flow through bone and presumably marrow. There is little firm evidence for a relationship between velocity of flow and cell release, but there is a relationship between blood supply and the level of hemopoiesis. Flow in the marrow sinuses remains pulsatile,[1] providing periods of lower intraluminal pressure that may contribute to cell egress (*see*, later in this chapter).

In a global sense, blood flow is required to deliver all mature hemopoietic cells from marrow to the systemic venous circulation but, there is no reason to believe that blood flow can determine selective release of cells. Specific hemopoietic cells are not positioned adjacent to specific sinuses; thus, recruitment of sinuses would not increase the delivery of cells in a specific manner. Since recruitment of cells is selective (i.e., if neutrophils are needed, their release is accelerated more or less specifically), an increase in blood flow could not explain this aspect of marrow cell release.

The Anatomical Process of Release

The process of cell egress from the hemopoietic compartment to the vascular sinus has been observed by both transmission and scanning electron microscopy. Characteristic features of egress have been confirmed in several laboratories.[9,14,17,19,20,26,136] First, cell migration occurs through channels that develop at the time of cell transit and do not preexist. Very few breaks in endothelial continuity are seen in the sinus wall of well-fixed preparations of animal marrow by transmission electron microscopy. Moreover, mature cells abutting the sinus ready for egress are pressed against intact endothelium. In some cases, small pseudopods of cells can be seen entering the cytoplasm of sinus endothelial cells without having broken through the luminal portion of the plasma membrane of the endothelial cell. Thus, it has been concluded that migrating cells make the hole that develops in the endothelial cell cytoplasm. Second, the diameter of migration channels is almost always much narrower than the spherical diameter of the cell, requiring substantial deformation of the cell during transit. The marked deformation of the migrating cell causes it to press laterally against the endothelial cell cytoplasm. This lateral pressure may prevent free communication from sinus to hemopoietic compartment, microhemorrhage, and platelet aggregation, or other injurious effects. Third, mature cells, but not immature cells, are found in the process of egress. Fourth, propulsion is presumably required for the cells to translocate across the sinus wall.

Adventitial reticular cell cytoplasm is absent at the site of penetration of the abluminal surface of the endothelial cell and the sinus wall may become attentuated at the site of cell egress. It is not known whether adventitial cell cover must be absent at the point of egress or the migrating cell could penetrate the reticular cell cytoplasm. Also, marked attentuation of the endothelial cell cytoplasm has not been established as being invariably necessary for a cell to penetrate the sinus wall.

It is not known how the exiting cell initiates egress. It is presumed that specific enzymes (e.g., glycosyltransferases) and acceptors (e.g., sugars) on the surface of the migrating cell interact with endothelium for a migration pore to develop. This process may be very similar to the invasion of metastatic tumor cells through the endothelium and into the tissues.

Ultrastructural Features of Reticulocyte Egress

Egress of cells may be initiated when cells detach from stromal anchoring sites. In vitro binding of marrow erythroid precursor cells to fibroblastoid cells derived from fetal liver can be inhibited specifically by antifibronectin antibodies.[134] Adherence to fibronectin persists until the perienucleation stage. Granulocyte precursors do not adhere to fibronectin-coated stroma in this system. Thus, cell surface features that anchor immature cells appear to be different when red and white cell precursors are compared. The maturation-associated detachment of precursors may contribute to the orderly regulation of the release of mature cells.

Studies of reticulocytes during migration have established that they do not traverse the sinus wall between endothelial cells, that is through junctions, rather they pass through migration pores in the endothelium.[17,22,28,135–137] These migration pores have been shown to be parajunctional in position during granulocyte egress and reticulocytes are usually in transit in a similar location (Fig. 6). Migration pores are thought to be made in the process of egress,[138,139] in part, because of studies indicating that the migration pores are rare unless cells are in them.[27] Our analysis (*see*, later in this chapter) suggests, however, that most pores would be filled whether they are permanent structures or not. The migration pore is usually very short, less than 1.0 µm, since reticulocytes usually pass through very attenuated areas of cytoplasm. Migration pores are usually less than one-third the diameter of the spherical cell, requiring the cell to deform markedly during transit (Fig. 7). The lateral pressure of the cell under deformation stress may provide functional closure for the migration pores.

Attenuation of endothelium is often observed at the site where a reticulocyte presses against the endothelium next to an endothelial cell junction. Adventitial reticular cell cytoplasm can provide a barrier to the approach of marrow reticulocytes to the abluminal surface of the endothelium (Fig. 8). Several stimuli that lead to accelerated egress of reticulocytes, including phlebotomy, phenylhydrazine-induced hemolytic anemia,

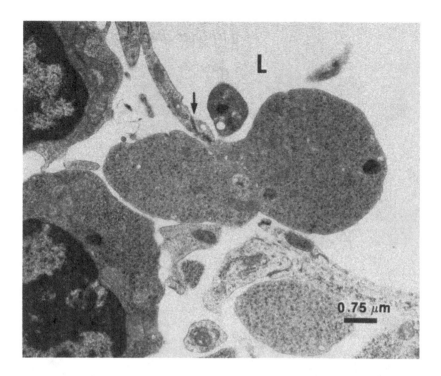

Fig. 6. TEM of a marrow sinus segment from the femur of a rat. An anucleate erythrocyte is in the process of egress into the lumen (L). The arrow indicates the location of an interendothelial cell junction.

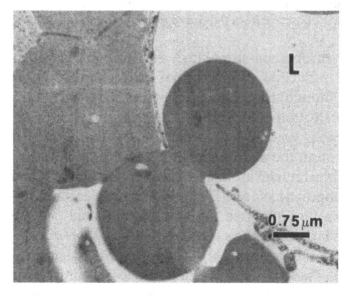

Fig. 7. TEM of a marrow sinus segment from the femur of a rat. An anucleate erythrocyte is in the process of egress into the lumen (L). There is characteristic marked deformation as the cell traverses the marrow migration channels.

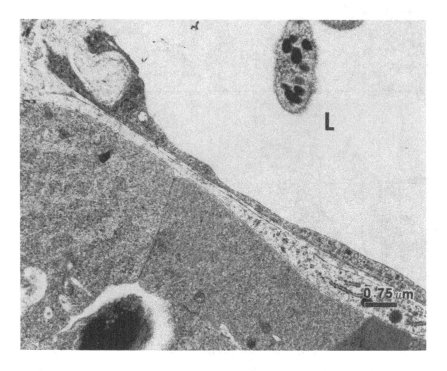

Fig. 8. TEM of a marrow sinus segment from the femur of a rat. A thin layer of adventitial cell cytoplasm separates the anucleate erythrocytes in the hemopoietic space from the endothelium of the sinus wall.

and erythropoietin-stimulated erythropoiesis, result in a marked reduction of adventitial cell cover of the sinus, a process thought to facilitate cell egress.[19,20]

Enucleation of erythroblasts occurs in most cases in the hemopoietic spaces leaving reticulocytes that must reach and pass through the endothelial lining of the sinus wall (Fig. 9). Erythroblast nuclei are ingested by perisinal macrophages in the hemopoietic spaces (Fig. 10). Erythroblasts can lose their nuclei as they traverse the sinus endothelial cell and rare erythroblasts enter the sinus before losing their nuclei. In the latter case, the erythroblast may enucleate in the marrow sinus (Fig. 11). These latter two events, nuclear pitting by the sinus wall and enucleation in the lumen, are presumably very in-

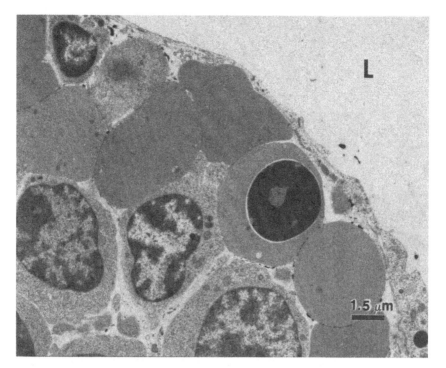

Fig. 9. TEM of a marrow sinus segment from the femur of a mouse. Several anucleate erythrocytes are evident in the hemopoietic space pressing against the abluminal surface of the sinus endothelium.

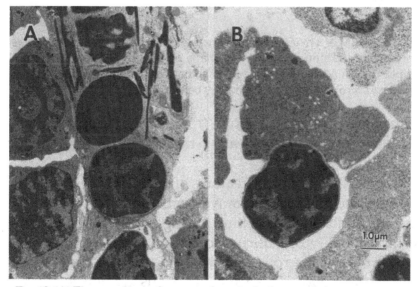

Fig. 10 (A) The cytoplasm of a macrophage in the hemopoietic space containing two erythroblast nuclei in different stages of karyorhexis. (B) The enucleation of an erythroblast in the hemopoietic space of marrow. A rim of cytoplasm containing hemoglobin surrounds the ejected nucleus.

115

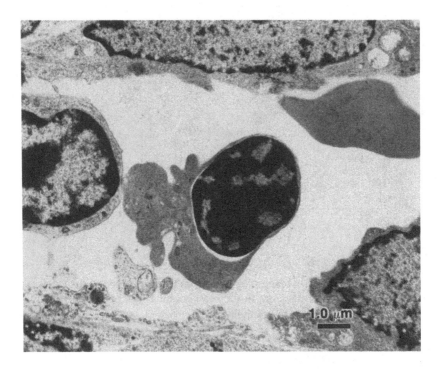

Fig. 11. TEM of a marrow sinus from the femur of a rat. An erythroblast is present in the sinus lumen. The shape of the cell and the thin rim of cytoplasm around the nucleus suggests that the nucleus is close to being extruded, a process that usually occurs before egress.

frequent ("accidents of nature") and do not represent the dominant timing of enucleation that occurs in the marrow hemopoietic spaces.

One of the perplexing features of reticulocyte egress is the source of the force for cell movement. Does the reticulocyte have for a short period of time during its stay in the marrow intrinsic motility of sufficient quantity and quality for it to crawl across the marrow sinus wall, or is the pressure gradient from the hemopoietic space to the sinus enough to push it across the sinus wall? The reticulocyte is presumably unable to use intrinsic motile forces analogous to the ameboid movement that can be generated by the leukocyte and megakaryo-cyte cytoplasm to leave the marrow. Furthermore, the spheri-cal contour of the portion of the cell in the sinus indicates that there is a pressure gradient across the membrane that could be driving the cell through the pore.

Modeling Reticulocyte Egress

The regulation of cell egress by physical parameters, such as membrane deformability, pore size, and pressure gradients has been analyzed.[140,141] The model was developed after exam-ining electron micrographs of reticulocytes passing through pores from the hemopoietic space into the marrow sinus. The pores in the endothelial cell wall, through which reticulocytes pass, range in size from slightly less than 0.5 μm to about 2.0 μm in diameter and from 0.1 μm or more in length. The geometry of the portion of the cell in the sinus was nearly always spher-ical. This finding suggests that egress might be driven by a hydrostatic pressure gradient since the pressure in the luminal portion of the reticulocyte should be nearly equal to the pres-sure in the abluminal portion which, in turn, should be similar to marrow pressure. The smooth, spherical appearance of the luminal portion of the reticulocyte indicates that the trans-mitted marrow pressure is greater than sinus pressure. The analysis considered the pressure-driven passage of a single cell through a pore of fixed dimensions.

Analytical Considerations

Egress is assumed to be driven by a constant pressure dif-ference across the spherical contour of the membrane in the sinus. The resistance to passage is owing to the deformation of the planar membrane in the hemopoietic compartment. The interaction between the cell and the pore is assumed to be fric-tionless and the radius of the pore is constant. The volume of the cell is allowed to change and the viscous resistance of the cytoplasm is neglected. Details of the analytical procedure have appeared elsewhere.[140]

Theoretical Expectations

The analysis predicts that there is a minimum pressure below which egress cannot occur. The minimum pressure needed to drive the cell into the sinus is strongly dependent on the pore radius. For pores 1.0 µm in diameter (0.5 µm radius) and larger, the minimum calculated pressure required for egress is less than 1.5 mm of mercury. These values are small compared to the pressures measured in rabbit bone marrow by Michelson,[132] who recorded differences in pressure on the order of 20 mm Hg between the marrow tissue and the emissary veins just outside the cortical bone. Based on Michelson's measurements, it is reasonable to hypothesize that there is sufficient pressure difference across the pores to move reticulocytes through the boundary.

The larger the difference between the driving and minimum pressures, the less time it takes the cell to enter the sinus. The functional relationships between egress time and driving pressure for different-sized pores indicate that a very short time is needed to complete egress when the minimum pressure gradient for egress is exceeded. For pores larger than 1.0 µm in diameter with pressures of about 3.0 mm Hg, the time for egress is less than three-tenths of a second. This is an important result, considering the fact that the pressures within the marrow are pulsatile and pressures sufficient to cause egress may be transient. There appears to be a correlation between transient increases in pressure within the marrow and an increase in the release of reticulocytes into the circulation in rabbits, indicating that the pulsatile nature of the pressure within the marrow may contribute to cell release.[144] Also, pulsatile flow in marrow can lead to dilatation of sinuses and an increase in tissue pressure because of the nondistensibility of the cortical bone.[32]

Experimental Results

Existing micropipet techniques are adequate for aspirating cells at precisely controlled pressures, but they do not simulate the geometry of marrow pores. In an attempt to approximate more closely the dimension of marrow pores, silicon wafers with a thickness of 0.5–1.5 µm, and with a single hole 1.5–2.0 µm in diameter, affixed with epoxy to the tip of a large (15.0 µm ID) micropipet have been used to test the predictions of the analytical model. Using a syringe attached to the air-filled side of a manometer, constant pressure can be imposed across the pore, and a cell can be observed as it passes through the opening. The experiments are recorded on videotape for subsequent analysis.

The experimental observations confirm two important results of the theoretical analysis. First, there is a threshold pressure below which cells will not pass through the pore. (For pores greater than 1.0 µm in diameter, this threshold is less than 2.0 mm Hg.) Second, when pressure across the pore exceeds the threshold pressure by 20% or more, the time required for the cell to complete egress is less than 0.5 s.

Implications for the Regulation of Reticulocyte Egress

These theoretical and experimental results have implications about mechanisms for the regulation of marrow egress. Electron micrographic examination of marrow sections reveals that nearly all of the pores that exist in the marrow are filled with cells. This observation is evidence for the hypothesis that pores only form when cells are in close contact with the hemopoietic face of the endothelial barrier.[27] This conclusion presumed that if the pores were permanent structures, a significant fraction would be empty at any given time. If the average pore diameter is about 1.5 µm, and the pressure difference across the pore is 4.0 mm of mercury, the fraction of pores filled at any time is 93%. This result does not disprove the hypothesis that pores only form when cells are in contact with the endothelium. However, it shows that the hypothesis is not established by the fact that most pores in the marrow are filled, because nearly all the pores would be filled, even if the pores were permanent structures. If one considers the presence of white cells in the marrow, the fraction of filled pores is even higher.[140]

The expression for the flux of cells at the endothelial boundary enables one to identify and evaluate potential mechanisms for the regulation and control of cell egress. Increasing the number of cells (and hence the volume fraction of cells) in the hemopoietic space is not an effective means of increasing the net flux of cells out of the marrow, because this requires an increase in the fraction of pores filled. Nearly all the pores are filled under normal conditions, so increasing the volume fraction of cells can only increase the flux by a few percent. A more effective way to increase the flux is to increase the number of pores per unit area. Doubling the pore number would double the flux without affecting the fraction of pores filled, assuming that the reservoir of cells in the hemopoietic space is not depleted.

Other possible mechanisms for increasing cell flux include increasing the driving pressure or the pore radius. These mechanisms work by decreasing the time for egress and increasing the flow per pore. These mechanisms may not work for actively migrating cells, because the active process may be insensitive to pore size or pressure difference.

Ultrastructural Features
of White Cell Egress

The shape of granulocytes, monocytes, and lymphocytes in egress through the sinus wall is similar to that of reticulocytes. Small portions of leukocyte cytoplasm can be seen penetrating sinus endothelium and micrographs of leukocytes partially translocated across endothelium indicate that marked deformation of the cells occurs as they penetrate the cytoplasm of the endothelial cell to enter the sinus lumen (Fig. 12). Moreover, their egress also occurs frequently adjacent to junctions of endothelial cells. The nucleus of the granulocyte, usually segmented, does not require marked deformation to traverse the migration pore (Fig. 13), whereas the nuclei of monocytes and lymphocytes require more deformation to traverse the narrow migration pores in the sinus wall (Fig. 14). Little is known of the changes in nuclear deformability with cell maturation. It is rare to see leukocytes invaginating endothelial cell cytoplasm, except for monocytes (Fig. 15). Presumably neutrophils penetrate very thin areas of endothelium, where migration pores are made, perhaps by fusion of the luminal and abluminal plasma membrane of the endothelial cell. Granulocytes in the hemopoietic spaces sometimes have pseudopods indicating that the cell has been caught during movement and, at times, these probes are invaginating or deforming portions of the sinus wall that are an impediment to egress (Fig. 16).

The transcellular passage of mature blood cells into the circulation is associated with the accumulation of a nonsialated anionic material at the advancing margin of diapedesis. This material first accumulates beneath the endothelium at an area of the blood cell surface during the initial phases of transcellular passage near the site of the migration pore formation, but disappears as passage progresses. This observation suggests that the anionic material may be associated with either the dis-

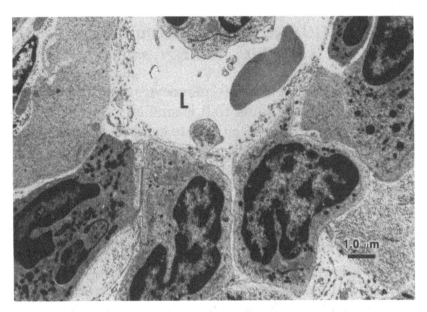

Fig. 12 TEM of a marrow sinus segment from the femur of a rat. A pseudopod of monocyte cytoplasm has penetrated the endothelial cell and entered the sinus lumen.

criminative recognition event, the formation of the migration pore, or both.[54] The observation that erythrocyte maturation is associated with a decrease in concanavalin A labeling concomitant with an increase in sialic acid and concanavalin A labeling on the granulocyte surface with cell development, further supports the role of carbohydrates on endothelial and blood cell surfaces as possible recognition determinants.[59]

The immature granulocytes in marrow make close contact with the processes of adventitial reticular cells and may be anchored to these cells through lectin-like interactions between the two cell surfaces. Thus, adhesion molecules on the surface of immature cells may favor attachment to stromal cells; loss of these molecules during maturation could permit egress from the marrow. Transient changes in surface glycoproteins of mature marrow granulocytes may also favor contact with endothelium.[98]

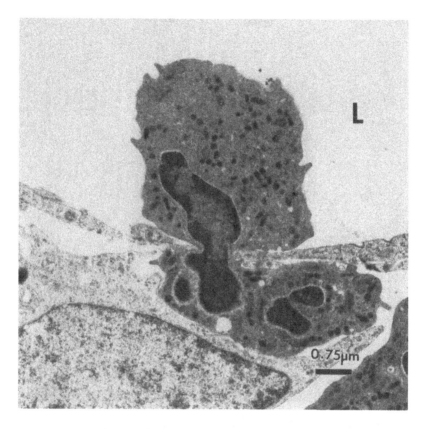

Fig. 13. TEM of a marrow sinus segment. A granulocyte is in the process of egress through the sinus wall. The characteristic marked deformation of the cell as it passes through a narrow migration channel is evident. The ease with which the segmented nucleus flows through the migration channel can be appreciated.

Ultrastructural Features of Platelet Release

In order to complete the process of platelet release, the megakaryocyte periphery invaginates the abluminal surface of the marrow sinus endothelial cell until a pore is made (Fig. 17). Cytoplasm flows through this pore into the marrow sinus (Fig. 18) and is eventually separated from the body of the megakaryocyte resulting in a multiplatelet fragment or proplatelet

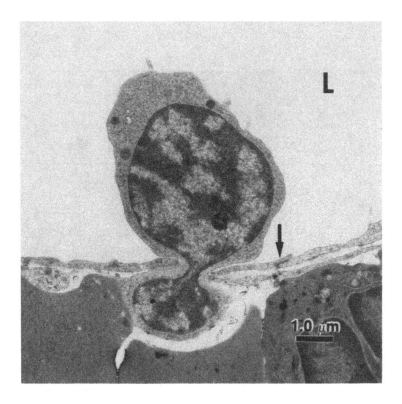

Fig. 14. TEM of a marrow sinus segment from the femur of a rat. A lymphocyte in the process of egress. Marked deformation of both the cell and the nucleus is required to traverse the narrow migration pore. An interendothelial cell junction is at the point of the arrow.

(Fig. 19). The proplatelets often are stringbean-shaped structures and are found in the marrow sinus lumen (Fig. 20). They contain constrictions that develop between future individual platelets. In transmission micrographs, the proplatelets in the marrow sinus may be sectioned transversely and appear to be large spherical structures, the size of red or white cells or may be sectioned longitudinally to show their long axis dimension. The proplatelets fragment further, usually in the marrow circulation, into single platelets.[23,29,144–148] Formation of proplate-

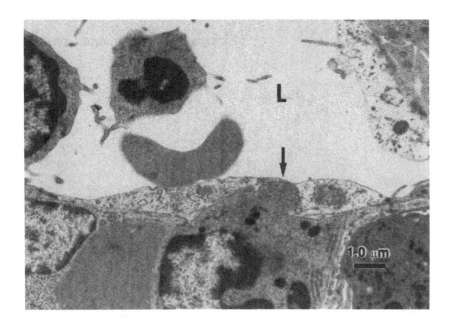

Fig. 15. TEM of a marrow sinus segment from the femur of a rat. A monocyte has invaginated the endothelial cell cytoplasm as shown by the arrow.

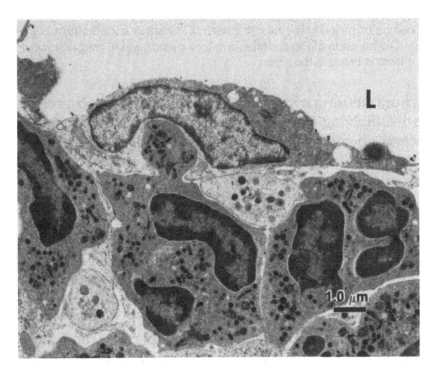

Fig. 16. TEM of a marrow sinus segment from the femur of a rat. Several granulocytes are present in the hemopoietic space and one can be seen with a pseudopod invaginating the perikaryon of an endothelial cell.

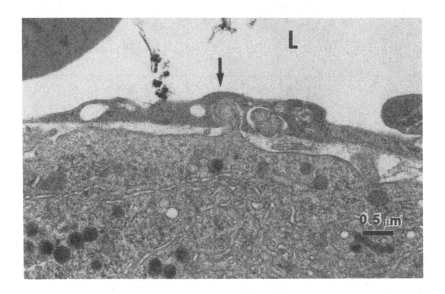

Fig. 17. TEM of a marrow sinus segment from the femur of a rat. The close apposition of megakaryocyte cytoplasm to the sinus endothelium is evident. The invasion of the endothelium by a pseudopod of megakaryocyte cytoplasm is beneath the arrow.

lets from mouse marrow megakaryocytes has been observed in vitro combining time-lapse cinemicrography and scanning electron microscopy.[149] Megakaryocyte filipod formation in vitro is enhanced when these cells are placed on surfaces coated with extracellular matrix.[150]

Megakaryocyte Remnants

It is presumed that most megakaryocyte nuclei are left in marrow after platelet release and that they are degraded and phagocytized (Fig. 21). The infrequency of nuclear remnants in unstimulated marrow could be the result of rapid nuclear ingestion and degradation by macrophages.[151] The erythroblast expels its nucleus in the hemopoietic compartment and, thereafter, the erythrocyte penetrates the sinus wall and enters the circulation. The megakaryocyte, however, expels its cyto-

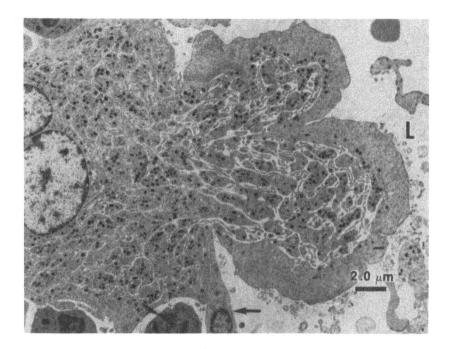

Fig. 18. TEM of a marrow sinus segment from the femur of a rat. The small arrow points to an endothelial cell body of the sinus wall. An enormous portion of megakaryocyte cytoplasm has broken through the endothelium and spewed into the sinus lumen (L).

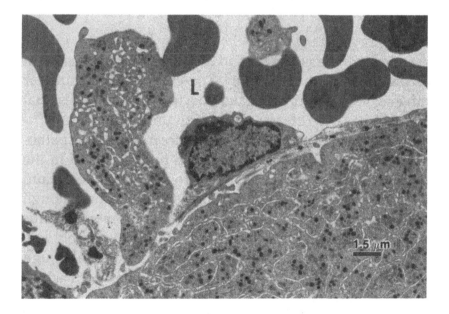

Fig. 19. TEM of a marrow sinus segment from the femur of a rat. The close proximity of megakaryocyte cytoplasm to the sinus wall is evident. A large piece of megakaryocyte cytoplasm (proplatelet) has entered the sinus lumen.

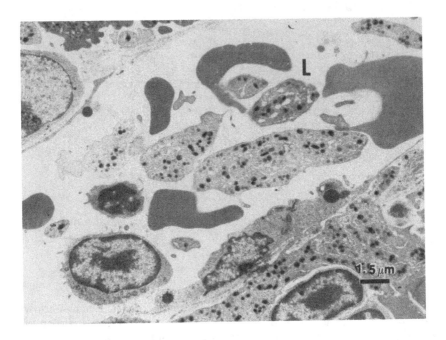

Fig. 20. TEM of a marrow sinus segment from the femur of a rat. Several proplatelets are present in the marrow sinus. Proplatelets undergo further fragmentation to form individual platelets.

plasm through the sinus wall and the nuclear remnant is left in the hemopoietic compartment. The entry of either nuclear remnants[152-154] or entire megakaryocytes with more residual cytoplasm has been observed, but is an uncommon event.[155]

In healthy individuals,[156,157] and more frequently in pathologic states,[158,159] megakaryocyte nuclei may be found in the blood. The delivery of platelets across sinus endothelium usually occurs through migration pores that are small enough to prevent egress of nuclei. Nuclei may enter the marrow sinus blood in the process of platelet release.[160] This presumably is an accident and does not represent a common event, although there are no firm kinetic data on the frequency with which nuclear escape occurs.

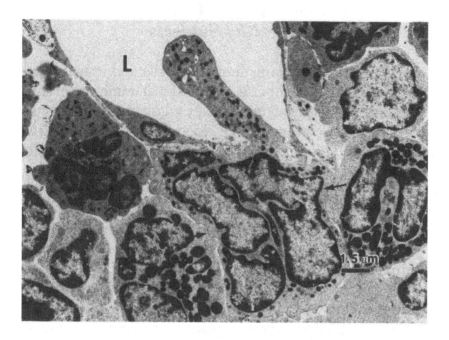

Fig. 21. TEM of a marrow sinus segment from the femur of a rat. A proplatelet is in the sinus lumen (L). The nucleus and small rim of surrounding cytoplasm of a spent megakaryocyte is in the hemopoietic space between the two arrows. Following shedding of cytoplasm into the sinus for the purpose of platelet delivery, the megakaryocyte nucleus takes on a cerebriform shape with chromatin condensation near the nuclear membrane. Occasionally, megakaryocyte nuclei or whole megakaryocytes enter the sinus lumen, presumably as an accident of nature without major functional significance.

Some megakaryocyte cytoplasm (potential platelets) may be left in marrow. A failure to accomplish release results in a small amount of ineffective thrombopoiesis. In pathological states, larger degrees of ineffective thrombopoiesis may occur as a result of megakaryocytes being in positions distant from a sinus wall or as a result of an abnormality in the structures that lead to cytoplasmic expulsion.

Release of Immature Cells
in Healthy Subjects

The system that retains immature cells and megakaryocytes in the marrow is imperfect. Occasional immature granulocytes and megakaryocyte nuclei or whole megakaryocytes are present in cell concentrates of blood.[156] Nucleated red cells are rarely seen and it is probable that few nucleated red cells escape the marrow. This is supported by the rarity of finding nucleated red cells in transit through the sinus wall or in the sinuses in marrow even after erythropoietin administration.[136] The absence of circulating erythroblasts also may be related, in part, to splenic sequestration and enucleation of the late erythroblast after release.[161]

The precise explanation for the small percentage of immature granulocytes in the blood is unknown. The late myelocyte and metamyelocyte have developed the capacity to move, respond to chemoattractants, and deform, albeit less well than the mature neutrophil, and thus may occasionally exit marrow by normal mechanisms. Alternatively, the sinus wall may undergo cyclic minor breakdowns, thereby allowing less mature cells to emerge.

One may find in micrographs of marrow occasional degenerating megakaryocytes that project into the sinus lumen as though they have broken through a sinus wall. This may account for their presence in the venous circulation.

Release of Immature Cells
in Pathological States

The exact mechanisms for the development of striking increases of immature cells in the blood under a variety of circumstances are not fully known. An increase in circulating nucleated erythroid cells occurs when there is intense stimulation of erythropoiesis such as during hypoxic states or hemolytic anemias. A similar slight increase in the proportion of immature granulocytes may occur when there is stimulation of granulopoiesis.

The presence of metastatic cancer, hemopoietic malignancies, or increased collagen deposition in marrow is associated with increased prevalence of immature cells in the circulation. It has been hypothesized that damage to the architecture of marrow, with a breakdown of the integrity of sinus walls, allows cells to enter the circulation less discriminantly. Animal studies of transplantable leukemia have indicated that sinusoidal wall damage is correlated to the prevalence of leukemic blast cells in the circulation.[162] Even when the marrow is replaced by leukemic cells, there is a difference in the ratio of immature to mature cells in the marrow and blood: blood tends to have a higher proportion of mature cells than marrow. This finding suggests discrimination in the release of cells in leukemia. The size of leukemic blast cells has also been suggested as one of several factors determining marrow release.[163]

In some pathological states such as leukemia, the ability of undifferentiated cells to penetrate the sinus wall is greater than that of their normal immature counterparts. Murine leukemic cells can penetrate the marrow sinus endothelial cells. Their mode of egress is similar to that of mature cells, since they deform and migrate through narrow migration pores formed in endothelial cell cytoplasm.[164–166]

Another factor in the release of immature cells in pathological states could be the inappropriate loss of anchoring surface molecules. A loss of appropriate surface glycoproteins or change in composition of surface complex sugars, for example, could free leukemic cells prematurely from attachment to marrow stroma permitting them to move toward and penetrate sinus endothelium.

Release from and Reentry into Marrow of Stem Cells and Progenitor Cells

Several lines of evidence indicate that stem cells circulate in the blood and can reenter marrow and reestablish hemopoiesis in the marrow cords. The development of a new vascular system prior to the recovery of hemopoiesis, when animal marrow fragments are transplanted to extramedullary sites, provides circumstantial evidence for the reentry of circulating stem cells into the reconstituted hemopoietic spaces.[167,168] Primitive hemopoietic cells with the capacity to differentiate into several cell lineages have been found in the blood of animals and man.[169] The experimental technique of endocloning, which involves whole body irradiation of an animal except for the shielding of one bone or a portion of one bone, and observing the repopulation of the irradiated marrow strongly implies release of stem cells from shielded marrow into the circulation and entry into hemopoietic spaces of irradiated marrow.[170–172]

In rodents, migration of intravenously transfused marrow cells into previously irradiated marrow has also been demonstrated.[173] An additional line of evidence supporting the migration of stem cells into established marrow tissue is provided by studies using rats joined by parabiosis. The hind limbs of one member of a parabiotic pair are shielded during the administration of 1000 cGy total body irradiation to both animals. The circulation between the animals is transiently interrupted while the shielded rat is labeled with ^{3}H-thymidine. Subsequently, circulation is reestablished and recovery of irradiated marrow in the nonlabeled, nonshielded animal is observed to occur predominantly via migration of labeled monocytoid cells.[174] To obviate the influence of irradiation, normal untreated of the CBA-T_6T_6 mice strain have been joined in parabiosis with normal male CBA recipients, with an exchange of marrow cells demonstrated.[175] The establishment of hemopoiesis in bone ossicles formed at sites of implantation of powdered, demineralized diaphyseal bone matrix also is compatible with the entry of circulating stem cells into reconstituted marrow stroma.[176] Most telling, in regard to stem cell reentry into marrow, is the ability to reconstitute the marrow of a human recipient by the intravenous infusion of marrow cells from a syngeneic or histocompatible allogeneic donor.

Little is known of the surface characteristics of stem cells that permit their release from the marrow or their attachment to the luminal surface of marrow sinuses and their penetration into the marrow spaces; but, it can be predicted that such specialization exists. For example, recent work has shown that hemopoietic stem cells agglutinated with lectins specific for galactosyl residues had a significantly reduced capacity to form spleen colonies. Endothelial cells have lectins that recognize galactosyl residues. This coincidence suggests that the entry of stem cells into the marrow could be mediated by a lectin–sugar interaction.[46] The entry of lymphocytes into lymph nodes through the high endothelium of lymph node venules provides a model for recognition sites acting as mediators of transvascular cell passage,[177] although no such ultrastructural modifications have been observed in marrow sinuses.

Acknowledgments

Patricia Santillo, Technical Supervisor of the Electron Microscope Laboratory in the Hematology Unit, University of Rochester School of Medicine provided the electron micrographs. Sandra Turner typed the manuscript and provided editorial assistance. Portions of this text were drawn from previously published articles or chapters on this subject by M. A. Lichtman.[28,136,160]

References

[1]Branemark, P. I. (1959) *Scand. J. Clin. Lab. Invest.* **11**, 5–82.
[2]Weiss, L. (1961) *Bull. Johns Hopkins Hospital* **108**, 171–199.

[3]Zamboni, L. and Pease, D. C. (1961) *J. Ultrastruct. Res.* **5**, 65–85.

[4]Weiss, L. (1965) *J. Morphol.* **117**, 467–537.

[5]Ito, U. (1965) *Bull. Tokyo Med. Dent. Univ.* **12**, 1–28.

[6]Watanabe, Y. (1966) *Tohoku J. Exp. Med.* **89**, 167–176.

[7]DeBruyn, P. P. H. (1966) *Anat. Rec.* **154**, 499 (abstract).

[8]Campbell, F. R. (1967) *J. Morphol.* **123**, 405–440.

[9]Weiss, L. (1967) *Clin. Orthop.* **52**, 13–23.

[10]Hudson, J. and Yoffey, J. M. (1968) *J. Anat.* **103**, 515–525.

[11]Tanaka, Y. (1969) *Acta Haematol. Jap.* **32**, 275–286.

[12]DeBruyn, P. P. H., Breen, P. C., and Thoms, T. B. (1970) *Anat. Rec.* **168**, 55–68.

[13]Fliedner, T. M., Calvo, W., Haas, R., Forteza, J., and Bohne, F. (1970) *Morphologic and Cytokinetic Aspects of Bone Marrow Stroma* (Stohlman, F., Jr, ed.), Grune & Stratton, New York, pp. 67–86.

[14]Weiss, L. (1970) *Blood* **36**, 189–207.

[15]Brookes, M. (1971) *The Blood Supply of Bone*, Butterworths, London.

[16]Samson, J. P., Hulstaert, C. E., Molenaar, I., and Nieweg, H. O. (1972) *Acta Haemtol.* **48**, 218–226.

[17]DeBruyn, P. P. H., Michelson, S., and Thomas, T. B. (1971) *J. Morphol.* **133**, 417–438.

[18]Aoki, M. and Tavassoli, M. (1981) *J. Ultrastruct. Res.* **74**, 255–258.

[19]Chamberlain, J. K., Leblond, P. F., and Weed, R. I. (1975) *Blood Cells* **1**, 655–674.

[20]Chamberlain, J. K., Weiss, L. and Weed, R. I. (1975) *Blood* **46**, 91–102.

[21]DeBruyn, P. P. H., Michelson, S., and Becker, R. P. (1975) *J. Ultrastruct. Res.* **53**, 133–151.

[22]Leblond, P. F., Chamberlain, J. K., and Weed, R. I. (1975) *Blood Cells* **1**, 639–651.

[23]Irino, S., Ono, T., Watanabe, K., Toyota, K., Unot, J., Takasugi, N., and Murakami, T. (1975) *Proceedings of the Eighth Annual Meeting* (Johari, O. and Corvin, I., eds.), ITT Research Institute, Chicago, pp. 268–273.

[24]Becker, R. P. and DeBruyn, P. P. H. (1976) *Am. J. Anat.* **145**, 183–206.

[25]Weiss, L. (1976) *Anat. Rec.* **186**, 161–184.

[26]Lichtman, M. A., Chamberlain, J. K., Weed, R. I., Pincus, A., and Santillo, P. A. (1977) *The Granulocytes: Function and Clinical Utilization*, Liss, New York, pp. 53–75.

[27]Chamberlain, J. K. and Lichtman, M. A. (1978) *Blood* **52**, 959–968.

[28]Lichtman, M. A., Chamberlain, J. K., and Santillo, P. A. (1978) *The Year in Hematology* (Silber, R., LoBue, J. and Gordon, A. S., eds.), pp. 243–279.

[29]Lichtman, M. A., Chamberlain, J. K., Simon, W., and Santillo, P. A. (1978) *Am. J. Hematol.* **4**, 303–312.

[30]DeBruyn, P. P. H., Michelson, S., and Becker, R. P. (1978) *J. Cell Biol.* **78,** 379–389.

[31]Shaklai, M. and Tavassoli, M. (1979) *J. Ultrastruct. Res.* **69,** 343–361.

[32]Tavassoli, M. and Shaklai, M. (1979) *Br. J. Haematol.* **41,** 303–307.

[33]Yoffey, J. M. (1962) *J. Anat.* **96,** 425.

[34]Tavassoli, M. (1974) *Acta Anat.* **90,** 608–616.

[35]Lichtman, M.A. (1981) *Exp. Hematol.* **9,** 391–410.

[36]Lichtman, M. A. (1984) *Long-Term Bone Marrow Culture* (Wright, D. G. and Greenberger, J. S., eds.), Liss, New York, pp. 3–29.

[37]Weiss, L. and Chen, L.-T. (1975) *Blood Cells* **1,** 617–638.

[38]Bradley, T. R., Hodgsen, G. S., and Rosendaal, M. (1978) *J. Cell Physiol.* **97,** 517–524.

[39]Maloney, M. A. and Patt, H. M. (1969) *Science* **165,** 71–73.

[40]Meyer-Hamme, K., Haas, R. J., and Fliedner, T. M. (1971) *Acta Hematol.* **46,** 349–361.

[41]Jaffe, E. A., Minick, R., Adelman, B., and Becker, C. G. (1976) *J. Exp. Med.* **144,** 209–225.

[42]DeBruyn, P. P. H., Michelson, S., and Bankston, P. W. (1985) *Cell Tissue Res.* **240,** 1–7.

[43]Geoffroy, J. S. and Becker, R. P. (1984) *J. Ultrastruct. Res.* **89,** 223–239.

[44]Pearse, B. M. F. (1976) *Proc. Natl. Acad. Sci. USA* **73,** 1255–1259.

[45]Bankston, P. W. and DeBruyn, P. P. H. (1974) *Am. J. Anat.* **141,** 281–290.

[46]Kataoka, M. and Tavassoli, M. (1985) *Blood* **65,** 1163–1171.

[47]Helenius, A., Mellman, I., Wall, D., and Hubbards, A. (1983) *Trends Biochem. Sci.* **8,** 245–250.

[48]Pastan, I. and Willingham, M. (1983) *Trends Biochem. Sci.* **8,** 250–254.

[49]Buys, C. H. C. M., DeJong, A. S. H., Bouma, J. M. W., and Gruber, M. (1975) *Biochem. Biophys. Acta* **392,** 95–100.

[50]Brouwer, A. and Knook, D. L. (1982) *J. Reticuloendothel. Soc.* **32,** 259–268.

[51]Soda, R. and Tavassoli, M. (1984) *J. Ultrastruct. Res.* **88,** 18–29.

[52]DeBruyn, P. P. H. and Michelson, S. (1979) *J. Cell Biol.* **82,** 708–714.

[53]DeBruyn, P. P. H. (1979) *J. Histochem. Cytochem.* **27,** 1174–1176.

[54]DeBruyn, P. P. H. (1981) *Sem. Hematol.* **18,** 179–193.

[55]Weiss, L., Mayhew, E., and Ulrich, K. (1966) *Lab. Invest.* **15,** 1304–1309.

[56]Goldstein, I. J., Hughes, R. C., Monsigny, M., Osawa, T., and Sharon, N. (1980) *Nature* **285,** 66 (letter).

[57]Barondes, S. H. (1984) *Science* **223,** 1259–1264.

[58]Soda, R. and Tavassoli, M. (1983) *J. Ultrastruct. Res.* **84,** 299–310.

[59]Pino, R. M. (1984) *Am. J. Anat.* **169,** 259–272.

[60]Holthofer, H., Virtanen, I., Kariniemi, A.-L., Hormia, M., Linder, E., and Miettinen, A. (1982) *Lab. Invest.* **47,** 60–66.

[61]Soda, R. and Tavassoli, M. (1984) *J. Ultrastruct. Res.* **87**, 242–251.

[62]Regoeizi, E., Chindemi, P. A., Hatton, M. W. C. , and Berry, L. R. (1980) *Arch. Biochem. Biophys.* **205**, 76–84.

[63]Knudtzon, S. and Mortensen, B. T. (1975) *Blood* **46**, 937–943.

[64]Knopse, W. H., Blom, J., and Crosby, W. H. (1968) *Blood* **31**, 400–405.

[65]Friedenstein, A. J., Chailakhyan, R. K., Latsinik, N. V., Panasyuk, A. F., and Keiliss-Borok, I. V. (1974) *Transplantation* **17**, 331–340.

[66]Westen, H. and Bainton, D. F. (1979) *J. Exp. Med.* **150**, 919–936.

[67]Demmler, K. (1975) *Clin. Hematol.* **4**, 331–351.

[68]Dexter, T. M. and Moore, M. A. S. (1977) *Nature* **269**, 412, 413.

[69]Dexter, T. M., Allen, T. D., and Lajtha, L. G. (1977) *J. Cell Physiol.* **91**, 335–344.

[70]Greenberger, J. S. (1978) *Nature* **275**, 752–754.

[71]Greenberger, J. S. (1979) *In Vitro* **15**, 823–828.

[72]Myoshi, I., Irino, S., and Hiraki, K. (1966) *Exp. Cell Res.* **41**, 220–223.

[73]Gordon, M. Y., King, J. A., and Gordon-Smith, E. C. (1980) *Br. J. Haematol.* **46**, 151,152.

[74]Mendelow, B., Grobicki, D., De La Hunt, M., Katz, J., and Metz, J. (1980) *Br. J. Haematol.* **46**, 15–22.

[75]Calvo, W. (1968) *Am. J. Anat.* **123**, 315–328.

[76]Calvo, A. and Forteza-Vila, J. (1970) *Blood* **36**, 180–188.

[77]Miller, M. L., and McCuskey, R. S. (1973) *Scand. J. Haematol.* **10**, 17–23.

[78]Donohue, D. M., Reiff, R. H., Hanson, M. L., Betson, Y., and Finch, C. A. (1958) *J. Clin. Invest.* **37**, 1571–1576.

[79]Harker, L. A. (1968) *J. Clin. Invest.* **47**, 452–457.

[80]Kaufman, R. M., Airon, R., Pollack, S., and Crosby, W. H. (1965) *Blood* **26**, 720–731.

[81]Sabin, F. R. (1928) *Physiol. Rev.* **8**, 191–244.

[82]Giordano, G. F. and Lichtman, M. A. (1973) *J. Clin. Invest.* **52**, 1154–1164.

[83]Lichtman, M. A. and Weed, R. I. (1972) *Blood* **39**, 301–316.

[84]Lichtman, M. A. and Weed, R. I. (1972) *Blood* **40**, 52–61.

[85]Bessis, M. (1973) *Living Blood Cells and Their Ultrastructure* (Bessis, M., ed.) Springer-Verlag, Berlin, pp. 85–183.

[86]Thiery, J. P. and Bessis, M. (1956) *Rev. Hematol.* **11**, 162–174.

[87]Behnke, O. (1969) *J. Ultrastruct. Res.* **26**, 111–129.

[88]Keyserlingk, D. G. and Albrecht, M. (1968) *Z. Zellforsch.* **89**, 320–327.

[89]Lichtman, M. A., Chamberlain, J. K., Simon, W., and Santillo, P. A. (1977) *Trans. Assoc. Am. Physicians* **90**, 313–323.

[90]Jahn, T. L. and Bovee, E. C. (1969) *Physiol. Rev.* **49**, 793–862.

[91]Pollard, T. D. and Weihing, R. R. (1974) *CRC Crit. Rev. Biochem.* **2**, 1–67.

[92]Sager, P. R., Cavanagh, J. B., and Clarkson, T. W. (1986) *The Cytoskeleton:*

A Target for Toxic Agents (Clarkson, T. W., Sager, P. K., and Syversen, T. L. M., eds.), Plenum, New York, pp. 3–21.

[93]Lichtman, M. A. (1973) *J. Clin. Invest.* **52**, 350–358.

[94]Lichtman, M. A. and Kearney, E. A. (1976) *Blood Cells* **2**, 491–506.

[95]Leblond, P. F., LaCelle, P. L., and Weed, R. I. (1971) *Nouv. Rev. Fr. Hematol.* **11**, 537–546.

[96]Leblond, P. F., LaCelle, P. L., and Weed, R. I. (1971) *Blood* **37**, 40–46.

[97]Lichtman, M. A. (1970) *N. Engl. J. Med.* **283**, 943–948.

[98]vanBeek, W., Tulp, A., Bolscher, J., Blanken, G., Roozendaal, K., and Egbers, M. (1984) *Blood* **63**, 170–176.

[99]Boggs, D. R. (1966) *Ann. Rev. Physiol.* **28**, 39–56.

[100]Dornfest, B. S. (1970) *Regulation of Hematopoiesis*, vol. 1, (Gordon, A. S., ed.), Appleton-Century Crofts, New York, pp. 237–267.

[101]Schultz, E. F., Lapin, D. M., and LoBue, J. (1973) *Humoral Control of Growth and Differentiation* (LoBue, J. and Gordon, A. S., eds.), Academic, New York, p. 51.

[102]Meuret, G., Bammert, J., and Gessner, U. (1976) *Blut* **33**, 389–402.

[103]Aster, R. H. (1967) *J. Lab. Clin. Med.* **70**, 736–751.

[104]Odell, T. T. and Murphy, J. R. (1974) *Blood* **44**, 147–156.

[105]Boggs, D. R., Cartwright, G. E., and Wintrobe, M. M. (1966) *Am. J. Physiol.* **211**, 51–60.

[106]Gordon, A. S., Neri, R. O., Siegel, C. D., Dornfest, B. S., Handler, E. S., LoBue, J., and Eisler, M. (1960) *Acta Haematol.* **23**, 323–341.

[107]Gordon, A. S., Handler, E. S., Siegel, C. D., Dornfest, B. S., and LoBue, J. (1964) *Ann. NY Acad. Sci.* **113**, 766–789.

[108]Alpers, C. A., Colten, H. R., Rosen, F. S., Rabson, A. R., MacNab, G. M., and Gear, J. S. S. (1972) *Lancet* **ii**, 1179–1181.

[109]Rother, K. (1972) *Eur. J. Immunol.* **2**, 550–558.

[110]Ghebrehiwet, B. and Muller-Eberhard, H. J. (1979) *J. Immunol.* **123**, 616–621.

[111]Bishop, C. R., Athens, J. W., Boggs, D. R., Warner, H. R., Cartwright, G. E., and Wintrobe, M. M. (1968) *J. Clin. Invest.* **47**, 249–260.

[112]Deinard, A. S. and Page, A. R. (1974) *Br. J. Haematol.* **28**, 333–345.

[113]Vogel, M. J., Yankee, R. A., Kimball, H. R., Wolff, S. M., and Perry, S. (1967) *Blood* **30**, 474–484.

[114]Boggs, D. R., Marsh, J. C., Chervenick, P. A., Cartwright, G. E., and Wintrobe, M. M. (1968) *Proc. Soc. Exp. Biol. Med.* **127**, 689–693.

[115]Kampschmidt, R. F. and Upchurch, H. F. (1980) *J. Reticuloendothel. Soc.* **28**, 191–201.

[116]Kampschmidt, R. F. (1984) *J. Leukocyte Biol.* **36**, 341–355.

[117]Mitchell, R. H., McClelland, R. M., and Kampschmidt, R. F. (1982) *Proc. Soc. Exp. Biol. Med.* **169**, 309–315.

[118]Fisher, J. W., Lajtha, G., Buttoo, A. S., and Porteous, D. D. (1965) *Br. J. Haematol.* **11**, 342–348.

[119]Gordon, A. S., LoBue, J., Dornfest, B. S., and Cooper, G. W. (1962) *Erythropoiesis* (Jacobsen, L. O. and Doyle, M., eds.), Grune & Stratton, New York, pp. 321–327.

[120]Herzog, G., Root, R., and Graw, R., Jr., (1977) *Blood* **39**, 554–567.

[121]Roy, A. J. (1980) *Cryobiology* **17**, 213–221.

[122]Dornfest, B. S., LoBue, J., Handler, E. S., Gordon, A. S., and Quastler, H. (1962) *J. Lab. Acta Haematol.* **28**, 42–60.

[123]Dornfest, B. S., LoBue, J., Handler, E. S., Gordon, A. S., and Quastler, H. (1962) *J. Lab. Clin. Med.* **60**, 777–787.

[124]Katz, R., Gordon, A. S., and Lapin, D. M. (1966) *J. Reticuloendothel. Soc.* **3**, 103–116.

[125]Lapin, D. M., LoBue, J., Gordon, A. S., Zanjani, E. D., and Schultz, E. F. (1969) *Proc. Soc. Exp. Biol. Med.* **131**, 756–762.

[126]Broxmeyer, H., Van Zant, G., Zucali, J. R., LoBue, J., and Gordon, A. S. (1974) *Proc. Exp. Biol. Med.* **145**, 1262–1267.

[127]Chikkappa, G., Chanana, A. D., Chandra, P., Commerford, S. L., and Cronkite, E. P. (1977) *Proc. Soc. Exp. Biol. Med.* **154**, 192–197.

[128]Rothstein, G., Christensen, R. D., Hugl, E. H., and Athens, J. W. (1971) *Blood* **38**, 820 (abstract).

[129]Wissler, J. H., Arnold, M., Gerlach, U., and Schaper, W. Z. (1980) *Physiol. Chem.* **361**, 351.

[130]Burdach, S. E., Wissler, J. H., Evers, K. G., and Godehardt, E. (1984) *Ric. Clin. Lab.* **14**, 565.

[131]Drinker, C. D., Drinker, K. R., and Lund, C. C. (1922) *Am. J. Physiol.* **62**, 1.

[132]Michelsen, K. (1967) *Acta Physiol. Scand.* **71**, 16–29.

[133]Michelsen, K. (1968) *Acta Physiol. Scand.* **73**, 264–280.

[134]Schickwann, T., Pactel, V., Beaumont, E., Lodish, H. F., Nathan, D. G., and Sieff, C. A. (1987) *Blood* **69**, 1587–1594.

[135]Tavassoli, M. (1978) *Exp. Hematol.* **6**, 257–269.

[136]Lichtman, M .A. and Waugh, R. E. (1985) *Humoral and Cellular Regulation of Erythropoiesis* (Zanjani, E. D., Tavassoli, M. , and Ascensao, J., eds.) Spectrum Publications, Jamaica, NY.

[137]Campbell, F. R. (1972) *Am. J. Anat.* **135**, 521–536.

[138]Campbell, F. R. (1982) *Anat. Res.* **203**, 365–374.

[139]DeBruyn, P. P. H. and Michelson, S. (1981) *Blood* **57**, 152–156.

[140]Waugh, R. E., Hsu, L. L., Clark, P., and Clark , A., Jr. (1984)*White Cell Mechanics: Basic Science and Clinical Aspects* (Meiselman, H. J., Lichtman, M. A., and LaCelle, P. L., eds.), Liss, New York, pp. 221–236.

[141]Waugh, R. E. and Sassi, M. (1986) *Blood* **68**, 250–257.

[142]Evans, E. A. and Skalak, R. (1979) *CRC Crit. Rev. Bioengr.* **3**, 181–330.

[143]Evans, E. A. and Hochmuth, R. M. (1976) *Biophys. J.* **13**, 941–954.

[144]Dabrowksi, A., Szygula, Z., and Miszta, H. (1981) *Acta Physiol. Pol.* **32**, 729–736.

[145]Wright, J. H. (1910) *J. Morphol.* **21**, 263–278.

[146]Radley, J. M. and Scurfield, G. (1980) *Blood* **56**, 996–999.

[147]Scurfield, G. and Radley, J. M. (1981) *Am. J. Hematol.* **10**, 285–296.

[148]Pennington, D. G. (1979) *Blood Cells* **5**, 5–10.

[149]Haller, C. J. and Radley, J. M. (1983) *Blood Cells* **9**, 407–418.

[150]Levin, R. F., Eldor, A., Hyam, E., Gamliel, H., Fuks, Z., and Vlodavsky, I. (1985) *Blood* **66**, 570–576.

[151]Radley, J. M. and Haller, C. J. (1983) *Br. J. Haematol.* **53**, 227–235.

[152]Behnke, O. (1969) *J. Ultrastruct. Res.* **26**, 111–129.

[153]Chen, L. T. and Weiss, L. (1980) *Anat. Embryol.* **159**, 277–288.

[154]Behnke, O. and Tinggaard-Pedersen, N. (1973) *Platelets: Production, Function, Transfusion and Storage* (Baldini, M. G. and Ebbe, S., eds.), Grune & Stratton, New York, pp. 21–31.

[155]Tavassoli, M. and Aoki, M. (1981) *Br. J. Haematol.* **48**, 25–29.

[156]Efrati, P. and Rozenszajn, L. (1960) *Blood* **16**, 1012–1019.

[157]Melamed, M. R., Cliffton, E. E., Meicer, C., and Koss, L. G. (1966) *Am. J. Med. Sci.* **252**, 301–309.

[158]Tinggaard-Pedersen, N. and Laursen, B. (1983) *Scand. J. Haematol.* **30**, 50–58.

[159]Hume, R., West., J. T., Malmgren, R. A., and Chu, E. A. (1964) *N. Engl. J. Med.* **270**, 111–117.

[160]Lichtman, M. A. and Brennan, J. K. (1987) *Hemostasis and Thrombosis* (Coleman, R., Hirsch, J., Marder, V. J. and Salzman, E., eds.), J. P. Lippincott, Philadelphia, pp. 395–417.

[161]Simpson, C. F. and Kling, J. M. (1967) *J. Cell Biol.* **35**, 237–245.

[162]Chen, L.-T., Handler, E. E., Handler, E. S., and Weiss, L. (1972) *Blood* **39**, 99–112.

[163]Stryckmans, P. A., Dubusscher, L., Ronge-Collard, E., Manaster, J., and Delalieux, G. (1977) *Leukemia Res.* **1**, 133–139.

[164]Campbell, F. R. (1975) *Am. J. Anat.* **142**, 319–334.

[165]DeBruyn, P. P. H., Becker, R. P., and Michelson, S. (1977) *Am. J. Anat.* **149**, 247–268.

[166]Cho, Y. and DeBruyn, P. P. H. (1979) *J. Ultrastruct. Res.* **69**, 13–21.

[167]Tavassoli, M. and Crosby, W. H. (1968) *Science* **161**, 54–56.

[168]Tavassoli, M., Maniatis, A., and Crosby, W. H. (1970) *Proc. Soc. Exp. Biol. Med.* **133**, 878–881.

[169]Schofield, R. (1979) *Clin. Haematol.* **8**, 221–237.

[170]Ford, C. E., Micklem, H. S., Evans, E., Gray, J. G., and Ogden, D. A. (1966) *Ann. NY Acad. Sci.* **129,** 283–296.

[171]Maloney, M. A. and Patt, H. M. (1972) *Blood* **39,** 804–808.

[172]Lambertsen, R. H. and Weiss, L. (1983) *Am. J. Anat.* **166,** 369–392.

[173]Congdon, C. C., Uphoff, D., and Lorenz, E. (1952) *J. Natl. Canc. Instit.* **13,** 73–93.

[174]Caffrey-Tyler, R. W. and Everett, N. B. (1966) *Blood* **28,** 873–890.

[175]Harris, J. E., Ford, C. E., Barnes, D. W. H., and Evans, E. P. (1964) *Nature* **201,** 886–887.

[176]Reddi, A. H. and Anderson, W. A. (1976) *J. Cell Biol.* **69,** 557–572.

[177]Woodruff, J. J. and Chin, Y.-H. (1984) *White Cell Mechanics: Basic Science and Clinical Aspects* (Meiselman, H. J., Lichtman, M. A., and LaCelle, P. L., eds.), Liss, New York, pp. 255–268.

Chapter 3

In Vivo Microscopy of Hemopoietic Tissue

Robert S. McCuskey

Introduction

In vivo microscopic studies of hemopoietic tissues and organs are limited in numbers and, to date, have been restricted to studies of the rabbit bone marrow,[1-6] the mouse spleen,[7-15] fetal liver,[16-19] and grafts of bone marrow or spleen into chambers implanted in the hamster cheek pouch or a dorsal skin flap of the mouse.[20,21] Nevertheless, these studies have provided valuable information concerning the microvascular compartment of the hemopoietic microenvironment.

The microvasculature within hemopoietic tissue is composed of arterioles, capillaries, sinusoids or sinuses, and venules, as well as associated neural elements, that may modulate or modify vascular mechanisms controlled locally or by hormones. This system is responsible for regulating everything that enters and leaves the hemopoietic site and, as a result, it regulates the delivery and release of blood cells and humoral substances, as well as influencing tissue oxygenation and pH. Since the microcirculation is dynamic, it is best studied using in vivo microscopic methods that permit the rate, duration, magnitude, and direction of dynamic events to be directly visualized, evaluated, quantified, and recorded continuously in life.

In Vivo Microscopic Methods

Basic Methods

The basic methods that have been used to study living organs with the light microscope include: examination of surgically exposed organs *in situ* or as isolated, perfused preparations and examination of organs *in situ* through windows contained within chambers implanted in ectopic sites. Each method has advantages as well as limitations.[22–24]

Microscopic study of surgically-exposed organs *in situ* usually permits high resolution examination of the microvasculature with its supplying vessels and nerve supplies intact. However, these preparations are subject to movements induced by the heart, respiratory, and gastrointestinal systems that, at times, can preclude critical microscopic study of the organ. Another limitation is the requirement to use anesthesia that limits the duration of the study to relatively short periods of time (2–12 h). Despite these limitations, the use of such methods has resulted in a better understanding of the structure and function of the microvasculature in the murine spleen under a variety of experimental conditions. Although most such studies have been of the intact spleen *in situ*, unpublished results in our laboratory indicated that the isolated, perfused spleen[25,26] also is a suitable candidate for high resolution in vivo microscopy. Such preparations are not subject to induced movements and permit critical control of blood pressure and flow. However, they usually are of very short duration since structural and functional deterioration frequently becomes evident after 1–2 h.

In contrast, bone marrow visualized through windows in the tibia or femur, as well as bone marrow and splenic tissue grafted into chambers in ectopic sites, can be studied chronically, frequently for several months, and often without the necessity for anesthesia.[1-6,20,21] However, grafts in ectopic sites are not in their normal anatomical position or environment and, like isolated perfused organs, are deprived of their normal vascular and nerve supply. Another limitation of these preparations is that the microscopic images of organs, contained in chambers or visualized through windows in bones, usually are not of as high definition as those obtained in acute preparations *in situ*. Details often are partially obscured by the presence of inflammatory exudate and granulation or connective tissue between the window and the underlying organ or graft. For certain types of studies, however, these latter preparations are extremely useful.

The spleens of a variety of small laboratory animals, including rats, mice, hamsters and guinea pigs, can be studied by light microscopy using transillumination of relatively thin (3–5 mm) areas of the organ. Thicker areas of the organs in these species, as well as the thicker organs of larger animals, such as cats, dogs, and monkeys, can be examined only by epi-illumination. It should be noted, however, that the resolution obtainable using epi-illumination usually is inferior to that realized with transillumination.[22-24]

Transillumination Methods

Two basic methods of transillumination have been used for light microscopy of the spleen. These include the use of quartz, glass or plastic light rods, or fiber optic light guides that generally are not focusable; alternatively, a focusable condenser contained on a modified compound microscope is used. Although the first method permits microscopic examination of the organ in its normal anatomical position, examination at high magnifications with good resolution rarely is possible. As a result, most in vivo microscopic studies of the microvasculature of the spleen during the past 25 years have used a modified compound trinocular microscope.[7-15, 22-24]

The compound trinocular microscope normally is equipped for both trans- as well as epi-illumination of the organ to be studied. After the animal is anesthetized, the spleen is exteriorized through a left subcostal incision and positioned over a window of optical grade mica or glass in a specially designed tray mounted on the microscope stage. The tray has provisions for the drainage of irrigating fluids; the window overlies a long working distance condenser. The spleen is covered with a piece of Saran or Mylar film that sometimes is cemented to a moveable "U"-shaped metal or plastic frame. The Saran or Mylar holds the organ in position and limits movement induced by the heart, respiration, and intestines, and yet it is flexible enough to avoid compression of the underlying splenic microvasculature. In addition, the plastic film helps to maintain homeostasis by limiting exposure of the organ surface to the external environment. Homeostasis is further insured by constant suffusion of the organ with Ringer's solution that is maintained at body temperature by proportional regulating heaters electronically clamped to rectal temperature. Once the organ is exteriorized and positioned on the window overlying the substage condenser, it is transilluminated with selected wavelengths of monochromatic light between 400–800 nm obtained by placing a monochromater in the light path between a broad spectrum xenon lamp and the substage condenser. The microscopic images of the microvasculature and its surrounding tissue are secured at magnifications up to 1500× using both dry and water immersion objectives. The resulting optical images are either studied and photographed directly or televised through a projection ocular (1.6–5.0×). A silicon or intensified silicon (SIT or ISIT) vidicon camera is used depending upon the sensitivity and resolution required, as well as the wavelengths of light to be imaged. The resulting video images are either videotaped or recorded on motion picture film using a camera whose motor is synchronized with the framing rate of the video system.

The use of specific wavelengths of monochromatic light enhance the definition of cellular detail through the selective absorption or transmission of these wavelengths by specific tissue and cellular components. When such monochromatic, microscopic images are televised, the contrast between tissue and cellular components can be enhanced further by readjustments of the brightness and contrast controls on the video monitor. Thus, the images of a particular structure(s) can be enhanced or supressed depending on the wavelength of light selected and the adjustments of the television system. For example, the use of wavelengths of light that are selectively absorbed by hemoglobin contained in the circulating erythrocytes aids in the study of patterns of blood flow or the overall morphological organization of a microvascular bed in the organ, particularly at low or moderate magnifications. However, for studying the highly vascular spleen at high magnifications, it is useful to transilluminate the organ at wavelengths of light between 575 and 750 nm to eliminate the absorption of light by the hemoglobin contained in the numerous erythrocytes flowing or sequestered in the microvasculature. This not only increases the amount of light transmitted through the spleen, but also enhances the definition of the endothelium and other cellular components. When such images are televised using a silicon vidicon that has a peak spectral response between 600 and 800 nm, the following usually can be observed: differentiation of the microvasculature into arterioles, capillaries or sinuosoids, and venules; patterns of blood flow in these vessels; the shape and deformation of individual blood cells; differentiation of the endothelium and smooth muscle of most vessels; identification of most cells contiguous with the microvasculature; and some cytoplasmic and nuclear detail. Under optimal conditions, the measured resolution is 0.3–0.5 μm when using 80–100× water immersion objectives.

Epi-illumination Methods

In addition to transillumination, the organ can be epi-illuminated through the objective lens using appropriate optics. As indicated above, the resolution obtained using this method of illumination is considerably less than that obtained by transillumination. However, epi-illumination is particularly useful for studying the patterns and distribution of fluorescent probes of microvascular and cellular function. Potential uses of fluorescent probes include the study of phagocytic properties of macrophages under a variety of conditions, differences in patterns between cellular and plasma flow, and entrapment of labeled leukocytes, tumor cells, and so on. For intensely fluorescing materials, epi- and transillumination can be combined to provide improved definition of the cellular localization of a variety of fluorescent probes. Alternatively, weakly fluorescing probes may first be imaged and recorded by epi-illumination and their localization subsequently identified by transillumination. In many cases, the use of intensified (SIT or ISIT) video cameras, coupled with digital image processing and/or filtered techniques, are necessary to obtain images of reasonable quality and for extraction of the desired information, especially if this information is to be quantified. Such techniques are just beginning to be used in studying the microvasculature of organs by in vivo microscopy.

In Vivo Microscopic Studies of Hemopoietic Tissue

Most reported in vivo microscopic studies of hemopoietic tissues and organs have been directed toward elucidating the relationship of the microvasculature to blood cell formation and release, especially erythropoiesis. Concommitantly, an improved understanding of microvascular architecture has resulted, as well as its neural and hormonal regulation.[1-21]

A number of investigations have demonstrated increases in blood flow through hemopoietic organs during periods when they contain active erythropoiesis and suggested that erythropoietin itself might be vasoactive and mediate these blood flow increases, as well as promote cellular release.[27] Using in vivo microscopic methods, increases were observed both in the microcirculation and vascularity in the fibular marrow of rabbits following stimulation of erythropoiesis by bleeding.[1,2] Other in vivo microscopic studies[18] demonstrated microvascular responses to erythropoietin applied topically to the erythropoietic fetal liver; these responses were not seen in the adult liver that lacked erythropoiesis. In fetal liver, erythropoietin caused the fetal hepatic sinusoids to dilate and, thus, release stored mature or maturing red blood cells. Normoblasts adherent to the sinusoid wall also were seen to be released. These responses were not immediate, suggesting that the effect might be indirect and that an intermediary substance, possibly a metabolite, might be elaborated from the erythropoietic tissue when stimulated by erythropoietin. Other experiments showed that erythropoietic stimuli or the administration of erythropoietin increased the vascularity of splenic grafts in the mouse back chamber,[20] and also in chronically implanted bone marrow chambers in rabbits.[5]

Further insight into the effects of erythropoietin on the microvascular system of hemopoietic tissue were derived from in vivo microscopic studies of the erythropoietic spleen of the mouse.[7-11] Regenerating erythropoiesis in the splenic red pulp of sublethally X-irradiated, anemic animals was accompanied by an elevation in blood flow through the red pulp when compared with unirradiated, normal mice.[7] In contrast, in polycythemic mice and in X-irradiated, polycythemic mice with suppressed erythropoiesis, splenic blood flow was decreased and there was a marked increase in the amount of blood being stored in the red pulp.[7] The effect was postulated to be related to the circulating levels of erythropoietin since it was assumed that the circulating levels of endogenous erythropoietin were elevated in the anemic mice and reduced in the polycythemic mice.

Subsequent experiments supported the contention that the microvascular responses described above were related to erythropoietin.[8] Administration of erythropoietin to transfused polycythemic mice resulted in increased blood flow through the splenic red pulp and a reduction in the storage of blood. This response was first seen 4–6 h after injection; it persisted for 48 h and was reduced markedly by 72 h. By 120 h, the spleens were indistinguishable from controls. That the response was due to erythropoietin and not to some contaminant in the hormone preparation was suggested by the duration of the response, which coincided closely with the time required for stem cells to differentiate into mature erythrocytes. In addition, when erythropoietin was incubated with antierythropoietin serum prior to injection, the vascular response was abolished, again suggesting that the microvascular response was a result of erythropoietin.[10]

To firmly establish that these responses in transfused, polycythemic mice were specific for erythropoietic tissues, not related to the transfusion of exogenous blood cells or a general microvascular response to increased circulating red blood cell mass, and that the restoration of flow was not owing to contaminants in the erythropoietin preparation, the splenic micro-circulation of polycythemic mice was examined after 0–210 h of hypoxia (erythropoietic stimulation) and also 6 d posthypoxia (erythropoietic suppression).[14] During the period of hypoxia, flow increased 30% above controls; 6 d posthypoxia, flow was reduced to 48% of controls. Examination of the effect of poly-cythemia on the microcirculation in several nonerythropoietic organs demonstrated no significant changes in blood flow in the microvasculature of the nonhemopoietic pancreas, skeletal muscle, and kidney and only slight changes in the liver.[10,14]

Although these studies strongly suggested a role for eryth-ropoietin in regulating blood flow through hemopoietic tissue, the precise mechanism of action was not clear. The 4 h delay before a response was seen suggested that the reaction was indirect and mediated by the release of some vasoactive substance(s) from the erythropoietic tissue.[8] The vascular re-sponse occurred prior to any significant incorporation of ^{59}Fe in these animals, and the response coincided with the time when early precursor cells were reported to be active, but prior to their differentiation in recognizable erythroid cells. Together with the observation of no vascular response in a number of anemic, lethally-irradiated animals that failed to develop eryth-ropoiesis,[8] it was suggested that the source of the intermediary substance was an early precursor cell of erythropoiesis, such as a colony-forming unit (CFU) or an erythropoietin responsive stem cell (ERC). Further support for this was obtained from in vivo microscopic studies of the genetically anemic W/W$_v$ mouse that has a defect in its stem cell compartment.[9] In the W/ W$_v$ anemic mouse, blood flow through the splenic microvascu-lature was half of that seen in normal, nonanemic (++) litter-mates. In contrast, blood flow through the red pulp of Sl/Sl$_d$ anemic mice having a microenvironmental defect in its stroma was found to be elevated significantly above normal, nonanemic littermates. When W/W$_v$ mice were transfused with a suspension of normal +/+ cells from either spleen or bone marrow to correct the anemia, the spleens of the recipients, 10 d after transfusion, were found to contain a near normal microcirculation. These results provided additional evidence that an early erythroid precursor, such as CFU or ERC, might be the source of a vasoactive substance(s) that locally regulated blood flow through erythropoietic tissue. Blood flow in the spleens of Sl/Sl$_d$ mice was elevated above normal, consistent with the presence of competent stem cells in these animals that were responding to elevated levels of circulating erythropoietin by releasing elevated levels of vasodilatory substance(s).

The cellular origin of vasoactive substance(s), and whether the vascular response induced by erythropoietin was dependent upon stimulation of ERC, was determined more precisely by examining the alterations in splenic microcirculation that accompanied the suppression and recovery of ERC and CFU in normal and polycythemic mice treated with Myleran.[11] Five days after administering Myleran to normal mice that have circulating erythropoietin, there was a significant reduction in blood flow through the red pulp that coincided with the reported interval of time of suppression of ERC by Myleran. After 10 d, when replacement of ERC had been initiated but CFU were still suppressed, the microcirculation returned to normal. These vascular responses were abolished in polycythemic animals having no circulating erythropoietin. Both ERC and erythropoietin were required to elicit these responses, supporting the hypothesis that the effect of erythropoietin on the microvasculature was indirect and mediated by some substance(s) released from ERC when stimulated by erythropoietin. Further experiments suggested that ERC triggered into replication by erythropoietin were the primary source of vasoactive substances(s).[11]

The identity of this substance(s), and the mechanism by which this substance(s) elicits blood flow increases through the red pulp, however, has not yet been completely defined although two mechanisms appear likely. First, the vasoactive substance(s) produces microvascular dilatation; second, the substance(s) increases the permeability of the walls of sinusoids and venules to blood cells, thus increasing the exit of mature circulating red blood cells from the red pulp, as well as promoting the release of reticulocytes and recently developed erythrocytes.

In this regard, the microvasculature of the erythropoietic mouse spleen was found to be responsive to numerous vasoactive substances and neural stimulation.[12,13,28,29] Based on these studies, utilizing a variety of vasoactive substances, adenosine formed from the degration of elevated levels of cAMP found in developing erythroid cells might elicit the hyperemia observed 4–6 h after erythropoietin stimulation.[12] Further support for this concept was suggested by unpublished results from our laboratory that demonstrated the abolition of vasodilation when polycythemic mice were treated with theophylline (an inhibitor of the breakdown of cAMP) in conjunction with the administration of erythropoietin.

Regarding changes in permeability, in vivo microscopic and electron microscopic studies demonstrated that arterial blood flows into the erythropoietic, murine splenic red pulp from "arterial" capillaries (Fig. 1) that deliver the blood into channels formed by the cytoplasmic process of reticular cells.[15] After flowing through this meshwork of reticular cell processes, the blood reenters the vasculature by penetrating the endothelial walls of venous sinuses (Fig. 2) or venules.[15] Thus, increases in blood flow through the red pulp also may be a reflection of increases in the number and size of open apertures in the endothelial walls of sinuses and venules.

In vivo microscopic studies revealed dramatic increases in the number of erythrocytes penetrating the endothelium of splenic sinuses and venules during erythropoietic stimula-

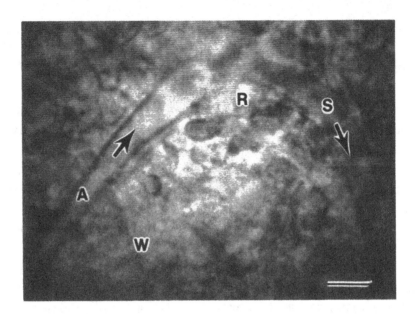

Fig. 1. In vivo photomicrograph of central arteriole (A) passing through the white pulp (W) to terminate in the red pulp (R). S is a venous sinus. Arrow indicates the direction of blood flow. Size marker is 10 μm.

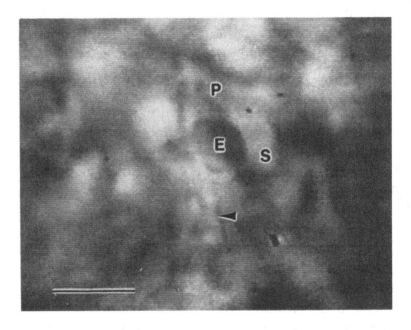

Fig. 2. In vivo photomicrograph of an erythrocyte (E) being deformed in passage through the endothelial wall (arrow) into a venous sinus (S). Two platelets (P) are adherent to the abluminal surface of the sinus endothelium. Size marker is 10 μm.

tion.[7,8,15] Electron microscopic studies of the spleens of erythro-
poietically-stimulated and nonstimulated polycythemic mice[15]
suggested an increase in the number of apertures through the
endothelial walls of sinusoids and venules during stimulation;
numerous reticulocytes, as well as mature erythrocytes, were
observed in transit from the red pulp into the venous circulation. Similar increases also have been reported in the porosity
of sinusoid walls in the marrow during erythropoietic stimulation.[30-32]

Prostaglandin(s) may be released during erythropoietic
stimulation.[27] These substances, particularly PGE_2, influence
the permeability of the endothelial walls of splenic sinusoids
and venules promoting cellular release and increased blood
flow through the red pulp[12] (and unpublished results). This
concept is supported further by other unpublished observations in our laboratory that treatment of polycythemic mice
with indomethacin (an inhibitor of prostaglandin synthesis),
prior to administering erythropoietin, reduced cellular egress,
as well as blood flow, through the red pulp.

It also was found that subthreshold levels of neurotrans-
mitter may modulate the sensitivity of the vascular wall to
various vasoactive substances including adenosine and prostaglandins E_2 and $F_{2\alpha}$.[12] In addition, a number of vasoactive
substances caused alpha-mediated arteriolar constriction by
releasing stored catecholamine from sympathetic nerves, in
addition to acting directly on the vascular wall. Although these
neurovascular phenomena may be important in the modulation of hemopoiesis by the central nervous system, they did not
appear to affect the changes in microcirculation exhibited in
polycythemic and erythropoietin-treated, polycythemic mice,
i.e., they did not affect the mechanism of action of the vasoactive substance(s) released from ERC upon stimulation with
erythropoietin. This was determined by evaluating the microcirculation in mice having functional and nonfunctional inner-
vation.[12]

In summary, all the studies reviewed above indicated that erythropoietin had no direct effect on the microcirculation within hemopoietic tissue, but that one or more vasoactive substances were released as a consequence of its action on ERC since removal of either erythropoietin or ERC abolished the microvascular response. These substance(s), possibly adenosine and/or one or more prostaglandins, locally elicited dilatation and increased the permeability of the microvasculature, resulting in increased blood flow and cellular release in erythropoietic sites. Although most of the in vivo microscopic studies have used the murine spleen as an experimental model, the results are probably applicable to all erythropoietic sites, e.g., bone marrow and fetal liver, since changes in blood flow, vascular permeability, and cellular release have been demonstrated in these sites following erythropoietic stimulation. Additional in vivo microscopic studies in the future hopefully will address these issues, as well as further elucidate the interrelationship between blood flow, tissue oxygenation and pH, and the chemical composition of the stromal compartment of the hemopoietic microenvironment.[7-11]

References

[1]Brånemark, P. I. (1959) *Scand. J. Clin. Lab. Invest.* **38**, 1–82.

[2]Brånemark, P. I., Breine, U., Johansson, B., Roylance, P. J., Rockert, H., and Yoffey J. M. (1964) *Acta Anat.* **59**, 1–46.

[3]Kinosita, R. and Ohno, S. (1961) *Bibl. Anat.* **1**, 106–109.

[4]McCuskey, R. S., McClugage, S. G., Jr., and Younker, W. J. (1971) *Blood* **38**, 87–95.

[5]McClugage, S. G., Jr., McCuskey, R. S., and Meineke, H. A. (1971) *Blood* **38**, 96–107.

[6]Paulo, L. G., McCuskey, R. S., Fink, G. D., Roh, B. L., and Fisher, J. W. (1973) *Proc. Soc. Exper. Biol. Med.* **143**, 986–990.

[7]McCuskey, R. S., Meineke, H. A., and Townsend, S. F. (1972) *Blood* **39**, 697–712.

[8]McCuskey, R. S., Meineke, H. A., and Kaplan, S. M. (1972) *Blood* **39**, 809–813.

[9]McCuskey, R. S. and Meineke, H. A. (1973) *Amer. J. Anat.* **137**, 187–198.

[10]McCuskey, R. S., Meineke, H. A., Kaplan, S. M., and Reed, P. A. (1973) *Microvas. Res.* **6**, 124, 125.

[11]McCuskey, R. S. and Meineke, H. A. (1977) *Proc. Soc. Exper. Biol. Med.* **156**, 181–185.

[12]Reilly, F. D. and McCuskey, R. S. (1977) *Microvas. Res.* **13**, 79–90.

[13]Reilly, F. D. and McCuskey, R. S. (1977) *Microvas. Res.* **14**, 293–302.

[14]McCuskey, R. S., Meineke, H. A., and McCuskey P. A. (1976) *Microcirculation*, vol. 1 (Grayson, J. and Zingg, W., eds.), Plenum, New York, pp. 359, 360.

[15]McCuskey, R. S. and McCuskey, P. A. (1985) *Experientia* **41**, 179–187.

[16]McCuskey, R. S. (1967) *Angiology* **18**, 648–653.

[17]McCuskey, R. S. (1967) *Bibl. Anat.* **9**, 71–75.

[18]McCuskey, R. S. (1967) *Life Sci.* **6**, 2129–2133.

[19]McCuskey, R. S. (1968) *Anat. Rec.* **161**, 267–280.

[20]Feleppa, A. E., Jr., Meineke, H. A., and McCuskey R. S. (1971) *Scand. J. Hematol.* **8**, 86–91.

[21]McCuskey, P. A., McCuskey, R. S., and Meineke, H. A. (1975) *Exp. Hematol.* **3**, 297–308.

[22]McCuskey, R. S. (1981) *Prog. Clin. Biol. Res.* **59**, 79–87.

[23]McCuskey, R. S. (1986) *The Science of Biological Specimen Preparation* (Muller, M., Becker, R., Boyde, A., and Wolosewick, J. J., eds.), SEM, Chicago, pp. 73–77.

[24]McCuskey, R. S. (1986) *Physical Techniques for Studying the Microvasculature of Internal Organs* (Baker, C. H. and Nastuk, W. F., eds.), Academic, New York, pp. 247–264.

[25]Cilento, E. V., McCuskey, R. S., Reilly, F. D., and Meineke, H. A. (1980) *Amer. J. Physiol.* **239**, H272–277.

[26]Stock, R. J., Cilento, E. V., Reilly, F. D., and McCuskey, R. S. (1983) *Amer. J. Physiol.* **245**, H17–21.

[27]McCuskey, R. S. and Meineke, H. A. (1977) *Kidney Hormones*, vol. II (Fisher, J. W., ed.), Academic, New York, pp. 311–327.

[28]MacKenzie, D. W. , Whipple, A. O. , and Wintersteinner, M. P. (1941) *Amer. J. Anat.* **68**, 397–456.

[29]Fleming, W. W. and Parpart, A. K. (1958) *Angiology* **9**, 294–302.

[30]Chamberlain, J. K., Weiss, L., and Weed, R. I. (1975) *Blood* **46**, 91–102.

[31]LeBlond, P. F., Chamberlain, J. K., and Weed, R. I. (1975) *Blood Cells* **1**, 639–654.

[32]Tavassoli, M. (1979) *Brit. J. Hemat.* **41**, 297–302.

Chapter 4

Fatty Involution of Marrow and the Role of Adipose Tissue in Hemopoiesis

Mehdi Tavassoli

Introduction

On gross examination, bone marrow may be red or yellow. Red marrow is hemopoietic and contains all cell lines normally considered to be associated with hemopoiesis. It derives its color from heme chromogen of erythrocytes and their pigmented precursors. By contrast, the major cell type in yellow marrow is the adipocyte (Fig. 1) that imparts a yellow color. Hence, yellow marrow is also known as fatty marrow. This marrow is not normally hemopoietic and is considered as a natural experimental model for marrow aplasia.[1]

Even in red marrow, there exists a large number of adipocytes, but their proportion is far less than in the yellow marrow. Adipocytes and hemopoietic cells are in a labile state and, under certain conditions, may rapidly displace one another.

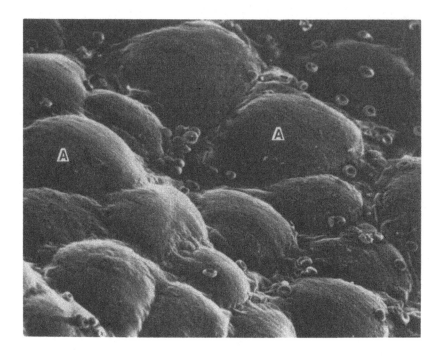

Fig. 1. Scanning electron micrograph of rabbit tibial marrow. Note the presence of numerous large adipocytes (A) compared to small disk shaped erythrocytes (×750).

In vivo, the association of hemopoiesis and adipocytes is restricted to the bone marrow and it is not seen in extramedullary hemopoiesis such as what may occur in liver, spleen, or yolk sac during mammalian embryogenesis, or in murine spleen after birth. This association is only one distinguishing characteristic of medullary hemopoiesis. Another feature is that hemopoiesis in the marrow, in contrast to extramedullary hemopoiesis, occurs within the confines of bone that provides a rigid frame for the hemopoietic tissue. These two features may be related: the volume contained within the frame of bone is fixed and does not expand or shrink. On the other hand, the volume of hemopoietically active marrow must expand and shrink in response to the fluctuating body requirement for blood cells. Therefore, the adipose component of marrow may serve as a "cushion," shrinking when hemopoiesis expands and expanding when hemopoiesis shrinks. This reciprocal relationship is evident in clinical examination of marrow: in aplastic anemias, marrow is replaced entirely by adipocytes whereas in polycythemias, it is entirely devoid of this component. Extramedullary hemopoiesis does not call for this "cushion" effect and, therefore, it is not associated with adipocytes.

Distribution of Red and Yellow Marrow

Ernst Neumann, who in 1868 identified the bone marrow as a seedbed of blood,[2] made another seminal discovery in 1882. In a classical contribution,[3] he noted that at birth all bones that contain marrow, have red marrow. With age, however, hemopoiesis undergoes regression in a centripetal direction so that, in adults, the more peripherally located marrow consists entirely of adipose tissue and does not take part in hemopoiesis (yellow or fatty marrow). During the ensuing 50 yr, other investigators substantiated this observation[3-12] that is now sometimes referred to as Neumann's law. Custer[8] carried out a systematic study and defined the pattern of distribution of red and fatty marrow in adults and changes that can occur in certain hematological disorders. Askanazi[4] suggested that premature vascular senescence of marrow may be responsible for its subsequent fatty involution.

In 1936, Huggins and his coworkers observed a parallel phenomenon: at birth, marrow temperature is comparable in all bones, but with maturity, a cooling of 4–8°C develops in a centrifugal direction.[13] This parallelism immediately suggested a relationship: thermal conditions in the bones of extremities are not optimal for hemopoiesis; thus, hemopoiesis regresses to be confined only to the central parts of the body where conditions are optimal. To test this hypothesis, these researchers "looped" the rat tail and placed the distal end of it inside the peritoneal cavity. The vertebrae in the adult rat tail normally contains yellow marrow, but after this experimental manipulation hemopoiesis resumed in the vertebrae of the intraperitoneally distal tail that was subjected to higher temperature. The marrow in the vertebrae of proximal tail (external to the peritoneal cavity) remained unchanged and was still yellow.[14,15]

This "temperature gradient" hypothesis was supported by the fascinating comparative observations of Weiss and Wislocki[16] in the nine-banded armadillo (*Dasypus novemcinctus*). Hemopoietic activity of the marrow in the dermal bones of these animals undergoes seasonal variations. In the winter months, hemopoiesis ceases and the marrow is replaced by adipose tissue.

As warmer weather returns in the spring, hemopoiesis resumes and during the summer months, the entire marrow cavities of the dermal bones are hemopoietic. A similar seasonal effect can also be noted in frogs and other amphibia in whom the marrow is initiated to the function of hemopoiesis during the course of evolution.[17] In these species, marrow is hemopoietic only in the spring and summer. During the winter, the spleen is the hemopoietic organ. Further evidence for a thermal effect on hemopoiesis comes from the observation that in equatorial countries hemolytic anemias are associated with a relatively higher reticulocyte count, compared to diseases of comparable severity in the inhabitants of cold countries.[17]

The Role of Bone

Not entirely consistent with the "temperature gradient" hypothesis is the observation that whereas the temperature in any one marrow cavity is probably the same, the distribution of hemopoiesis is not uniform. This can best be appreciated in

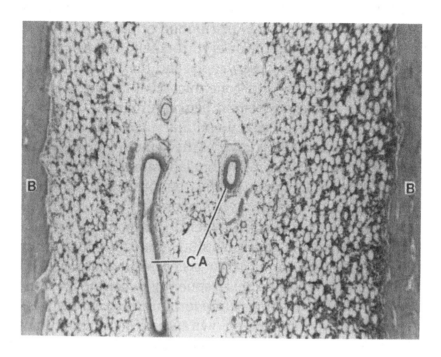

Fig. 2. Horizontal section of bone marrow cavity in rabbit femur. The bone (B) is seen in both side and the central artery (CA) is at the middle. Note the increasing gradient of adipocytes toward the central artery and increasing gradient of hemopoiesis toward the bone (×16).

tubular bones where, in microscopic examination, hemopoiesis forms a gradient with the highest intensity in the subendosteal area (Fig. 2). The area surrounding the central artery consists almost entirely of adipose tissue. This pattern of distribution would not be expected if the temperature were the sole determinant of the intensity of hemopoiesis. The relative spatial distribution of hemopoietic precursor cells (CFU-S, CFU-C, BFU-E, and CFU-E) in a marrow cavity also forms gradients regarding the bone.[18-21]

In discussing the mechanism whereby elevation of temperature may facilitate hemopoiesis, Huggins et al.[13] suggested a combination of primary effect on tissue metabolism and a secondary vasomotor effect. Van Dyke[22] also found a remarkable similarity between the distribution of blood flow in the bone and the distribution of erythropoietic marrow in the skeleton. Based on his observations and the anatomical considerations of marrow and bone microcirculation, he postulated a local portal circulation between marrow and bone analogous to the hypothalamic-pituitary axis. He suggested that this portal circulation governs the hemopoietic activity of marrow through a humoral factor elaborated by bone.

This hypothesis could certainly be consistent with short-range interactions regulating hemopoiesis. Long-term bone marrow culture (discussed elsewhere in this volume) provides a suitable experimental model to study this sort of interaction. Van Dyke's hypothesis is also consistent with anatomical observation that marrow vessels frequently penetrate the bone, only to reenter the marrow before forming vascular sinuses.[17] From this observation and their own autoradiographic studies, Patt and Maloney[23] concluded that Haversian canals in the bone may serve as a reservoir for hemopoietic progenitor cells, a hypothesis that is also consistent with spatial distribution of marrow and hemopoietic progenitor cells relative to the bone. This hypothesis has recently found some experimental support as well.[24]

The relation of bone and hemopoiesis is further emphasized by the observation that, in the absence of gravity during spaceflight, cessation of bone formation is associated with a reduction in the magnitude of erythropoiesis.[25] Conversely, conditions associated with a higher activity in bone turnover may enhance hemopoiesis. Thus, from observations in osteoporotic patients, Little[26] has suggested that active hemopoiesis is seen in those bones where resorption is highly active and that breakdown products of bone may be used to stimulate hemopoiesis.

Although all these hypotheses require experimental evidence for their proof, one may safely conclude that bone may in someway modulate the intensity of hemopoiesis and thereby the distribution of red and yellow marrow. This relatively unexplored area deserves more attention.

Ectopic Implantation of Bone Marrow

The "temperature gradient" hypothesis is both attractive and plausible and certainly the experimental evidence provided by Huggins and coworkers is compelling. Nonetheless, when Petrakis[27] directly measured the temperature of tail vertebrae in the rat, he found that the temperature gradient did not exactly coincide with the transition zone from red to yellow marrow. Furthermore, several investigators[5,6,28-29] have shown that under conditions of intense hemopoietic stimulation, hemopoiesis does expand into areas where normally the yellow marrow resides. With the advent of modern radiotherapy in ablative doses for malignant lymphomas, a similar observation has been made when the normally hemopoietic areas of marrow are ablated.[30] Were the local temperature of the marrow the sole determinant of hemopoietic activity, one would not have expected extension of red marrow into the areas where yellow marrow normally resides and where thermal conditions are presumably suboptimal. Nor would one have expected to see a gradient of hemopoiesis in a single bone (*vide supra*). Temperature gradient is therefore an oversimplified explanation for the distribution of red and yellow marrow. Moreover, many years after Huggins et al. reported on their observations, Maniatis et al.[31] attempted to reproduce their results. They were unable to do so.

Successful transplantation of marrow stroma to extramedullary sites helped to further clarify those factors involved in determining the intensity of hemopoiesis in the marrow. In this model, bits of marrow are removed from the bony cortex and autotransplanted in ectopic sites. The pattern of regeneration, recapitulating the ontogeny of marrow, has been de-

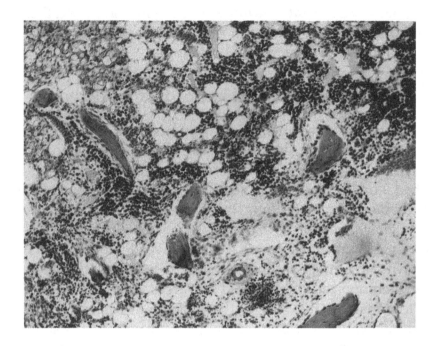

Fig. 3. Implant of yellow marrow in the subcutaneous tissue of the rabbit at 6 wk. Regenerative process has led to the formation of a hemopoietic nodule that is now undergoing fatty involution. Note the development of many adipocytes, replacing hemopoietic tissue (×40).

scribed and need not be repeated.[32-36] The final product is a reorganized hemopoietic nodule surrounded by a shell of bone. Ectopic implantation of yellow marrow affords comparative studies on the growth behavior and final cellularity of red and yellow marrow under different thermal conditions. When bits of red and yellow marrow are implanted side by side, they both undergo a similar regenerative process to form hemopoietic nodules.[37] In the case of red marrow, the nodule remains hemopoietic. In the case of yellow marrow, the transiently hemopoietic nodule undergoes fatty involution (Fig. 3), similar to postnatal involution, and forms a yellow marrow nodule surrounded by a shell of bone (Fig. 4).

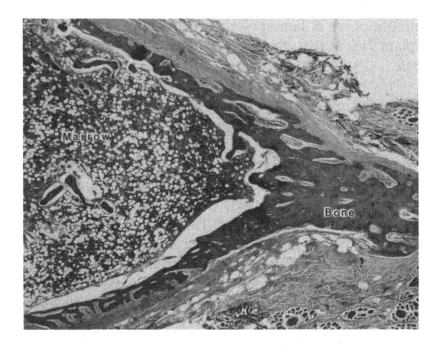

Fig. 4. Implant of rabbit red marrow in the subcutaneous tissue in retromalleolar area where the adjacent bone normally contains yellow marrow and has a temperature of 28.5°C. Regeneration has resulted in the establishment of a red marrow nodule at 8 wk, showing considerable hemopoietic activity (×16).

Actually, fatty involution also occurs in the implants of red marrow, but here the number of adipocytes is not so great that it entirely replaces the hemopoietic tissue. In fact, quantitative studies have indicated that the proportion of adipocytes in these implants correlate well with the marrow from which they are derived.[38] Thus, the difference in the behavior of red and yellow marrow implants appears to be a quantitative one, translating into quality. This type of observation leads us to conclude that the proportion of adipocytes in the final product (the reconstituted nodule) is *predetermined* and is a reflection of the proportion of their precursors in the initial implant. Only because the development of adipocytes is a slow process, a transient phase of hemopoiesis occurs in the yellow marrow implant before it is superceded by the developing adipose tissue.

This type of observation is in conflict with Huggins et al.,[14,15] for it indicates that the fate of red and yellow marrow implants does not depend solely on their thermal environment. When both types of marrow are implanted side by side in the splenic bed (temperature 37°C), or subcutaneous tissue of the lower leg (temperature 28.5°C), hemopoietic activity of the recovered nodules reflects the original tissue (Figs. 4–6), irrespective of its environment.[39] The disparate behavior of the two tissues, placed in similar environments, represents a fundamental intrinsic difference: as Abercrombie[40] has suggested, they are of different epigenotypes. Epigenotype is defined as a self-reproducing regulatory mechanism that characterizes each of the different tissue types of an organism. Further support for this concept is derived from an experiment of Patt et al.[41] These investigators grew fibroblasts derived from the rabbit red and yellow marrow. These fibroblasts are stromal-derived and, upon reimplantation in vivo, can reconstitute marrow nodules. Transplantation of these fibroblasts in the subcapsular area of the kidney resulted in the formation of marrow nodules, the cellularity of which reflected the cellularity of the original marrow: red marrow nodule from red marrow-derived fibroblasts and yellow marrow nodule from yellow marrow-derived fibroblasts. Here again, morphologically nonidentifiable fibroblasts of the same genetic constitution, implanted in similar environments, yield tissues with different characteristics.

How are we then to reconcile these observations with those of Huggins et al.?[13] Are we to dismiss the observations of these investigators, particularly in view of the fact that Maniatis et al.[31] could not reproduce them? Not exactly. The

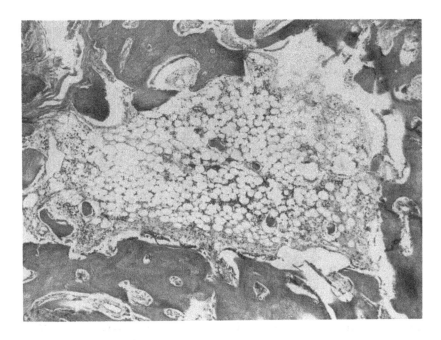

Fig. 5. Implant of rabbit yellow marrow after 8 wk in abdomen where the temperature is 37°C. The implant has been established as a yellow marrow consisting mostly of adipocytes with little or no hemopoiesis (×40).

apparent irreconcilability of the two sets of observation only indicates the complexity of those mechanisms involved.

It is clear that the yellow marrow, or at least part of it, despite its intrinsic differences with the red marrow, can transform into red marrow upon demand. For this to occur, a heightening of demand is required. When a hemopoietic stimulus is given to an animal harboring yellow marrow implants in the proper thermal environment, the implants are activated. This is evident in another experiment by Maniatis et al.[31] who repeated the experiments of Huggins et al. with the "looped" rat tail, but this time a hemopoietic stimulus was given in the form of phenylhydrazine-induced hemolysis. Under this experimental condition, the marrow in the distal

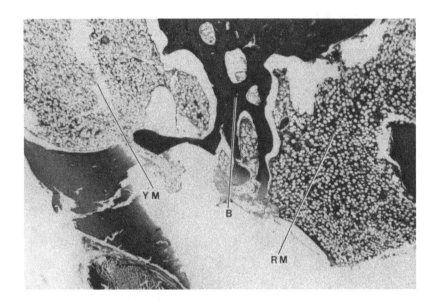

Fig. 6. Implants of rabbit red (RM) and yellow (YM) marrow, side by side, in the subcutaneous tissue of the abdomen (temperature, 33°C). The surrounding shells of bone (B) have merged. But the hemopoietic activity of marrow reflects that of the originally implanted tissue (×16).

vertebrae of rat tail (subjected to a higher temperature) converted to red marrow. Enhanced demand for hemopoiesis is also a major factor in preventing fatty transformation of regenerating marrow in ectopic implant model, or after evacuation of marrow cavity. But it can not cause conversion of fatty to red marrow once the fatty marrow is established.[42–44]

At this juncture, it should be mentioned that the experiments of Huggins et al. were done in 1936 when experimental rats were generally Bartonella-infested. Bartonella produces a compensated hemolytic disease in this species that, in the presence of the spleen, is not symptomatic.[45] Bartonella-free species became available to research only after the Second World War.

Therefore, it is likely that the animals used by Huggins et al. had already a hemopoietic stimulus, a possibility that can reconcile his observations with those of Maniatis et al.

Thus, it appears that the thermal factor and the magnitude of hemopoietic demand act synergistically to determine the hemopoietic activity of marrow. The hemopoietic stimulus appears to be more influential than the thermal environment. This is evident from the following observations

1. Sustained stimulation is required. Otherwise, with the cessation of the stimulus, the hemopoietic marrow reverts again to yellow marrow.[39]
2. Implants made in the thermal environment of less than 37°C (e.g., subcutaneous tissue of the abdomen, 33°C) can also be converted.[39] Thus, there may here be a permissive temperature of less than 37°C that can nonetheless permit hemopoiesis in the presence of adequate stimulus.
3. Even in the tibia, with a temperature of 28.5°C, hemopoiesis can be sustained with hemopoietic stimulation, provided that the adipose cells are first ablated.[42] These cells have been shown to be relatively stable and do not yield to hemopoietic expansion. Resumption of hemopoiesis may also provide a more intense circulation that can raise the temperature to a permissive level.
4. Hemopoietic expansion into some bones, normally containing yellow marrow, is seen after irradiation of red marrow-bearing bones (e.g., in patients with Hodgkins disease or other lymphomas).[30] Irradiation of these bones may provide the needed hemopoietic stimulus. However, hemopoiesis does not expand in all the limb bones. Presumably, the bone in which hemopoiesis expands has a permissive temperature.

Marrow Adipocyte

The difference between red and yellow marrow is primarily a quantitative one that is translated into a qualitative difference (*vide supra*). Yellow marrow consists entirely of adipocytes that, upon development, completely obliterate hemopoiesis. But adipocytes are also present in the red marrow, interspersed with hemopoietic cells in almost equal proportion.

Development

Although the development of marrow itself is a prenatal event, occurring during the last part of gestation, the development of marrow adipocytes is a postnatal event.[46,47] In the rabbit, the most intensely studied species, fat cells begin to appear 2 wk after birth and the adult pattern is attained by 3–4 mo. Its cellular origin appears to be the adventitial cells of bone marrow sinuses.[46-48] Thus, the first lipid inclusions appear in elongated cells, 20–25 µm, that have a tendency to spread on the outside surface of the marrow sinus endothelium. The nucleus contains numerous pores and prominent nucleoli. The abundant cytoplasm that may branch out, contains numerous small dense mitochondria, large numbers of ribosomes, and a prominent and well-defined Golgi zone. Lysosomes are not seen. The cell membrane contains numerous vesicles. Lipid inclusions, few and small at first, gradually coalesce to form larger droplets. Thus, both the cell and its lipid inclusions increase in size, reaching a maximum diameter of 140–160 µm. The coalescence of these small inclusions leads to the formation of a very large inclusion, although a few additional small inclusions are always present. In this process, the nucleus and cytoplasmic organelles (including smaller lipid inclusions) are displaced to the periphery, giving the cell a typical "signet-ring" morphology. During this maturation process, few, if any, glycogen granules are seen in the cell, and the cell is not associated with collagen fibers, these last two characteristics being associated with extramedullary adipocyte cell development.

Structure

In its fully mature form,[49] the cell is very large, with a peripherally located nucleus and a markedly attenuated cytoplasm that forms a narrow band at the periphery and is best seen in the perinuclear area. It contains mitochondria, ribosomes, and a few profiles of endoplasmic reticulum, but no glycogen or lysosomes. The cell membrane shows few, if any, invaginations or pinocytic vesicles normally seen in lipid-exchanging adipocytes. This suggests a low rate of lipid turnover in the steady state. The bulk of cytoplasm is occupied by a large and homogeneous fat globule. The cell shows a complete basement membrane that gives a positive reaction with PAS and reticulin stain. Association with collagen fibers is not seen.

Cytochemically,[50] the cell stains positively with esterases irrespective of the substrate used. This reaction is resistant to the inhibitory function of fluoride, a fact that distinguishes this cell from a monocyte, another potential fat-accumulating cell. The cell gives a negative reaction with alkaline and acid phosphatases, as well as peroxidase. It is, however, positive with PAS.

Histochemically,[49] the lipid substance in the cell stains with oil red O and Sudan black B, but not with acid hematin. This pattern of staining indicates that the lipid substance consists largely of neutral fat with little or no phospholipid. Moreover, the lipid substance stains purple with Nile blue sulfate in 1% concn., but the reaction product is deep blue with a 0.2% concn. of this stain. This differential reaction suggests the relative paucity of the 18-carbon unsaturated oleic acid.

Direct analysis of lipid composition also indicates that the bulk of lipid in these cells consists of the 16-carbon palmitate (almost 40%) and 18-carbon saturated stearate (about 30%), oleate being only 25% of the lipid.[51]

Function

The exact function of the marrow adipocyte is obscure. However, several facts have been established by clinical and experimental observations.

1. In the bone marrow, adipocytes bear a reciprocal relationship to the hemopoietic tissue. After hemopoietic stimuli, as the hemopoietic tissue expands, the lipid substance in the adipocytes undergoes resorption.[8,43,52-58] This is also the case with hyperproliferative disorders such as hemolytic diseases, polycythemia, and leukemias. Conversely, in induced or clinical aplasias, lipid-engorged cells are increased, replacing the hemopoietic tissues.[59-64] This reaction appears to involve only the lipid substance, whereas the cells, with or without lipids, may remain in the marrow. Thus, the metabolic behavior of marrow adipocytes seems to be "coupled" to the hemopoietic activity of the marrow. It is not known how this coupling comes about. Two possibilities may be considered: hemopoietic regulatory factors (e.g., erythropoietin) may affect, reciprocally, the metabolic behavior of adipocytes in a systemic manner; or local microenvironmental factors may bring about such reactions in the marrow adipocytes. Certain hormones may affect the behavior of marrow adipocytes. It has been shown by Cohen and Gardner[54] that massive doses of triamcinolone can blunt the erythropoietic response of the marrow to phenylhydrazine-induced hemolysis and retain adipocytes. Later, Greenberger[65] demonstrated that the differentiation of marrow preadipocytes is corticoster-

oid-dependent. This is in contrast to extramedullary pre-adipocytes that are insulin-dependent.

2. The anatomic position of marrow adipocytes suggests that they may have a function in controlling cell egress into the circulation.[66,67] In a perisinal position, these cells supplant the adventitial cells of marrow sinuses.[46] The extent of coverage of sinus endothelium is a function of cell traffic across the sinus wall.[68] When cell traffic is enhanced, adventitial cells retract, permitting more extensive inter-action of migrating cells with the sinus endothelium. It is possible that the marrow adipocytes, which originate from adventitial cells,[46,48] are not capable of retraction and thereby limit the access of migrating cells to the endo-thelium. Mature cells can then remain in the hemopoietic compartment of the marrow, leading to a certain degree of ineffective hemopoiesis.

3. It is possible that the adipocytes may serve as the store of energy required for hemopoiesis. This may explain the depletion of lipid substance in the state of stimulated hemopoiesis and its reaccumulation when hemopoiesis is suppressed.

4. In murine systems, granulopoiesis is generally associated with marrow, whereas erythropoiesis is generally associated with spleen that lacks adipose tissue. This pattern may suggest a function for adipocytes in providing an environment favorable to granulopoiesis. In this context, it is interesting that in long-term marrow culture, where lipid-containing cells are present, granulopoiesis also occurs, but not erythropoiesis.

At any rate, elucidating the function of marrow adipocytes requires focusing investigative efforts on this area and, in particular, the role of hemopoietic regulatory factors in the modulation of marrow adipocytes.

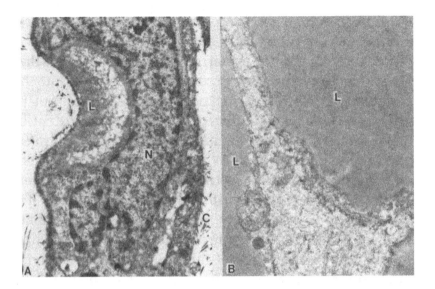

Fig. 7. Electron micrographs showing epididymal (A) and marrow (B) adipocytes after 10 d of total starvation. Epididymal adipocyte shows almost complete loss of lipid. As a result, the cell size shrinks. Only a small lipid inclusion (L) displaying a "fluffy" appearance remains in the vicinity of the nucleus (N). In contrast, marrow adipocytes do not undergo lipid mobilization. The large lipid inclusion is maintained and retains its homogeneous appearance. Note also collagen fibers (C), typically associated with extramedullary adipocyte, but not marrow (both figures ×17,500).

Distinct From Extramedullary Adipocytes

Marrow adipocytes should be considered entirely different entities from their extramedullary counterparts. The two cell types differ in many respects.

1. Structurally, extramedullary adipocytes are associated with a large amount of collagen (Fig. 7).[69-71] This is not the case for marrow adipocytes that are associated with the collagen-related reticulin fibers that can be recognized by PAS and reticulin stains.[46-49]

2. The progenitor of extramedullary adipocytes is a fibroblast-like cell.[69,70] Its salient feature is the presence of nu-

merous profiles of rough endoplasmic reticulum (RER) evidently forming collagen. On the other hand, the progenitor of marrow adipocytes appears to be a "reticular cell" closely resembling the adventitial cells of marrow sinuses;[46-48] it contains but a few profiles of RER. It is probable that the two cells bear a kinship, since the reticular cell is thought to be the origin of reticulin fibers in the marrow that are related structurally to collagen. Nonetheless there exist certain differences as well.

3. In the course of their development, extramedullary adipocytes contain large amounts of glycogen,[69,70] a feature absent in marrow adipocytes.[46] This difference, however, may be more apparent than real. Glycogen is a constant feature of brown adipose tissue where deposition and resorption of fat occurs rapidly and constantly to provide heat and to maintain the body temperature. Glycogen is seldom seen in mature white adipose tissue where the rate of fat deposition and resorption is not rapid. Its presence in developing white adipose tissue is thought to be an important step in the formation of lipid and may be related to its rate of deposition.[69] It also appears in mature adipocytes from animals that have been refed after a period of starvation. Formation of the lipid substance in white adipocytes, however, is a relatively rapid phenomenon, occurring within 10 d.[69] This process is much slower in marrow adipocytes, occurring over a period of months.[46] The difference in the rate of lipid deposition may account for the absence of glycogen deposition in marrow adipose cells.

4. There are certain differences in the cytochemistry of the two cell types.[50] Naphthol esterase and chloracetate esterase, present in marrow adipocytes, are absent in their extramedullary counterparts, and nonspecific esterase (α-naphthyl-butyrate-reacting) is fluoride-resistant in the marrow, but sensitive in extramedullary cells.

5. The mean volume of the extramedullary adipocyte is about 10× larger than its marrow counterpart, in rabbits being about 500 and 50 pL respectively.[72] This difference is primarily in the size of the major lipid inclusion.

6. The palmitate turnover rate is 5× higher in marrow adipocytes, indicating a higher basal metabolic activity.[72]

7. There appears to be a difference in hormonal response of the two cell types. Lipogenesis occurs in the marrow adipocyte in response to corticosteroids, but this process is primarily insulin-dependent in the extramedullary cell.[65,73]

8. Another difference between the two cell types is shown after reimplantation of adipocytes grown in vitro. Both the marrow and extramedullary cells lose, in vitro, their lipid inclusions and develop into fibroblast-like cells indistinguishable from each other.[50,74] Upon reimplantation in vivo, the cells derived from extramedullary sites regain their inclusions and develop into a nodule of adipose tissue; marrow-derived cells form a fibrotic nodule.[74]

Functional Differences

The most convincing evidence yet that the two cell types are indeed different is derived from their pattern of response. In response to acute and total starvation (10–15 d), lipolysis occurs in the extramedullary cell, but not in marrow adipocytes[73-75] (Fig. 7) that continue to esterify fatty acids at an unaltered rate.[75] With partial starvation over a long period, lipolysis occurs in marrow adipocytes that then become devoid of fat.[76] Under these conditions, the inverse relationship between hemopoietic cells and adipocytes is lost. Hemopoiesis does not intensify to replace the volume lost by lipolysis. In fact, hemopoiesis is also reduced under these conditions. The volume lost by lipolysis is occupied by increased polysaccharides of the ground substance that are PAS positive. As a result, the marrow attains a gelatinous appearance.[76] Alteration in hemopoiesis is thought to result from a shift of these mucopolysaccharides from neutral to acidic. Acidic mucopolysaccharides are thought to provide an unfavorable environment for hemopoiesis.[77] Similar findings have been reported in chronic starvation in humans[78-81] (in anorexia nervosa, kwashiorkor, marasmus, and survivors of Nazi concentration camps) in whom gelatinous transformation of marrow is associated with hemopoietic alterations.

In contrast to its remarkable resistance to starvation, the marrow adipocyte is highly sensitive to hemopoietic stimuli.[43,52-55] This has been best studied by using phenylhydrazine-induced hemolysis. Whereas extramedullary adipocytes show no significant response to this experimental procedure,[58] marrow adipocytes mobilize their lipid content readily, and their volume is reduced, although their esterification capacity (measured by labeled palmitate turnover) remains unchanged.[58] Fat mobilization appears to be preferentially of polyunsaturated fatty acids. A similar, but less dramatic, response is seen after chronic phlebotomy and in hypoxia. Lipid mobilization from marrow adipocytes is also seen in humans with hyperproliferative disease (hemolytic anemias, polycythemia, and myeloproliferative diseases).

By contrast, experimentally-induced reduction in the volume of hemopoiesis is expected to be associated with increased lipogenesis, particularly triglycerides.[59-64] This is apparently owing to an increase in esterification and inhibition of the oxidation of fatty acid. Most studies have used radiation-induced aplasia, but unfortunately no comparison with extramedullary adipocytes has been done. Lipogenesis has also been noted in animals recovering from hypoxia when adipocytes are again formed. Thus, the differences in the reaction pattern of the two cell types suggest fundamental differences in their function and regulatory mechanisms: those of marrow adipocytes relating to the hemopoietic function and extramedullary cells relating to the nutritional state of the organism.

Heterogeneity of Marrow Adipocytes

There is, in addition, some evidence to indicate that even within the adipocyte population of the marrow, there exists at least two different subpopulations, and the distribution of these two subpopulations is congruent with the distribution of red and yellow marrow contained within the bones of the trunk and extremities, respectively.[82] Cohen and Gardner[54] reported that the yellow marrow fat defends itself partially against starvation, whereas the red marrow fat is mobilized as readily as extramedullary fat. The stability of the yellow marrow adipocyte is also evident after intense hemopoietic stimulation, using phlebotomy or phenylhydrazine-induced hemolysis. Under these conditions, the yellow-marrow adipocyte is not mobilized as readily as its counterpart in the red marrow.[31,42,44,82] It is the latter that yields readily to expanding hemopoietic tissue.

Furthermore, in the course of studying lipid histochemistry of marrow, it was noted that the performic acid-Schiff reaction (PFAS) can be used to differentiate between two populations of adipocytes; the lipid substance in one gives a positive reaction and in the other, a negative reaction. The distribution of these two populations is congruent with the distribution of red and yellow marrow. After hemopoietic stimulation, using phenylhydrazine-induced hemolysis, only PFAS-negative cells remain.[82] This observation suggests a relation between the chemical composition of lipid contained within adipocytes and their relative stability during the expansion of hemopoietic tissue. Indeed, gas chromatographic analysis of fatty acids in adipocytes of red and yellow marrow (Fig. 8) shows a consistent and highly significant shift from

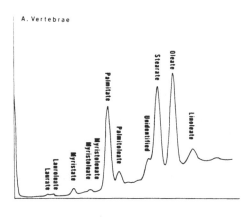

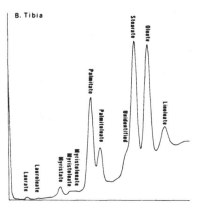

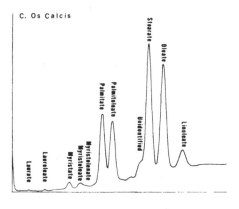

Fig. 8. Gas chromatographic pattern of rabbit bone marrow adipose tissue: (A) Vertebrae (representative red marrow); (B) Tibia (intermediate zone); (C) or calcis (representative of yellow marrow). Note the shift from palmitate to palmitoleate in the direction of red to yellow marrow (Varian Aerograph, 12 × 10.8" stainless steel mesh column packed with 20% diethylglycosuccinate on Chromosorb W, 60/80 mesh at temperature 20°C. N₂ carrier gas at flow rate of 25 mL/min).

179

myristate and palmitate (in red marrow) to myristoleate and palmitoleate (in yellow marrow), with an intermediate pattern in the tibia.[51]

Although there is no evidence that these differences bear any relationship to hemopoietic activity of red and yellow marrow, a good correlation may suggest more than a chance relationship. It is possible that these differences may represent an epiphenomenon caused by local differences in the temperature or other such factors. But it is also possible that the lipid composition of marrow adipocytes may contribute to their relative stability during the expansion of hemopoiesis.

Marrow Adipocytes in Culture

When marrow adipocytes are separated by centrifugation, placed in McCoy's medium, and supplemented with 20% fetal calf serum, they lose their lipid inclusions and develop into spindle-shaped, fibroblast-like cells.[50,74] In long-term marrow cultures, lipid-containing cells develop, and they are particularly prominent when the cultures are supplemented with hydrocortisone.[65,73,83] Several lines of evidence suggest that these lipid-containing cells are different from marrow adipocytes.

1. Although the marrow adipocyte in a single lipid inclusion dominates, giving the cell a "signet-ring" morphology,[46-49] in long-term marrow cultures lipid-containing cells have multiple inclusions.[83] In this regard, their morphology is more comparable to brown adipocytes.[84-86] This similarity is further substantiated by the presence, in some cells, of multiple rod-shaped mitochondria also characteristic of brown adipocytes.[85] Yet, cells with signet-ring morphology have also been described in these cultures,[87] and it is possible that cells with multiple inclusions merely represent an early developmental stage of signet-ring cells.

2. The lipid-containing cells of long-term cultures are hetero-geneous. Both epithelioid cells and macrophages can accumulate lipid inclusions.[83] Lipid accumulation may, therefore, be a culture epiphenomenon. Thus, it appears that a distinct adipocyte cell type does not exist in these marrow cultures, although the presence of such a cell type cannot be ruled out. The major problem here is the lack of objective criteria to identify the in vivo marrow adipocyte in cultures. It is possible that this cell may be present in long-term marrow cultures with or without lipid inclu-sions, but we do not have objective criteria by which to recognize it.

3. In addition, lipid accumulation has been demonstrated in a variety of cell types both in vivo and in vitro.[65,73,83,88–92] Thus, lipid accumulation, *per se,* does not warrant the iden-tification of a cell as an adipocyte.

4. There is no evidence that marrow adipocytes, recogniz-able in vivo, remain viable in long-term marrow cultures. The lipid-containing cells, therefore, should not be con-sidered related to marrow adipocytes and should not be called so.

The lipid-containing cells are thought to contribute to the maintenance of hemopoietic progenitor cells in long-term cul-tures. This interpretation originates from the fact that hydro-cortisone can potentiate both lipogenesis in these cells and the maintenance of progenitor cells.[65,73,83] However, recent evi-dence indicates that these two effects are not coordinated and may therefore be totally unrelated.[93,94] This conclusion appears to be supported by earlier work of Greenberger et al.,[95] who reported that 25% fetal calf serum with corticosteroids main-tains stability of adherent cells, decreases lipogenesis (which is deleterious after 10 wk), and increases proliferation of hemo-poietic stem cells. Moreover, long-term cultures of hamster bone marrow occurs in the absence of a lipid-containing adher-ent layer.[96–98]

Conclusions

On the basis of the facts discussed above, we may construct three frames of reference for understanding the function of adipocytes, their association with hemopoiesis, and their relation to the extramedullary adipose tissue.

1. The first frame of reference should be constructed on the basis of a reciprocal relationship between adipocytes and hemopoietic cells in the marrow. As discussed above, within the rigid frame of bone where the volume is fixed, hemopoietic tissue expands and shrinks in response to the fluctuating body requirement for blood cells. The adipose component of the marrow may then serve as a "cushion," having a reciprocal relationship to the hemopoietic component.

2. A second frame of reference is constructed on the basis of heterogeneity of adipose tissues and the physiological differences between the marrow and extramedullary white adipocytes. Certain similarities in lipid composition have led to the assumption that the marrow adipocyte is a typical adipose tissue.[99] This proposition is not valid. The primary function of white adipose tissue relates to energy conservation, its development and degradation being controlled by the nutritional state of the organism through a complex endocrine and neuroendocrine system. In contrast, the primary function of a marrow adipocyte appears to be regulating the intensity of hemopoiesis; development and degradation of these cells are controlled by factors related to the regulation of hemopoiesis and, only to a lesser degree, to the nutritional state of the organism.

   Moreover, both the marrow and the white extramedullary adipocytes may be heterogeneous. These cells are distributed widely in the body, and the cells in one part may behave differently from those in other parts. In this context, it should be remembered that in certain species—notably sheep, rats, and mice—there exists a third type of adipocyte known as the brown adipocyte. These cells are both morphologically and functionally distinctive and can be readily distinguished from both the marrow and extramedullary white adipocytes. Their function is in rapid generation of heat in response to cold, a function equivalent to a shivering mechanism in those species that lack this mechanism.[84]

3. A third frame of reference is particularly relevant to the observations made in long-term marrow culture. This relates to the definition of the adipocyte and is constructed on the basis of the ability of many cell types from a variety of sources to accumulate lipid inclusions, both in vivo and in vitro, e.g., monocytes, hepatocytes, and so on. Thus, the presence of lipid inclusions in a cell does not in itself warrant its identification as an adipocyte. On the other hand, preadipocytes have certain characteristics of adipocytes (e.g., surface receptors for insulin) without having lipid inclusions.[100] It is only after the exposure to insulin that they develop lipid inclusions and other metabolic characteristics of adipocytes, and can be so recognized morphologically. Even cultured mature adipocytes, both from the marrow and extramedullary sources, lose their lipid inclusion under certain culture conditions, but retain other characteristics of the cells of origin. Extramedullary adipocytes actually increase their number of surface receptors for insulin,[101] a process that may be related to receptor down regulation. But these cultured cells should still be considered adipocytes, because not only do they have metabolic characteristics of adipocytes, but also because upon reimplantation in vivo, they develop into adipose tissue.[74]

References

[1]Tavassoli, M. (1978) *Aplastic Anemia* (Hibino, S., Takaku, F., and Shahidi, N. T., eds.), University of Tokyo Press, Tokyo.

[2]Tavassoli, M. (1980) *Blood, Pure and Eloquent* (Wintrobe, M. M., ed.), McGraw-Hill, New York.

[3]Neumann, E. (1882) *Centr. Med. Wissensch.* **20**, 321–323.

[4]Askanazy, M. (1927) *Handbuch der Speziellen Pathologischen Anatomie und Histologie* (Henke, F. and Lubrasch, O., eds.), Springer, Berlin, 1, 2, 775.

[5]Peabody, F. W. (1926) *Am. J. Pathol.* **2**, 487–502.

[6]Oehlbeck, L. W. F., Robscheit-Robbins, F. S., and Whipple, G. H. (1932) *J. Exp. Med.* **56**, 425–448.

[7]Hashimoto, M. (1962) *Acta Hematol.* **27**, 193–216.

[8]Custer, R. P. and Ahlfeldt, F. E. (1932) *J. Lab. Clin. Med.* **17**, 960–962.

[9]Uchida, M. (1958) *J. Kyu. Hem. Soc.* **8**, 905.

[10]Nagahama, M. (1959) *J. Kyu. Hem. Soc.* **9**, 299, 300.

[11]Tateno, K. (1957) *J. Kyu. Hem. Soc.* **7**, 150.

[12]Higuchi, T. (1959) *J. Kyu. Hem. Soc.* **9**, 613.

[13]Huggins, C. B., Blocksom, B. H., and Noonan, W. J. (1936) *Am. J. Physiol.* **115**, 395–401.

[14]Huggins, C. B. and Blocksom, B. H. (1936) *J. Exp. Med.* **64**, 253–274.

[15]Huggins, C. B. and Noonan, W. J. (1936) *J. Exp. Med.* **64**, 275–280.

[16]Weiss, L. P. and Wislocki, G. B. (1956) *Anat. Rec.* **126**, 143–163.

[17]Tavassoli, M. and Yoffey, J. M. (1983) *Bone Marrow: Structure and Function* Liss, New York.

[18]Frassoni, F., Testa, N. G., and Lord, B. I. (1982) *Cell Tissue Kinet.* **15**, 447–455.

[19]Lord, B. I., Testa, N. G., and Hendry, J. H. (1975) *Blood* **45**, 65–72.

[20]Lord, B. I., and Hendry, J. H. (1972) *Br. J. Radiol.* **45**, 110–115.

[21]Lambersten, R. H. and Weiss, L. (1984) *Blood* **63**, 287–297.

[22]Van Dyke, D. (1967) *Clin. Orthop.* **52**, 37–51.

[23]Patt, H. M. and Maloney, M. A. (1970) *Hemopoietic Cellular Proliferation* (Stohlman, F., ed.), Grune and Stratton, New York, pp. 55–66.

[24]Gong, J. K. (1978) *Science* **199**, 1443, 1444.

[25]Tavassoli, M. (1982) *Blood* **60**, 1059–1067.

[26]Little, K. (1969) *Gerontologia.* **15**, 155–170.

[27]Petrakis, N. L. (1966) *Am. J. Phys. Anthrop.* **25**, 119–130.

[28]Hamazato, Y. (1968) *J. Kyu. Hem. Soc.* **8**, 25.

[29]Sheard, A. (1924) *Prenicious Anaemia and Aplastic Anaemia*, Williams Wood, New York.

[30]Knospe, W. H., Rayudu, V. M. S., Cardello, M., Friedman, A. M., and Fordham, E. W. (1976) *Cancer* **37**, 1432–1442.

[31]Maniatis, A., Tavassoli, M., and Crosby, W. H. (1971) *Blood* **37**, 581–586.

[32]Tavassoli, M. and Crosby, W. H. (1968) *Science* **161**, 54–56.

[33]Sahebekhtiari, H. A. and Tavassoli, M. (1978) *Cell Tissue Res.* **192**, 437–450.

[34]Sadr, A. M., Cardenas, F., and Tavassoli, M. (1980) *Experientia* **36**, 605, 606.

[35]Tavassoli, M. and Khademi, R. (1980) *Experientia* **36**, 1126, 1127.

[36]Tavassoli, M. (1984) *Long-Term Bone Marrow Culture* (Wright, D. G. and Greenberger, J. S., eds.), Liss, New York.

[37]Tavassoli, M. and Crosby, W. H. (1970) *Science* **169**, 291–293.

[38]Maloney, M. A., Flannery, M. L., and Patt, H. M. (1980) *Proc. Soc. Exp. Biol. Med.* **165**, 309–312.

[39]Bigelow, C. L. and Tavassoli, M. (1984) *Exp. Hematol.* **12**, 581–585.

[40]Abercrombie, M. (1967) *Cell Differentiation* (DeReuck, A. V. S. and Knight, J., eds.), Little, Brown, Boston.

[41]Patt, H. M., Maloney, M. A., and Flannery, M. L. (1982) *Exp. Hematol.* **10**, 738–742.

[42]Tavassoli, M., Maniatis, A., and Crosby, W. H. (1974) *Blood* **43**, 33–38.

[43]Tavassoli, M., Maniatis, A., and Crosby, W. H. (1972) *Br. J. Haematol.* **23**, 707–711.

[44]Tavassoli, M., Watson, L. R., and Khademi, M. R. (1979) *Cell Tissue Res.* **200**, 215–222.

[45]Weiman, D. (1944) *Trans. Am. Philos. Soc.* **33**, 243–350.

[46]Tavassoli, M. (1976) *Acta Anat.* **94**, 65–77.

[47]Bigelow, C. L. and Tavassoli, M. (1984) *Acta Anat.* **118**, 60–64.

[48]Weiss, L. (1965) *J. Morphol.* **117**, 467–538.

[49]Tavassoli, M. (1974) *Arch. Pathol.* **98**, 189–192.

[50]Tavassoli, M. (1978) *Scand. J. Haematol.* **20**, 330–334.

[51]Tavassoli, M., Hanchin, D. N., and Jacob, P. (1977) *Scand. J. Haematol.* **18**, 47–53.

[52]Evans, J. D., Baker, J. M., and Oppenheimer, M. J. (1955) *Am. J. Physiol.* **181**, 504–512.

[53]Evans, J. D. and Oppenheimer, M. J. (1955) *Am. J. Physiol.* **181**, 509–512.

[54]Cohen, P. and Gardner, F. H. (1965) *J. Lab. Clin. Med.* **65**, 88–101.

[55]Krause, R. F. (1943) *J. Biol. Chem.* **149**, 395–505.

[56]Dietz, A. A. and Steinberg, B. (1953) *Arch. Biochem.* **45**, 1–9.

[57]Lee, M. Y. and Rosse, C. (1979) *Anat. Rec.* **195**, 31–46.

[58]Bathija, A., Davis, S., and Trubowitz, S. (1978) *Am. J. Hematol.* **5**, 315–321.

[59]Lewis, G. M., Efstratiadis, A. A., Mantzos, J. D., and Miras, C. J. (1975) *Radiat. Res.* **61**, 342–349.

[60]Ahlers, I., Ahlersova, E., Sedlakova, A., and Praslicka, M. (1973) *Folia. Biol.* **19**, 130–134.

[61]Snyder, F. (1965) *Nature* **206**, 733.

[62]Pfleger, R. C. and Snyder, F. (1967) *Radiat. Res.* **30**, 325–328.

[63]Snyder, F. (1966) *Radiat. Res.* **27**, 375–383.

[64]Dietz, A. A. and Steinberg, B. (1950) *Arch. Biochem.* **26**, 291–298.

[65]Greenberger, J. S. (1979) *In Vitro* **15**, 823–828.

[66]Tavassoli, M. (1979) *Br. J. Haematol.* **41**, 297–302.

[67]Tavassoli, M. (1978) *Exp. Hematol.* **6**, 257–269.

[68]Tavassoli, M. (1977) *Br. J. Haematol.* **35**, 25–32.

[69]Napolitano, L. (1963) *J. Cell Biol.* **18**, 663–679.

[70]Slavin, B. G. (1972) *Int. Rev. Cytol.* **33**, 297–334.

[71]Tavassoli, M. (1974) *Experientia* **30**, 424, 425.

[72]Trubowitz, S. and Bathija, A. (1977) *Blood* **49**, 599–605.

[73]Greenberger, J. S. (1978) *Nature* **255**, 752–754.

[74]Tavassoli, M. (1982) *Exp. Cell Res.* **137**, 55–62.

[75]Bathija, A., Davis, S., and Trubowitz, S. (1979) *Am. J. Hematol.* **6**, 191–198.

[76]Tavassoli, M., Eastlund, D. T., Yam, L. T., Neiman, R. S., and Finkel, H. E. (1976) *Scand. J. Haematol.* **16**, 311–319.

[77]McCuskey, R. S., Meinke, H. A., and Townsend, S. F. (1972) *Blood* **39**, 696–712.

[78]Helweg-Larsen, P., Hoffmeyer, H., Kieler, J., Thaysen, H. E., Thaysen, J. S., Thaysen, P., and Wulff, M. H. (1952) *Acta Med. Scand.* **274**, 170–173.

[79]Kondi, A., McDougall, L., Hoy, H., Mehta, S., and Mliaya, V. (1963) *Arch. Dis. Child.* **38**, 267–275.

[80]Allen, D. W. and Dean, R. F. A. (1965) *Trans. R. Soc. Trop. Med. Hyg.* **59**, 326–341.

[81]Mant, M. J. and Faragher, B. S. (1972) *Br. J. Haematol.* **23**, 737–749.

[82]Tavassoli, M. (1976) *Arch. Pathol. Lab. Med.* **100**, 16–18.

[83]Tavassoli, M. and Takahashi, K. (1982) *Am. J. Anat.* **164**, 91–111.

[84]Hull, D. and Segall, M. M. (1966) *Nature* **212**, 469–472.

[85]Hull, D. (1966) *Br. Med. Bull.* **22**, 92–96.

[86]Napolitano, L. and Fawchett, D. (1958) *J. Biophys. Biochem. Cytol.* **4**, 685–692.

[87]Dexter, T. M., Allen, T. D., and Lajtha, L. G. (1977) *J. Cell Physiol.* **91**, 335–344.

[88]Chase, W. H. (1959) *J. Ultrastruct. Res.* **2**, 283–287.

[89]Barnett, R. J. and Ball, E. G. (1960) *J. Biophys. Biochem. Cytol.* **8**, 83–100.

[90]Cushman, S. W. (1970) *J. Cell Biol.* **46**, 326–341.

[91]Gerrity, R. G. (1981) *Am. J. Pathol.* **103**, 181–190.

[92]Zucker-Franklin, D., Grusky, G., and Marcus, A. (1978) *Lab. Invest.* **38**, 620–628.

[93]Touw, I. and Lowenberg, B. (1983) *Blood* **61**, 770–774.

[94]Sakakeeny, M. A. and Greenberger, J. S. (1982) *J. Natl. Cancer Inst.* **68**,

305–317.

[95]Greenberger, J. S., Sakakeeny, M. A., and Parker, L. M. (1979) *Exp. Hematol.* **7,** 135–148.

[96]Eastment, C., Denholm, E., Katznelson, I., Arnold, E., and Tso, P. O. P. (1982) *Blood* **60,** 123–135.

[97]Eastment, C. E., Ruscetti, F. W., Denholm, E., Katznelson, I., Arnold, E., and Tso, P. O. P. (1982) *Blood* **60,** 495–502.

[98]Eastment, C. E. and Ruscetti, F. W. (1982) *Blood* **60,** 999–1006.

[99]Zakaria, E. and Shafrir, E. (1967) *Proc. Soc. Exp. Biol. Med.* **124,** 1265–1268.

[100]Soda, R. and Tavassoli, M. (1983) *Int. J. Cell Cloning* **1,** 79–84.

[101]Takahashi, M. and Tavassoli, M. (1983) *J. Ultrastruct. Res.* **83,** 233–241.

Chapter 5

Hematopoiesis on Artificial Membranes

William H. Knospe

The use of artificial membranes to study the hematopoietic microenvironment began with Seki and his colleagues who implanted cellulose membranes intraperitoneally (ip) in mice. After 7 d, the membranes became coated with adherent cells of peritoneal origin. They then exposed the mice to 700 rad total body irradiation to reduce the stem cell pool, followed by injecting the membrane implanted mice with 10^6 bone marrow cells. Seven days later, the mice were killed and the implanted membranes were observed to have hematopoietic colonies that were primarily granulocytic (90% or more) with an occasional colony being erythroid (10% or less). Megakaryocytic colonies were not seen. Colony formation occurred only when the mice received lethal whole body irradiation followed by the infusion of bone marrow cells ip. Colony formation did not occur when the membrane implanted mice were irradiated and then received bone marrow cells intravenously (iv). The cell layer developing upon the ip implanted cellulose membranes was only a few cell layers thick, yet it was able to provide a simplified hematopoietic microenvironment capable of engrafting hematopoietic stem cells (lodgment) and then providing an environment conducive to commitment and differentiation of stem cells along a primarily granulocytic lineage[1,2] (Figs. 1 and 2).

Hematopoiesis on Flat CEM

Seki's work inspired my colleagues and me to study the characteristics of the cells coating cellulose membranes, using simple surface markers as well as tests for phagocytic capacity. Using monocyte markers for the complement 3b and IgG receptors, we showed that the makeup of the cells coating the membranes was heterogeneous, at least in terms of monocyte markers. A maximum of 52% of the cells carried monocytic markers 1–2 wk after implantation. Similarly, a maximum of 57% of the cells were able to phagocytose yeast particles 3 d after implantation. This fraction fell off to 13% by 17 d after implantation.[3] We also showed that iron[59] and technetium sulfur colloid[99] were taken up by the membrane and colony stimulating factor was produced by the cells on the Cellulose Ester Membrane (CEM)[3] (Table 1).

We interpreted these results to mean that either the population of cells having their origin from the peritoneum was heterogeneous or, if homogeneous, was capable of rapid transformation into other cell types such as fibroblasts, vascular cells, and so on. Even the rather artificial and simplified hematopoietic microenvironment developing on the ip implanted cellulose membranes showed a rather complex cellular makeup. These results were not dissimilar to the cellular complexity developing on the adherent layers of the long-term culture system developed by Dexter.[4]

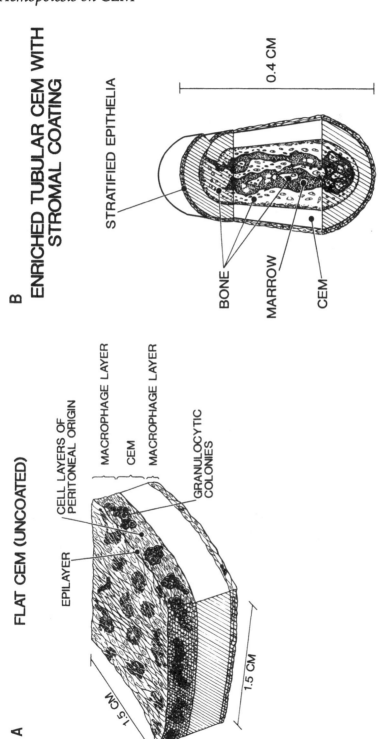

Fig. 1. Diagrams of methods.

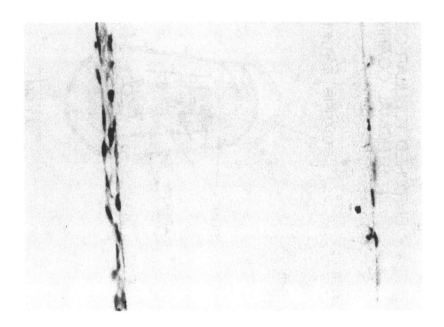

Fig. 2. Cellulose ester membrane removed from peritoneal cavity after 7 d. Hematoxylin and eosin stain. Original magnification 200 × (Ref. 3).

Table 1

Nucleated Cells Eluted from ip Implanted CEM with Receptors for C3b and Fc and with Phagocytic Properties

% of Cells From CEM at Various Days Postimplantation,			
	1	3	7	7
EA (Fg 6) rosettes	35 ± 2	32 ± 10.4	28 ± 6.4	21 ± 4.8
EA C rosettes	31 ± 3.8	48 ± 5.1	22 ± 4.1	27 ± 9.6
Yeast ingestion	27 ± 1.5	55 ± 4.9	26 ± 4.0	13 ± 3.6

Several years later, we returned to the use of flat cellulose membranes to study the hematopoietic microenvironment of Sl/Sl^d mice. This congenitally anemic mouse strain carries a defect in the hematopoietic stroma, but has normal pluripotent hematopoietic stem cells.[5-7] Our studies showed that the cell layer developing on CEM implanted ip in Sl/Sl^d mice had a defective capacity for colony development compared to similar experiments with CEM implanted in the nonanemic and coisogeneic Sl$^+$/Sl$^+$ littermates. Thus, the cell layer of peritoneal origin in Sl/Sl^d mice, which developed the hematopoietic microenvironment on the CEM, carried the genetic defect for a defective hematopoietic stroma.[8]

These studies confirmed similar results reported by Miyano et al. and Lai et al.[9,10] We also repeated studies done by Lai et al.[10] who implanted CEM into Sl/Sl^d or Sl$^+$/Sl$^+$ mice for 1 wk and then transferred the CEM into a mouse of opposite type: CEM implanted ip in Sl/Sl^d mice after 1 wk were transferred into mice of Sl$^+$/Sl$^+$ and CEM placed ip in Sl$^+$/Sl$^+$ mice after 1 wk were transferred into Sl^d/Sl^d mice. The mice receiving transferred CEM were irradiated 3 d later with bone marrow cells from either Sl/Sl^d or Sl$^+$/Sl$^+$ mice. The capacity to support colony development depended primarily upon the cell layer contributed by the last host. Thus, CEM coated originally in Sl/Sl^d mice, then transferred to Sl$^+$/Sl$^+$ mice, had a capacity for relatively normal colony development. Conversely, CEM placed in Sl$^+$/Sl$^+$ mice, then transferred to Sl/Sl^d mice had a defective hematopoietic microenvironment for colony development resembling the Sl/Sl^d mouse.[8] There was no difference between the number of colonies developed on CEM from bone marrow cells of Sl/Sl^d and Sl$^+$/Sl$^+$ mice. We also confirmed the results reported by Tavassoli et al. who reported that colony formation on ip implanted CEM depended upon the most superficial cell layers on the membrane. Tavassoli also reported that the most superficial layer developed cilia on the abdominal surface.

Hematopoietic progenitor cells then interacted with the cilia-bearing-surface-layer of cells and, by endocytosis, traversed the superficial layer to form a colony just below an epilayer usually only one cell layer thick.[8,11]

We also studied the phagocytic character of cells gently scraped from the CEM. Cells from CEM, implanted into Sl/Sl^d mice, phagocytosed fewer yeast particles than cells removed from CEM and implanted into Sl$^+$/Sl$^+$ mice.[8] These results were interesting in relation to Tavassoli's electron microscopic studies of the spleen in Sl/Sl^d mice. He observed small central macrophages with few or no interdigitations with erythroid cells and without crystalloid inclusions.[12]

Finally, and most importantly, we observed that the number of cell layers developing on CEM implanted into Sl/Sl^d mice were fewer than those developing on CEM implanted into Sl$^+$/Sl$^+$ mice.[8] These studies indicate that Sl/Sl^d mice have abnormal (structural) hematopoietic stromal macrophages. Furthermore, these abnormal macrophages have defective phagocytosis and an impaired ability to form layers on CEM. For the first time, definite defects of structure and function are identified in hematopoietic stromal cells in the Sl/Sl^d mouse.

Hematopoiesis On Stromally-Enriched, IP-Implanted Tubular CEM

The ip-implanted, flat CEM developed by Seki et al. and studied by ourselves in the forgoing experiments were of great interest in defining selected aspects of stromal function particularly regarding the primarily granulopoietic colony formation occurring in this model.[1,3] However, this model was of limited value in studying the more complicated hematopoietic stroma found in the bone marrow in vivo. The stroma of the bone marrow is able to support trilineal hematopoiesis and not the restricted granulopoiesis developed on the ip-implanted, flat CEM.

We developed a modified CEM that was coated with stromal cells from bone marrow, bone, regenerating endosteal cells, or spleen. Previous experiments with femurs transplanted to subcutaneous sites showed that the hematopoietic cells died, but that *in situ* stromal cells regenerated to form a hematopoietic microenvironment capable of attracting and circulating pluripotent hematopoietic stem cells that reestablished trilineal hematopoiesis. We intended to examine the interdependence of hematopoiesis and bone by examining the capacity of stromal cells from bone to develop a hematopoietic microenvironment and conversely, the osteogenic potential of stromal cells from marrow and spleen. We also studied the capacity of regenerating endosteal cells to form a hematopoietic microenvironment.[13] Our interest in endosteal cells stemmed from previous studies of bone marrow curettage in which removal of all hematopoietic tissue and flushing from the medullary cavity of murine femurs, resulted in a stimulation of endosteal cellular proliferation. The single layer of endosteum became mitotically active and filled the medullary cavity with a primitive mesenchyme-like tissue in 7–10 d. Over the next 14 d, this tissue differentiated into fully functioning hematopoietic stroma with sinusoidal structures, macrophages, fibroblasts, and fat cells. Within 3 wk, the stroma permitted the lodgment of circulating pluripotent hematopoietic stem cells that reestablished trilineal hematopoiesis in the regenerated hematopoietic stroma.[14-16]

Stromal cells from marrow or diaphyseal bone (flushed free of all marrow), spleen, or regenerating endosteal tissue were coarsely homogenated to preserve intact cells and spread on one surface of a CEM 1.5 cm². This was then folded into thirds or into an open-ended tubular structure with the stromal cell-bearing surface folded into the interior of the tube and stapled. The enriched CEM was then implanted ip and examined after intervals of 1, 3, and 6 mo[13] (Fig. 3).

The CEM coated with splenic stromal cells regenerated stroma and developed trilineal hematopoiesis within 6 wk. New bone formation was absent and involution of hematopoietic support capacity occurred after 3 and 6 mo. The CEM coated with stromal cells from marrow or bone showed regeneration of stroma and developed trilineal hematopoiesis after 3–6 mo ip implantation, and there was no involution of hematopoiesis. Stromal regeneration on CEM enriched with marrow or bone stromal cells was associated with new bone formation. In fact, the presence of trilineal hematopoiesis was almost always associated with, and in close proximity to, new bone formation (Fig. 3). Initial studies of CEM enriched with regenerating endosteal cells in tissue culture were devoid of hematopoiesis and bone.[13] However, later studies modified the source of endosteal cells, permitting the endosteal regeneration to occur in vivo after curettage and flushing. The endosteal cells were harvested from the femur at 7 d postcurettage. The endosteal cells, when harvested in vivo and applied to ip implanted CEM, regenerated a fully capable hematopoietic stroma with trilineal hematopoiesis and new bone formation similar to stromal cells from marrow and bone. Uncoated, control CEM, implanted ip, never developed hematopoiesis or bone and became progressively more fibrotic and collagen-laden with time[13,15] (Fig. 4). These studies suggested that hematopoietic stromal cells from these several sources had the capacity to inhibit fibroblasts and collagen deposition on the CEM.

Additional studies of CEM were performed using marrow or bone stromal cells or endosteal tissue, leaving the CEM implanted for 9 and 12 mo. Hematopoiesis on the CEM appeared to be permanent with no evidence of involution. The population of stromal cells, identified on the CEM with a capacity to support trilineal hematopoiesis, included sinusoidal

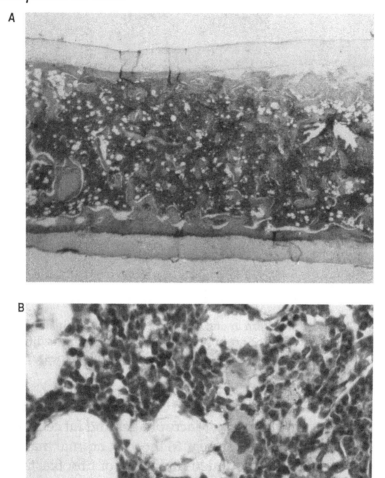

Fig. 3. (A) CEM pore size 3 μm enriched with bone after 12 mo ip; original magnification 10×; hematoxylin and eosin stain; diffuse trilineal hematopoiesis is present with scattered fat; extensive bone formation is present along membrane surface as well as scattered bony trabeculae within the membrane cavity (Ref. *53*). (B) CEM 8 μm; enriched with bone stoma after 12 mo ip; original magnification 160 × ; hematoxylin and eosin stain; trilineal hematopoiesis is present (Ref. *18*).

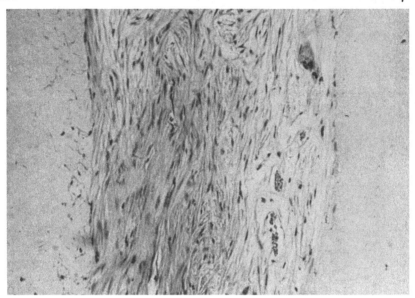

Fig. 4. CEM pore size 3 μm unenriched after 12 mo ip; original magnification 52×; hematoxylin and eosin stain; the membrane cavity is diffusely fibrotic without hematopoiesis; scattered sinusoid-like capillaries are present (Ref. 53).

endothelial cells usually distributed in an even and diffuse pattern similar to bone marrow. Macrophages and fat cells were also observed in numbers similar to those in normal marrow. We also observed the continued inhibition of fibroblasts and collagen deposition after 12 mo implantation, whereas control, uncoated CEM had become densely fibrotic and massively collagen-laden.[17]

We then desired to extend our use of hematopoiesis on artificial membranes by examining stromal cell regeneration and developing a hematopoietic microenvironment for trilineal hematopoiesis by using other types of artificial membranes with a variety of pore sizes. Our initial studies used Millipore filtration membranes with a composition of mixed nitrate and acetate esters of cellulose (CEM) and a pore size of 0.4 μm. Long-term studies of CEM with pore sizes of 0.4 μm showed a tendency for hematopoietic involution, perhaps because of "clogging" of the membrane pores. We selected CEM with pore sizes of 3 and 8 μm and also studied polytetrafluoroethylene (Teflon or Mitex), pore sizes 5 and 10 μm; polyvinylchloride (Polyvic), pore size 2 μm; cellulose acetate (Celotate), pore size 1 μm; polycarbonate (Nuclepore), pore sizes 3 and 8 μm; and linear polyethylene, pore sizes 30 and 70 μm.

We were interested in determining whether an artificial membrane with large lacuna-like pore sizes, approximating the lacunar structure of bone, would provide a better supporting structure and environment for stromal regeneration. CEM with pore sizes of 3 and 8 μm were clearly superior to CEM with a pore size of 0.4 μm, and these stromally enriched CEM showed no signs of stromal or hematopoietic involution after 1 yr of ip implantation. Teflon membranes that were relatively hydrophobic turned out to be superb scaffolds for stromal cell regeneration. These hydrophobic membranes seemed to stimulate both stromal cell regeneration and new bone formation. Stromal cells and bone actively infiltrated, and even split, the Teflon membranes that "bulged" with regenerating stromal cells, hematopoietic tissue, and new bone formation. These Teflon membranes were the best of all the artificial membranes examined in terms of supporting stromal cells. Celotate and Polyvic membranes coated with stromal cells from bone and Polyvic membranes coated with marrow promoted stromal regeneration, bone growth, and trilineal hematopoiesis. However, Celotate and Polyvic membranes coated with stromal cells from marrow or endosteal tissue showed no stromal cell regeneration.

Polycarbonate membranes coated with marrow stromal cells had good hematopoietic, stromal cell, and bone regeneration. But the same membranes coated with bone showed no hematopoiesis and when coated with endosteal cells, showed an inconstant, unpredictable, or minimal stromal regeneration, trilineal hematopoietic support capacity, and new bone formation. The polyethylene membranes of 30 and 70 μm pore sizes showed no stromal regeneration, hematopoiesis, and little or no new bone formation. The membranes without stromal cell regeneration, hematopoiesis, or new bone formation were densely fibrotic and heavily laden with collagen. These studies suggested that hematopoietic stromal cells from different sources—bone marrow or bone, or regenerating endosteal mesenchyme—interacted with artificial membranes in a variable manner suggesting significant metabolic and membrane differences between these stromal cell populations.[18] It is possible that membranes with varying physical characteristics, such as surface charge, hydrophobic vs hydrophilic character, and chemical composition, may attract or interact with stromal cells in a variable manner. One set of stromal cells may secrete a matrix protein that might interact or adsorb onto an artificial membrane and positively affect subsequent stromal cell differentiation or transformation. Other artificial membranes may inhibit or destroy stromal cells because of a different physical and chemical composition. These several kinds of interactions between hematopoietic stromal cells from different tissue sources and artificial membranes, may provide methods to separate stromal cells or better understand the cellular differences mediating these responses.[18]

Pore size did not appear to be critical with respect to the development of a hematopoietic support capacity or bone formation, except for the smallest pore size of 0.4 μm for the CEM membranes. CEM with pore sizes of 0.4 μm frequently involuted between 6 and 12 mo of ip implantation. We are uncertain why this occurred and suspect that "clogging" of pores may have interfered with the function of the hematopoietic stroma. CEM and the other membranes with pore sizes between 1 and 10 μm were functionally capable of supporting hematopoiesis and did not show late involution between 6 and 12 mo. Very large pore sizes of 30 and 70 μm were only available with poly-ethylene membranes and supported no hematopoiesis or bone formation. We do not know why polyethylene inhibited hematopoietic stromal cell growth and bone formation, but suspect it may be a toxic effect of the polyethylene on stromal and osteogenic cells.[18]

The mechanism of inhibition of stromal cell growth by several of the membranes remains unknown. It is known that filtration membranes can inactivate erythropoietin and col-ony-stimulating factor. It is possible that the "toxic" mem-branes injure a crucial stromal cell transferred to the membrane or inactivate a product of a transferred, live stromal cell crucial to the process of forming a hematopoietic microenvironment capable of supporting trilineal hematopoiesis and bone for-mation.[19-22]

Hematopoiesis and Proteoglycans

Investigations from several different centers have sug-gested that matrix proteins such as proteoglycans (PG) or glycosaminoglycans (GAGs) play an important role in the functioning of the hematopoietic microenvironment as well as mediate or positively influence hematopoiesis.[23-33] McCuskey et al. had previously reported histochemical studies suggest-ing PG favored erythropoiesis, whereas the absence of PGs were associated with granulopoiesis.[23-27] It seemed appropri-ate to use the same techniques to study stromal cell regener-ation on CEM and determine if PG or GAG species could be correlated with induction of specific hematopoietic lineages in terms of specialized microniches or microenvironments favor-ing one or another hematopoietic lineage. Histochemical stain-ing of marrow-enriched CEM were examined after intervals of ip implantation from 6 wk to 6 mo. Sections were stained with High Iron Diamine (sulfated acidic GAGs and sulfated PGs),

Alcian Blue (nonsulfated acidic GAGs), Periodic Acid Schiff (PGs), and Periodic Acid Phenylhydrazine Schiff (acidic nonsulfated PGs). PGs and nonsulfated acidic GAGs accumulated at the membrane surface. The remainder of the CEM and the interior cavity contained only limited amounts of sulfated and nonsulfated GAGs. The CEM developing new bone and trilineal hematopoiesis showed an accumulation of acidic and nonsulfated PGs, possibly sialoglycoproteins. The stroma supporting trilineal hematopoiesis also contained nonsulfated acidic GAGs, but not sulfated acid GAGs. Control CEM without stromal cell enrichment contained both sulfated and nonsulfated GAGs. It was concluded that the primitive regenerating stromal cells interact with the membrane surface and secrete several species of matrix proteins that accumulate in the portion of the membrane adjacent to the surface. These secreted matrix proteins (which may include species unidentified by the techniques used in these studies) may then effect further changes in stromal cell differentiation or transformation and also may contribute to hematopoietic differentiation and proliferation.[34]

These events of stromal cell regeneration on CEM were studied with the techniques of electron microscopy. Ultrastructural analysis of these events after intervals of 4 wk to 6 mo of ip implantation showed that stromal cell regeneration on the membranes occurred primarily at the CEM surface and appeared to be a surface mediated event. Primitive mesenchyme-like cells developed a secretory apparatus and, after a few months, took on the appearance of osteogenic cells[35] (Fig. 5).

Role of Bone and Tooth Matrix Proteins in Hematopoiesis

Reddi and Huggins, as well as Urist, described the use of demineralized, nonviable bone matrix proteins to induce new bone formation and a hematopoietic microenvironment in rats.[36,37] Rat bone was ground in a tissue mill to produce a fine powder with particles varying from 70 to 800 μm. This was then demineralized with 0.5M HCI and further extracted with ether and ethanol. The residue contained matrix proteins with a content of more than 90% collagen I, 3% PG, and less than 1% trace proteins.[38] This powder, when placed sc, was highly chemotactic for circulating mononuclear cells that rapidly infiltrated the surfaces and interstices of the bone powder explant. Within 3 wk, new bone formation was induced around the surfaces of the matrix protein particles. Within the interstices of the matrix particles, hematopoiesis developed indicating the induction of a hemopoietic microenvironment that attracted circulating pluripotent hematopoietic stem cells. These lodged into the hematopoietic stroma and differentiated into erythropoietic, granulopoietic, and megakaryocytopoietic lineages.

We attempted to repeat the studies of Reddi and Huggins in mice. We wished to study stem cell kinetics in the developing bony hematopoietic ossicles as well as study stromal cell functions. We were disappointed to observe that mouse bone powder, prepared according to Reddi's techniques and placed on CEM ip or sc, does not induce new bone formation or a hematopoietic microenvironment in the mouse. Although qualitatively the same types of hematopoietic stromal cells develop on mouse bone matrix powder implants (sinusoid-like structures, fibroblasts, macrophages, and fat cells) hematopoiesis did not develop.[39] At Reddi's suggestion, we used demineralized murine tooth powder. Tooth matrix powder was active in inducing new bone formation and a hematopoietic microenvironment, but with only two lineages represented— megakaryocytopoietic and granulopoietic, but not erythropoietic and only at subcutaneous, but not on ip CEMs. We also investigated hematopoietic stem cell kinetics in tooth and bone matrix subcutaneous and ip implants. Small numbers of CFU$_s$,

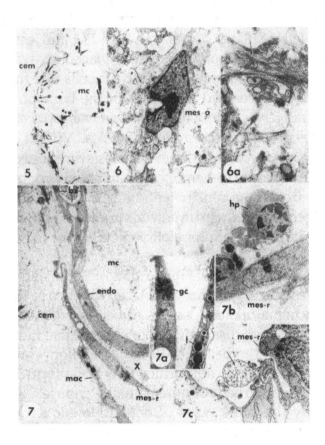

Fig. 5. (5–7) Bone marrow-enriched CEM 1 mo after implantation. (5) Light micrograph of the network of longutudinally oriented, spindle-shaped stromal cells near the CEM surface. Some cells branch into the medullary cavity (mc) (arrows); original magnification 242 ×. (6a) A transitional osseous–mesenchymal cell (mes-o) with large, prominent, euchromatic nucleus and developing secretory apparatus residues within an intramembranous site filled with collagenous fibers, granular material, and cellular debris (arrows); original magnification 9600 ×. (6b) An intramembranous site filled with collagenous fibers and cell debris (arrows); original magnification 25,020 × (7a) Essential cellular components of developing hematopoietic sites (x) are in close association near the CEM surface: mono-

CFU_{GM}, and CFU_E were found in the subcutaneous implants beginning at 3 wk, but not in the ip-implanted CEM.[40] These findings were reminiscent of the findings in Dexter long-term marrow cultures where CFU_s, CFU_{GM}, and BFU_E were found and only granulopoiesis developed without terminal erythropoiesis.[41] We have no explanation for the difference between rat bone matrix implants that foster trilineal hematopoiesis and murine tooth matrix implants that foster only bilineal hematopoiesis. We recently investigated the possibility that tooth matrix powder inactivated erythropoietin. However, incubation of tooth bone matrix powder and erythropoietin in tissue culture media for several hours resulted in no loss of erythropoietin activity.[42]

Another fascinating aspect of these studies was the observation that hematopoiesis only occurred within a surrounding shell of new bone. The close spatial dependence of hematopoiesis upon functioning bone in these implants represent a dramatic example of the interdependence of these two tissues[40] (Fig. 6).

We studied the serial histochemistry of PGs and GAGs in the tooth and bone matrix implants of mice. Significant differences in PG and GAG species were observed in the two kinds of implants. Tooth matrix implants developed acidic and nonsulfated PGs and nonsulfated acidic GAGs, but not sulfated

---

cytoid-like cells (mon), transitional mesenchymal–reticular cells (mes-r), and endothelial cells (endo) in early stages of blood sinus (bs) formation; original magnification 3068 ×. (7b) Transitional mesenchymal–stromal cells, exhibiting phase-specific cytoplasmic lipoid (l) and glycogen (gc) inclusions; original magnification 5760 ×. (7c) Rudimentary hematopoietic sites contain early hematopoietic progenitors (hp) in association with transitional mesenchymal–reticular cells (mes-r); original magnification 4091 × (7d) Cell processes of transition mesenchymal–reticular (mes-r) cell with pronounced variation in cytoplasmic density (dark to light electron density) (arrow); original magnification 7320 × (Ref. 35).

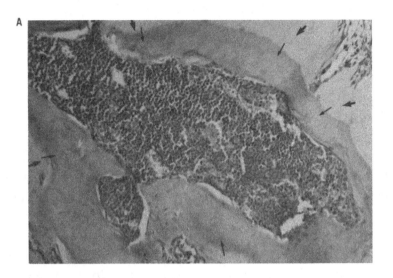

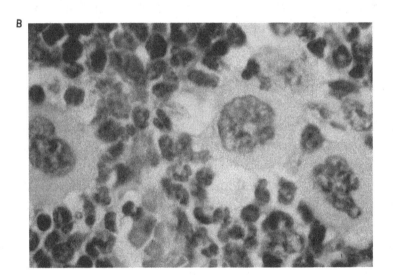

Fig. 6 (A) Tooth matrix implanted sc and removed after 6 wk. An intense hematopoietic focus is seen surrounded by a narrow zone of darker new bone formation (smaller arrows). The noncalcified matrix material stains lighter (larger arrows). Only granulocytopoiesis and megakaryo-cytopoiesis are present; hematoxylin and eosin stain; magnification 40 ×. (B) Same as (A), but a higher magnification to show that only granulocytopoiesis and megakaryocytopoiesis are present; hematoxylin and eosin stain; magnification 400 ×. (C) CEM-coated stromal cells from bone and irradiated with 4000 rad in vitro, following which ip implantation occurred for 6 mo. Hematopoietic cellularity and new bone formation are decreased, about 50% of that observed in (A) and (B). Fibrosis is also present in areas of diminished hematopoietic cellularity. Original magnification 10 ×; hematoxylin and eosin stain (Ref. 40).

acidic GAGs. Sulfated and nonsulfated GAGs were identified in the bone matrix powder implants.[43]

These results indicate that the nonviable tooth matrix powder in the mouse (and bone matrix powder in the rat) has the capability of transforming mononuclear cells residing in the skin of the host into cells of the osteogenic and hematopoietic stromal type. In this experimental model, bone cells and hematopoietic stromal cells derive from transformed mesenchymal cells of the host.

Irradiation of Stromal Cells

These results lead us to again take up the question of which cell forms the regenerated hematopoietic microenvironment on CEM—donor or host stromal cells. Previous studies in my laboratory and in Fried's had examined the radiation sensitivity of hematopoietic stromal cells.[44,45] Rat bone marrow was locally irradiated with x-irradiation doses from 1000 to 10,000 rad. An initial wave of aplasia at 1 wk, owing to destruction of hematopoietic cells, was followed by regeneration at 2 wk and then a secondary wave of aplasia at 1–3 mo. The secondary wave of aplasia was related to delayed destruction of marrow sinusoidal cells. Late regeneration of sinusoids occurred up to 2000 rad doses after 6–12 mo, but permanent destruction of sinusoids and permanent aplasia occurred with doses of 4000 rad and higher.[44]

We applied stromal cells from bone marrow or bone to CEM, irradiated the enriched CEM in vitro with doses of 1000, 2000, or 4000 rad of gamma irradiation, and implanted the irradiated CEMs ip. The CEMs were removed after intervals of 3, 6, and 12 mo and examined histologically. Irradiation of bone marrow stromal cells with 1000 rad or higher resulted in complete prevention of new bone formation or hematopoiesis. Irradiation of bone stromal cells placed on CEM just prior to ip implantation led to rather surprising and different results. Irradiation of bone stromal cells with 1000 rad had no significant effect on new bone formation or the development of hematopoiesis at 6 or 12 mo. Hematopoietic cellularity was abundant and perhaps even somewhat increased. A dose of 2000 rad inhibited regeneration of new bone and hematopoiesis up to 50% of development on unirradiated CEM enriched with stromal cells of bone or bone marrow. A 4000 rad dose to the bone-enriched CEM completely ablated the capacity for new bone formation or hematopoiesis. These results clearly indicated that the development of new bone and hematopoiesis, upon ip implanted CEM enriched with stromal cells, was dependent upon the transfer of a living stromal cell.[46]

We have no explanation for the difference in radiation sensitivity of stromal cells from these two closely related tissues. The differing response to radiation may reflect the same underlying stromal cell differences that resulted in various interactions with artificial membranes of varying physical and chemical properties.[46,18]

Complementary studies have been done to determine relations between donor and host cells on the CEM. Most of our studies have been done in CAF_1 mice. We repeated our studies in CBA/Ca and CBA/T_6/T_6 mice that are coisogeneic to each other, except for the difference in presence or absence of the T_6/T_6 marker chromosome in one strain. Stromal cells from bone of CBA/T_6/T_6 mice were placed on CEM and implanted in CBA/Ca mice and conversely CBA/Ca mice were used for donor marrow and bone stromal cells to be placed on CEM and implanted ip into CBA/T_6/T_6 mice. After 6 and 12 mo, CEM were removed and cells on the CEM (primarily hematopoietic, but including some stromal cells) were examined cytogenetically for ratios of CBA/Ca and CBA/T_6/T_6 cells. All cells on CEM were of host type. These studies indicate all hematopoietic tissue derived from the host, but do not answer the origin of stromal cells (Knospe, W. H., unpublished observations).

Studies of Scraped, Devitalized, and Reimplanted CEM

We wished to study the role of matrix protein enrichment of CEM by living stromal cells. The aforementioned studies of adsorption of matrix proteins upon superficial CEM layers following stromal cell enrichment suggested that PGs, GAGs, or some related species of matrix protein might play a positive role in the process of stromal cell regeneration. The previously described electron microscopic (EM) studies indicated the evolution and differentiation of a primitive stromal cell into a much more differentiated cell with osteogenic and secretory properties. The following experiments were designed to investigate varying tenures of transferred stromal cells on CEM upon the accumulation of matrix proteins. The experiments were designed to determine if CEM, conditioned with matrix proteins by living stromal cells and then sterilized by radiation, had the capacity to induce a hematopoietic microenvironment. Bone-enriched CEM were implanted ip for intervals of 1, 3, and 6 mo, removed from the peritoneal cavity, opened, and scraped free of all stromal, bone, and hematopoietic tissue.

Following CEM scraping, the membranes were irradiated in vitro to 4000 rad to assure destruction of any stromal cells that infiltrated into the CEM beneath the membrane surface. The CEM then were folded again into a tubular structure and reimplanted ip or sc for intervals of 1, 3, or 6 mo. Histological analysis of the reimplanted CEM revealed that new bone formation and trilineal hematopoiesis developed at 1 and 3 mo after secondary implantation but only at sc sites. These results indicated that the secondarily implanted CEM without any living stromal cells, but abundantly laden with adsorbed matrix proteins, was able to induce host cells that migrated onto the CEM from sc sites to be transformed into cells of osteogenic and hematopoietic stromal capacity. Furthermore, these secondarily implanted CEM developed new bone formation and hematopoiesis much faster than the primary CEM implants carrying living stromal cells.[46,47] With these maneuvers, we were able to make the CEM behave in a manner similar to the devitalized, demineralized bone and tooth matrix powders implanted sc. We are uncertain which matrix protein is the agent of the bone and hematopoietic stromal cell induction or whether more than one protein is involved. Reddi is currently attempting to isolate and characterize the bone-inducing principle. His preliminary results indicate that it is a trace protein, possibly a glycoprotein, present at a concn. of 1 ppm in the bone matrix powder.[48] These studies indicate that stromal cell regeneration upon ip implanted CEM is a highly complex process dependent initially upon the placement of living stromal cells from bone marrow. Our studies indicate that this stromal cell(s) is a unique cell found only in marrow or bone or regenerating endosteum.

The transferred stromal cell acquires secretory properties and produces a variety of PGs and GAGs of which the non-sulfated acidic PGs and GAGs appear to be most important, but we do not know whether this class of proteins carries the bone-inducing or hematopoietic stroma-inducing properties. Our studies suggest that a secreted factor (PG or other) then induces a transformation of sc host mononuclear cells into bone cells and hematopoietic stromal cells that produce a definitive hematopoietic microenvironment. At this point, host circulating, pluripotent hematopoietic stem cells invade the prepared "soil" of the induced hematopoietic stroma and establish trilineal hematopoiesis upon the CEM.

Overall Perspective and Significance of Hematopoiesis on CEM

Cellulose ester and other artificial membranes have provided a useful technique to study hematopoietic stroma. The studies using the flat, unenriched CEM provided a way to simplify and dissect the hematopoietic microenvironment, particularly for granulopoiesis. The use of marker studies permitted the identification of the proportions of monocytic–macrophage-type of cells adhering to the CEM. These studies indicated that the simplified hematopoietic microenvironment was not a homogeneous population of monocyte–macrophage cells, but included other cell types including fibroblasts and vascular cells. The same flat CEM was used to study the defective microenvironment of Sl/Sl^d mice that was expressed in the simplified stroma developing on CEM. We were able to make unique observations on stromal cells removed from the membrane and identified a phagocytic defect on cells adhering to the CEM implanted in Sl/Sl^d mice. We also identified an additional defect of deficient or reduced cell layering of peritoneal origin on the CEM.[49]

Studies of modified CEM with added stromal cells from several sources including spleen, bone marrow, bone, and regenerating endosteal mesenchyme permitted us to restructure and concentrate the stroma on a circumscribed scaffold. This provided a way to study the histogenesis of stromal regeneration by light and electron microscopy and identify the details of stromal cell differentiation on the CEM. We were able to show that this is a surface-active process that provided a way to study matrix proteins adsorbed selectively onto the CEM. Irradiation of the stroma on CEM identified differences in stromal cell sensitivity to irradiation, depending upon whether the stromal cells derived from bone or bone marrow, and these studies indicated that living cells were required to transfer the hematopoietic microenvironment to the CEM. By combining scraping of the implanted CEM with ablative irradiation, followed by reimplantation, we were able to show that matrix proteins secreted by the transferred donor stromal cells were able to induce new bone and an sc hematopoietic microenvironment in CEM independently of living donor stromal cells.

This provided unique insight into the function of matrix proteins upon stromal and bone cell transformation of migrating host mononuclear, mesenchymal cells of sc origin. These studies have also clarified similarities and differences between the subcutaneous bone and tooth matrix models of new bone formation, hematopoietic microenvironment induction developed by Reddi and Huggins, and the enriched CEM model developed by me and my colleagues.

The enriched CEM provides a way to examine in vivo, with a highly reproducible technique, the hematopoietic support capacity of a hematopoietic stromal cell population. We have used it to show that the adherent layer of Dexter cultures, although only able to support granulopoiesis in vitro, when transferred to CEM and implanted ip, can express a retained osteogenic potential and stromal support of trilineal hematopoiesis.[50] It also provides a way to study stromal cell integrity after cytotoxic injury from irradiation, chemotherapy, or other drug or immunologic injuries.

The close proximity of the nests of hematopoiesis in the tooth matrix implants to the surrounding "shell" of new bone formation suggests a nurturing or supportive role of bone to hematopoiesis. A similarly close association of bone to hematopoiesis is seen on the tubular CEM enriched by hematopoietic stromal cells. Hematopoiesis, when present on the CEM, was almost invariably associated with new bone formation. Our studies of hematopoiesis on CEM, as well as the studies of Tavassoli and Crosby[51] and Friedenstein et al.,[52] indicate that some hematopoietic stromal cells carry the potential to develop into bone-forming cells. And contrarily, mesenchymal cells of osteogenic potential carry the capability to develop stromal cells that support trilineal or bilineal hematopoiesis as in the rat or murine bone, or tooth matrix subcutaneous implants.

Ershler and Shahidi reported a case of congenital anemia of unknown cause in a young woman. Culture of the bone marrow stem cells (CFUc and CFUe) in dispersed culture systems revealed exuberant growth. Nondispersed marrow obtained by biopsy failed to produce heme in culture compared to a sample of bone and marrow obtained by biopsy from a normal subject. This interesting experiment of nature strongly indicates an inhibitory effect of bone cells upon hematopoietic cells and argues for a defect in the hematopoietic microenvironment.[53]

The elegant studies of Brookes on the vascular anatomy of rat bone indicated that nutrient arteries pierce the diaphysis of bone, arborize in a subendosteal manner, and then reenters bone to form a portal-like circulation that then reenters the medullary cavity to form the sinusoidal circulation of bone marrow.[54] This peculiar, portal-like circulation of bone that may sustain the marrow is consistent with the hypothesis that bone provides some nurturing factor for hemopoiesis. Our experimental studies suggest that this nurturing factor may act on hematopoietic stromal cells as well as on hematopoietic stem cells.

The close relationship of bone and hematopoiesis throughout vertebrate evolution provides dramatic support for the dependence of hematopoiesis upon bone. Our studies and those of others provide further clues for this dependence. These studies are at least consistent with the hypothesis that primitive stromal cells residing in bone and bone marrow elaborate matrix proteins that can induce sc mononuclear cells of mesenchymal lineage to become osteocytes and hematopoietic stromal cells. We do not know whether the active agent of cellular induction is a proteoglycan (consistent with our observations) or a matrix protein in trace concentration, as suggested by the studies of Reddi.[48] The close association of hematopoiesis and bone absorbed on enriched CEM was paralleled by a similar association of hematopoiesis and bone in the studies of sc implanted tooth matrix powder. In those studies, hematopoiesis was invariably found surrounded by a thin ossicle of new bone formation. The hematopoiesis developing on enriched CEM is permanent, persisting without involution for a year or longer and incorporates the newly induced extramedullary sites on CEM into the total hematopoietic organ of bone marrow and spleen.[55]

These studies also showed that sinusoid-like vascular structures were essential to the functioning of the hematopoietic stroma and were invariably present in the regenerated hematopoietic stroma. The sinusoidal microcirculation linked up with larger efferent and afferent vascular structures that connected with the systemic circulation, permitting this island of extramedullary hematopoiesis to be regulated by the homeostatic influences acting upon the total hematopoietic organ. The studies of stromal cell interactions with other artificial membranes identified differences in stromal cell response depending upon the tissue origin of the stromal cells. The basis of this variability in stromal cell interaction with artificial membranes remains unknown.

Studies are currently in progress to investigate the ability of cloned stromal cell lines to develop a hematopoietic microenvironment and bone following placement on ip implanted CEM. These cloned stromal cell lines established by Zipori et al. (and discussed elsewhere in this volume) have features of fibroblasts, fibroblast–endothelial-like, preadipocyte, and epithelioid cells. Each of these cell types is represented among stromal cells existing in bone marrow and each type has been identified among the complex adherent cell layers developing in long-term marrow cultures. It is not known which is the crucial cells necessary to establish the hematopoietic microenvironment in vitro or in vivo or whether a mixture of several stromal cells is necessary.

CEM have been coated with cloned stromal cells. Four cloned cell lines have been used: 14 F1.1 (adipocyte); MBA 2 (endothelial); MBA 1 (fibroblast); and MBA 13 (fibroblastoid and endothelial-like). CEM have been examined after 3 and 6

mo of ip implantation. Only the adipocyte (14 F1.1) and endothelial–fibroblast cell lines showed new bone formation and
only after 6 mo of ip implantation. Our previous experience
with CEM would suggest that new bone formation is associated with the capacity to support trilineal hematopoiesis. We
would expect these latter two cell types to develop hematopoiesis, perhaps after 6 and 12 mo of implantation. The removal
and histologic analysis of implanted CEM, coated with these
cloned cell lines after 9 and 12 mo of implantation, will be done
in the near future (Knospe, W. H., unpublished observations).

A final and unexpected benefit of hematopoiesis studies
on enriched CEM has been the evidence for a heretofore unrecognized role for marrow stromal cells. Control and uncoated
CEM implanted ip become densely fibrotic after 3–6 mo residence ip. However, when CEM are coated with viable stromal
cells, fibroblastic proliferation and collagen deposition are inhibited. When hematopoietic stromal cells are injured or killed
by interaction with some types of artificial membranes by
irradiation, dense fibrosis develops. These results suggest that
marrow stromal cells regulate fibroblastic proliferation and
when such cells fail or involute myelofibrosis may result.
These experimental results may provide new insights for understanding the nature of diseases like agnogenic myeloid meta-
plasia with myelofibrosis.

Acknowledgments

The author acknowledges the following publishing com-
panies for granting permission to reproduce figures that originally appeared in their respective journals: Munksgaard
International (1978) *Exp. Hematol.* **6**, 233–245; Allen Press (1983)
Exp. Hematol. **11**, 512–521; Springer-Verlag (1986) *Exp. Hematol.*
14, 108–118; Alpha Med Press (1984) *Int. J. Cell Cloning* **2**, 99–
112; and (1985) *Int. J. Cell Cloning* **3**, 320–329. The author also

acknowledges the secretarial assistance of Patricia G. Konieczny in the preparation of this manuscript.

References

[1]Seki, M. (1973) *Transplantation* **16**, 544–549.

[2]Kawata, T., Katamura, Y., Okano, K., Asayama, S., and Seki, M. (1975) *Exp. Hematol.* **3**, 117–123.

[3]Knospe, W. H., Mortenson, R., Husseini, S., and Trobaugh, F. E., Jr. (1978) *Exp. Hematol.* **6**, 233–245.

[4]Dexter, T. M., Allen, T. D., Lajtha, L. G., Schofield, R., and Lord, B. I. (1973) *J. Cell. Physiol.* **82**, 461–474.

[5]Bernstein, S. E., Russell, E. S., and Keighley, G. (1968) *Ann. NY Acad. Sci.* **149**, 475–485.

[6]McCulloch, E. A., Siminovich, L., Till, J. E., Russell, E. S., and Bernstein, S. E. (1965) *Blood* **26**, 399–410.

[7]Altus, M. S., Bernstein, S. E., Russell, E. S., Carsten, A. L., and Upton, A. C. (1971) *Proc. Soc. Exp. Biol. Med.* **138**, 985–98.

[8]Knospe, W. H., Husseini, S. G., and Adler, S. S. (1985) *Exp. Hematol.* **13**, 652–657.

[9]Miyano, Y., Tamai, M., and Kitamura, Y. (1978) *Cell Tissue Kinet.* **11**, 103–109.

[10]Lai, P. -K., Boggs, D. R., Boggs, S. S., and Turner, A. R. (1980) *Exp. Hematol.* **8**, 264–270.

[11]Tavassoli, M. (1984) *Br. J. Haematol.* **57**, 71–80.

[12]Shaklai, M. and Tavassoli, M. (1978) *Am. J. Pathol.* **90**, 633–640 .

[13]Knospe, W. H., Husseini, S., and Trobaugh, F. E., Jr. (1978) *Exp. Hematol.* **6**, 601–612.

[14]Knospe, W. H., Blom, J., and Crosby, W. H. (1968) *Blood* **31**, 400–405.

[15]Knospe, W. H., Gregory, S. A., Husseini, S. G., Fried, W., and Trobaugh, F. E., Jr. (1972) *Blood* **39**, 331–340.

[16]Knospe, W. H., Gregory, S. A., Fried, W., and Trobaugh, F. E., Jr. (1973) *Blood* **41**, 519–527.

[17]Knospe, W. H., Husseini, S. G., and Adler, S. S. (1983) *Exp. Hematol.* **11**, 512–521.

[18]Knospe, W. H., Husseini, S. G., and Adler, S. S. (1984) *Int. J. Cell Cloning* **2**, 99–112.

[19]Shadduck, R. K., Boegel, F., Pope, F., and Waheed, A. (1978) *Exp. Hematol.* **6**, 355–360.

[20]Motoyoshi, K., Takaku, F., and Miura, Y. (1983) *Exp. Hematol.* **11**, 389–393.

[21]Berman, I. and Newby, E. J. (1967) *Nature* **213**, 300, 301.

[22]Lowry, P. H. and Keighley, G. (1968) *Biochim. Biophys. Acta* **160**, 413–419.

[23]McCuskey, R. S., Meineke, H. A., and Townsend, S. F. (1972) *Blood* **39**, 697–712.

[24]McCuskey, R. S., Meineke, H. A., and Kaplan, S. M. (1972) *Blood* **39**, 809–813.

[25]McCuskey, R. S., and Meineke, H. A. (1973) *Am. J. Anat.* **137**, 187–191.

[26]McCuskey, P. A., McCuskey, R. S., and Meineke, H. A. (1975) *Exp. Hematol.* **3**, 297–308.

[27]Schrock, L. M., Judd, J. T., Meineke, H. A., and McCuskey, R. S. (1973) *Proc. Soc. Exp. Biol. Med.* **144**, 593–595.

[28]Ploemacher, R. E., Vant Hull, E., and Van Soest, P. L. (1978) *Exp. Hematol.* **6**, 311–320.

[29]Spicer, S. S. (1961) *Am. J. Clin. Path.* **36**, 393–407.

[30]Noordegraaf, E. M., Erkens-Verslius, E. A., and Ploemacher, R. E. (1981) *Exp. Hematol.* **9**, 326–331.

[31]Spooncer, E., Gallagher, J. T., Krizsa, F., and Dexter, T. M. (1983) *J. Cell Biol.* **96**, 510–514.

[32]Robinson, H. C., Brett, M. J., Tralaggan, P. J., Lowther, D. A., and Okayama, M. (1975) *Biochem. J.* **148**, 25–34.

[33]Zuckerman, K. S. and Wicha, M. S. (1983) *Blood* **61**, 540–547.

[34]McCuskey, R. S., Meineke, H. A., Pinkstaff, C. A., and Knospe, W. H. (1984) *Exp. Hematol.* **12**, 25–30.

[35]Seed, T. M., Husseini, S. G., and Knospe, W. H. (1986) *Exp. Hematol.* **14**, 108–118.

[36]Urist, M. R. (1965) *Science* **150**, 893–899.

[37]Reddi, A. H. and Huggins, C. B. (1975) *Proc. Natl. Acad. Sci. USA* **72**, 2212–2216.

[38]Reddi, A. H. (1976) *Biochemistry of Collagen* (Ramachandran, G. N. and Reddi, A. H., eds.), Plenum, New York, pp. 449–478.

[39]Knospe, W. H., Husseini, S. G., Adler, S. S., and Reddi, A. H. (1983) *Exp. Hematol.* **11**, 1021–1026.

[40]Knospe, W. H., Husseini, S. G., Adler, S. S., and Reddi, A. H. (1985) *Int. J. Cell Cloning* **3**, 320–329.

[41]Dexter, T. M., Testa, N. G., Allen, T. D., Rutherford, T., and Scolnick, E. (1981) *Blood* **58**, 699–707.

[42]Knospe, W. H. and Fried, W. (unpublished observations).

[43]McCuskey, R. S., Reddi, A. H. and Knospe, W. H. (1985) *Blood* **66**, 132a (abstract).

[44]Knospe, W. H., Blom, J., and Crosby, W. H. (1966) *Blood* **28**, 398–415.

[45]Fried, W., Husseini, S., Knospe, W. H., and Trobaugh, F. E., Jr. (1973) *Exp. Hematol.* **1**, 29–35.

[46]Knospe, W. H. and Husseini, S. G. (1986) *Exp. Hematol.* **14**, 975–980.

[47]Knospe, W. H. and Husseini, S. G. (1984) *Exp. Hematol.* **12**, 417 (abstract).

[48]Sampath, T. K., Muthukumaran, N., and Reddi, A. H. (1987) *Proc. Natl. Acad. Sci. USA* **84**, 7109–7113.

[49]Seed, T. M., Husseini, S. G., and Knospe, W. H. (1988) *Exp. Hematol.* **16**, 705–711.

[50]Adler, S. S., Husseini, S. G., and Knospe, W. H. (1988) *Int. J. Cell Cloning* **6**, 281–289.

[51]Tavassoli, M. and Crosby, W. H. (1968) *Science* **161**, 54–56.

[52]Friedenstein, A. J., Petrakova, K. V., Kurolesova, A. I., and Frolova, G. P. (1968) *Transplantation* **6**, 230–247.

[53]Ershler, W. B., Ross, J., Finlay, J. L., and Shahidi, N. T. (1980) *N. Engl. J. Med.* **302**, 1321–1327.

[54]Brookes, M. (1971) *The Blood Supply of Bone: An Approach to Bone Biology,* Butterworths, London.

[55]Knospe, W. H., Husseini, S. G., and Adler, S. S. (1983) *Exp. Hematol.* **11**, 512–521.

Chapter 6

Cellular Components of Stroma In Vivo In Comparison With In Vitro Systems

Mati Shaklai

Introduction

Hemopoiesis normally occurs in certain specific tissues that vary according to the class and order of animals observed. In lower animals, hemopoiesis may occur in different areas in the body.[1] In mammals, the site of hemopoiesis changes during the fetal life in the following sequence: from yolk sac to liver and spleen and then to the bone marrow, which remains the principal site of hemopoiesis postnatally.

The marrow residues within the bone consist of three main components: vascular and cellular elements and extracellular matrix. The latter two are in the extravascular and intersinu-

soidal space, known as the hematopoietic cord or compartment.[2-5] The cellular elements are made up of hematopoietic
and stromal cells. The stromal cells form an intricate network,
consisting of fibroblastic reticular cells, macrophages, and fat
cells, all embedded in a ground substance. It is upon this network that hematopoietic stem cells lodge, proliferate, differentiate, and mature.[6-11] This chapter deals with the cellular elements of stroma in vivo in comparison to the in vitro systems.

Cellular Components of the Stroma

Reticular cells and macrophages are the two major stromal
components in the marrow and other hematopoietic organs.
Additional cellular components include the adipocytes, endothelial cells, "branched stromal cells" and the stromal cells that
can be recognized by its preferential uptake of lanthanum.

Reticular Cells In Vivo

Reticular cells are histogenetically recognizable from
hematopoietic cells.[1] There are two types of reticular cells of the
hematopoietic cord: adventitial and fibroblastic. They are distinguished by their topographic location and minor ultrastructural features. Fibroblastic reticular cells are fixed cells, rarely
seen in smears of bone marrow obtained by aspiration. This is
a large cell with a diameter of 30 to 40 μm. Its cytoplasm is basophilic gray and contains azurophilic granules. The nucleus is
round or oval and voluminous, its chromatin is fine without
clumps, and contains one or two nucleoli.[12] Cytochemical
stainings have shown that these cells are alkaline phosphatase
positive.[13-15] In light microscopy of biopsy specimens, these
cells are characterized by their long cytoplasmic processes that
radiate into the marrow parenchyma and along the venous sinuses. In alkali phosphatase-stained sections, these cells can be

seen in large numbers near the endosteum and in close association with myeloid precursors.[16] These reticular cells are frequently associated with argentophilic fibers that can be seen by light microscopy in reticulin stain preparations. In electron microscopy, reticular cells have distinct structural features. The cytoplasm is frequently highly rarefied so that, without the use of extracellular tracers, its branches may be confused with the extracellular space[3,17] (Fig. 1). It contains a moderate to high number of profiles of rough endoplasmic reticulum and a large number of ribosomes (Fig. 2), usually in the perinuclear area suggestive of extensive protein synthesis. Filamentous structures 5–9 nm in diameter are dispersed through the cytoplasm thicker bundles filaments are sometimes seen in submembranous locations. Occasionally, microtubules, smooth and coated vesicles, are seen within the cytoplasm.[2,5]

Adventitial Reticular Cells

Adventitial reticular cells are located around the venous sinuses, partially covering the endothelium's abluminal side (Fig. 3).[3,18] Their slender cytoplasmic processes extend deep into the hematopoietic compartment and form a continuous anastomosing bridgework between sinuses. Their nucleus is seldom included in the electron microscopic sections and, when seen, it is predominately located near sinuses, although it may also be seen within the hematopoietic cords particularly when these reticular cells are associated with foci of myeloid cells.[5,16]

Adventitial reticular cells form a discontinuous layer covering a variable portion of the endothelium's abluminal surface. The proportion of the endothelial coverage depends on the traffic of mature blood cells from the hematopoietic compartment into the circulation.[18,19] The adventitial cells are thought to be contractile, and contain bundles of microfilaments that,

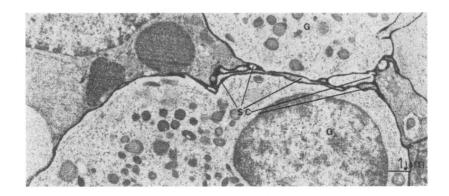

Fig. 1. Thin section micrograph of a lanthanum impregnated area of granulopoiesis. Lanthanum has delineated numerous very small projections of cytoplasm of stromal cells (SC) running between two neighboring granulocytes (G). Note the lucency of these cytoplasmic projections of the stromal cell (× 10,000) (Shaklai and Tavassoli, 1979, courtesy of Academic Press).

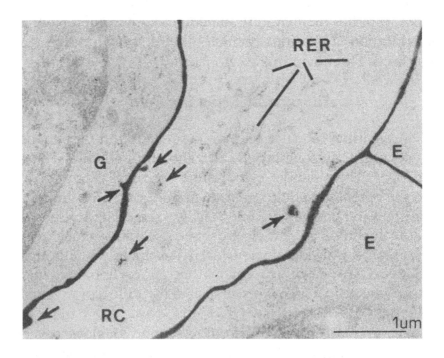

Fig. 2. This section of lanthanum-impregnated marrow tissue showing a reticular cell (RC) containing profiles of rough-surfaced endoplasmic reticulum (RER), ribosomes, and endocytic vesicles penetrated by lanthanum (three arrows). The cell bordered by two erythroid (E) and one granulocytic (G) cells (× 26,500) (Tavassoli et al., 1980, courtesy of Springer-Verlag).

222

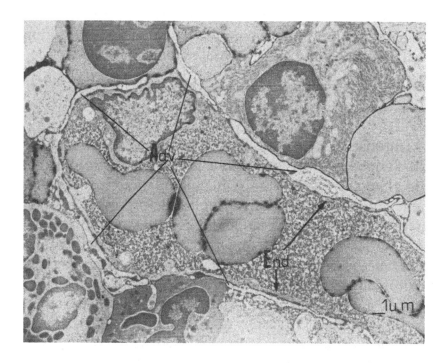

Fig. 3. Thin section micrograph of lanthanum-impregnated, tannic acid-treated marrow. A sinus passes diagonally in this figure and contains many red cells and a lymphocyte. Endothelium (End) has either dense or light cytoplasm. Adventitial layer (Adv) is lucent and covers most of the abluminal surface of the endothelium (× 4800).

under appropriate stimuli, may modulate the volume of the cell.[20-22] Intercellular contacts between adventitial cells and macrophages, and adventitial and endothelial cells, have been described.[23,24] These contact areas are seen in the mouse bone marrow fixed with glutaraldehyde and tannic acid. Morphologic features of these contact areas are similar to gap junctions in other organs. However, using techniques such as freeze fracture and lanthanum impregnation, gap junctions have not been demonstrated between similar cells in rat bone marrow.[3,24,25] Since intercellular junctions are heterogeneous, the possibility exists that the intercellular contact areas disclosed by tannic acid fixation in the mouse bone marrow are morphologic variants of gap junctions, or simply densities due to apposition of cell plasma membranes, resembling gap junctions.

Fibroblastic Reticular Cells
of the Hematopoietic Cord

Fibroblastic reticular cells of the hematopoietic cord are characterized by their long, thin cytoplasmic extensions that radiate haphazardly into the cellular population of the hematopoietic cord. Their rarefied cytoplasmic processes envelop each of the maturing hematopoietic cells in the compartment (Fig. 1).[3] The nucleus is largely euchromatic with a regular rim of heterochromatin. The endoplasmic reticulum is sparse and difficult to visualize. However, when the fixative contains tannic acid, a granular material has been revealed in the cisternae of the rough endoplasmic reticulum.[1,3,4,16,23] The space between the stromal cells is loosely packed with a collagenous matrix, consistent of fibers and ground substance. The ground substance contains water that is bound by proteins, glycosaminoglycans, and complexes of these substances. There is evidence that stromal cells are a major source of glycosaminoglycans of the ground substance.[26–30] Reticular cells also produce collagen types I and III, that are important constituents of the intercellular matrix (for detailed information on extracellular matrix, *see* Chapters 10 and 11).

In addition to morphologic, ultrastructural, and cytochemical characterization of the fibroblastic reticular cell, an attempt has been made to disclose possible antigenic properties that distinguish them from stromal cells in other hematopoietic organs and fibroblast populations in the body. A monoclonal antibody against murine bone marrow-derived fibroblasts has been produced. This antibody, called ER-HR1, reacts strongly with more than 90% of fibroblasts from spleen and marrow.[31] In bone marrow, the distribution pattern of reactive cells correlated with the distribution pattern of reticular cells. Similar correlations has been noted in the spleen. These cells are located directly under the splenic capsule.[31] In addition to this antigenic determinant that marrow and spleen reticular cells share, the two cell types lack Thy-1 antigen that can be detected in fibroblasts derived from thymus, blood, and skin.[32] These differences between stromal reticular cells of different organs is in line with the concept that fibroblasts from various origins, although morphologically indistinguishable, carry organ-specific properties. Such specific properties are preserved, even in several in vitro cell culture passages, following transplantation into different organs.[33,34]

Fibroblastic Reticular Cells in Long-Term Cell Culture

The major in vitro counterpart of reticular cells of the bone marrow is a fibroblastic cell. It belongs to a fraction of slowly proliferating and highly adherent bone marrow cells.[33-36,38] Methods are available to clone this cell.[39] On light microscopy, it has pale, elongated cytoplasm with tonofibrils and a nucleus containing large nucleoli.[34] This cell stains positively for the membrane-bound enzyme, alkaline phosphatase and manifests species-specific differences. In the mouse, human, and hamster, the fibroblastic colonies are strongly alkaline phosphatase positive; but in rabbit and guinea pig, alkaline phosphatase activity is very low.[31,40,41] Despite a great number of studies on these cells, they are not fully characterized morphologically. Different terms have been applied to them, raising the possibility of their heterogeneity. Fibroblast-like cells,[40] fibroblasts,[39] epithelioid cells,[37,42] and mechanocytes[33] are some of these terms. A common feature is their tendency to adhere.

Similar to reticular cells of the bone marrow, these fibroblastic cells of murine long-term marrow culture (LTMC) are capable of producing collagen types I and III, as well as fibronectin.[43-45] They stain positively for alkaline phosphatase, non-specific esterase, and lipids.[45] They do not have a Fc receptor that is characteristic of phagocytic mononuclear cells,[44] however, in appropriate culture conditions, these cells may exhibit facultative phagocytosis.[44] Phagocytic activity of reticular cells in bone marrow in vivo has also been described, although this is not a usual feature.[46] Two epithelioid cell types have been described in LTMC. They appear similar on scanning electron microscopy. They are elongated with flattened ends that are spreading to form veil-like structures with irregular fronts (Fig. 4). In transmission electron microscopy, however, marked differences are noted between them. One type is a synthesizing cell with numerous profiles of dilated, rough endoplasmic reticulum. Its cytoplasm is rich in filamentous structures of 5 to 7 nm in diameter, located under the cell membrane, and arranged in bands. Coated pits and vesicles may be seen throughout the cytoplasm (Figs. 5 and 6). This cell may be related to the in vivo adventitial reticular cell.[38,42] The second epithelioid cell is similar in size, but contains multisegmented euchromatic nucleus, filamentous bands, as well as numerous storage granules, and a variable number of fat globules (Fig. 7).[42] This cell has some resemblance to the fibroblastic reticular cell in bone marrow that accumulates lipids and secrets the type I banded collagen.[47] Giant fat cells of 80 to 100 μm diameter have been described in mouse LTMC.[48,49] They are associated with active and granulocytopoiesis, thus being reminiscent of the fat cells associated with myelopoiesis in the bone marrow.[2-4,88] The origin of these fat cells is not clear, although some investigators have suggested that fibroblastic reticular cells, adventitial reticular cells, and macrophages can all accumulate fat under culture conditions.[50,51] By using a macrophage-specific monoclonal antibody, the giant fat cells have been nonreactive and, therefore, they may not be of macrophage origin. Recently, another stromal cell type has

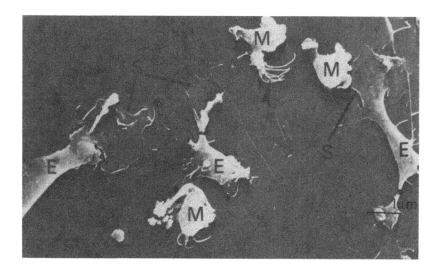

Fig. 4. Scanning electron micrograph of disaggregated stromal cells in a long-term culture. Two cell types can be seen. Epithelioid (E) are elongated with flattened ends that are spreading (S) to form veil-like structures with irregular fronts. Elongated microvilli are seen on the surfaces not yet flattened. The second cell type (M), probably corresponding to macrophages seen in transmission electron microscopy, are not elongated and show multiple microvilli (arrowhead) usually at one pole of the cell. These microvilli may be the means of spreading or may serve to establish contact with other cells (× 14,750) (Tavassoli and Takahashi 1982, courtesy of Liss Inc.).

been described in LTMC. It has been termed "blanket cell." It is adherent, large and is always associated with granulopoiesis. It overlays tightly packed foci of granulocytes and macrophages[42,75,86,95] and apparently produces a "niche" that supports active granulopoiesis.[86,95] Such intimate association of reticular cell with granulopoiesis also exists in vivo.[2-4,16]

A number of investigators have reported the establishment of continuous culture of stromal cell lines from murine bone marrow that can support hemopoiesis in vitro.[53-55] One of these lines, MBA-1,[55] resembles the fibroblastic reticular cells of hematopoietic stroma.[16] Similar to reticular cells, this cell is

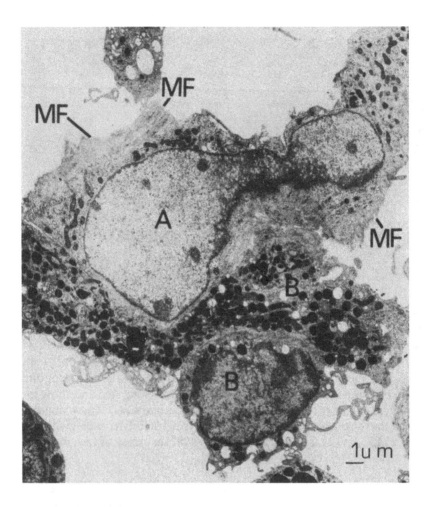

Fig. 5. Thin section through the adherent stroma layer. Two cells are seen. (A) is larger with a large indented nucleus showing a euchromatin pattern and multiple small nucleoli and the cytoplasm displays bands of microfilaments (MF) at the cell border where the cell appears to be spreading. Numerous thin rod-shaped mitochondria, often with angulation and profiles of endoplasmic reticulum, are the salient features of the cell. This is a synthesizing cell. The second cell (B) is smaller, has a more rounded nucleus with considerable heterochromatin, and the cytoplasm is often vesiculated and contains numerous dense granules. The cell surface shows microvilli. This cell is identified as macrophage. The two cells are in close association (× 5100) (Tavassoli and Takahashi, 1982, courtesy of Liss, New York).

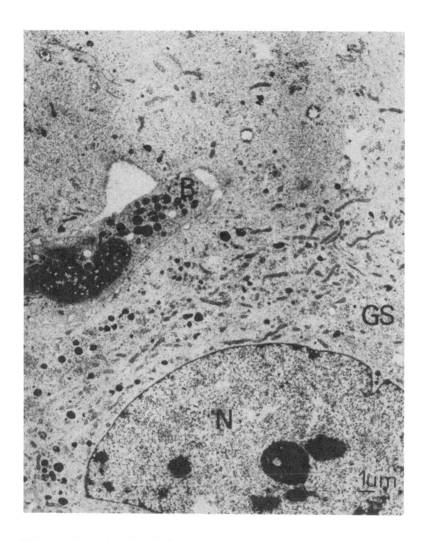

Fig. 6. Part of an epithelioid cell with its euchromatic nucleus. The cytoplasm contains numerous mitochrondria, ribosomes, granules, and the Golgi system (GS). Within the relatively organelle-free part of the cytoplasm, a small cell (B), most probably a macrophage, is engulfed by the cytoplasm of the epithelioid cell. Note the frequent membrane contact between the two cells (× 4500) (Tavassoli and Takahashi, 1982, courtesy of Liss, New York).

flattened and synthesizes collagen types I and III, stains positive for alkaline phosphatase, and produces colony stimulating activity.

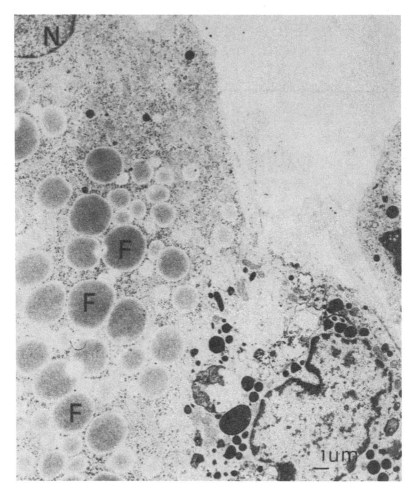

Fig. 7. Part of an epithelioid cell with a portion of its nucleus (N). The cytoplasm contains numerous lipid inclusions (F) is a storage cell. The cell is in close contact with a second cell type, part of which is seen in the right lower corner (× 5300) (Tavassoli and Takahashi, 1982, courtesy of Liss, New York).

Macrophages

The second cell type that is recognized as a major cellular component of hematopoietic stroma is the macrophage. Topographically, it is found in three sites in the bone marrow as a central macrophage in the erythroblastic island, perisinal macrophage on the abluminal side of the sinus endothelium, and also dispersed between the developing myeloid cells of the hematopoietic cord.

Central Macrophage

The central macrophage is usually surrounded by maturing red cells, thus forming an anatomic unit commonly referred to as an erythroblastic island.[2-4,11,23,56-61] Such units have been described in human marrow,[56,62] guinea pig yolk sac,[61] embryonic liver,[64] rat and mouse spleen,[57-70] ectopic marrow implants,[71,72] and adult mouse liver.[65,73] In bone marrow smears studied by light microscopy, the central macrophage cannot be appreciated because anatomical integrity of the erythroblastic island is not retained. In electron microscopy, central macrophages have only one nucleus, though occasionally a binucleated cell may be seen. The cytoplasm contains lysosomal structures, both primary and secondary, and displays various stages of digestion of ingested nuclei.[74] In cytochemical studies, the central macrophage gives a positive reaction for acid phosphatase and nonspecific esterase.[16,74,75] By electron microscopy, when rat bone marrow is fixed by intracavity perfusion, the central macrophage appears star-shaped, with the points of the star giving rise to long cytoplasmic processes extending irregularly in all directions and embracing the maturing erythroid cells with which they come in close contact (Fig. 8 and 9). Thinness of the cytoplasmic processes and the rarefaction of their cytoplasm prevents the appreciation of their extensiveness in the hematopoietic cord.[57,58] The association of macrophages with erythroid cells may be better perceived by using thin sections of bone marrow impregnated with lanthanum or freeze fracture replica of the tissue (Fig. 9 and 10)[17,23] or when membrane-enhancing agents, such as tannic acid, are used.[3,17]

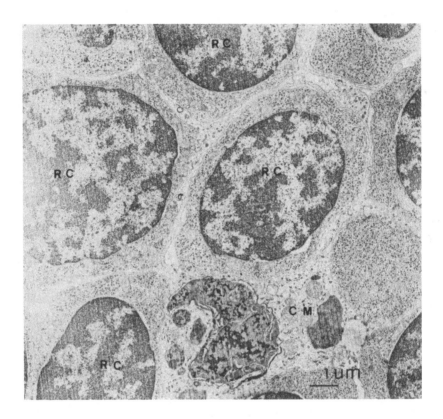

Fig. 8. Intracavitary perfusion fixed, tannic acid-treated thin section of an erythroblastic island. The central macrophage (CM) contains some cellular debris, including the remnants of some nuclei. Note that the small thin cytoplasmic processes of this cell run between the erythroid cells completely embracing one red cell (RC). Treatment with tannic acid has considerably increased the contrast of cell membrane in this preparation permitting the perception of the cytoplasmic processes of the central macrophage. Without this or similar treatment the perception of extremely attenuated and often lucent cytoplasmic processes may be difficult (×7800) (Shaklai and Tavassoli, 1979, courtesy of Academic Press).

In addition to extensive interdigitation of the macrophage processes with the erythroid cells, these processes also frequently invaginate into the cytoplasm of the developing erythroid cells. This interrelationship is emphasized when lanthanum is used to define the extracellular space (Fig. 11). The

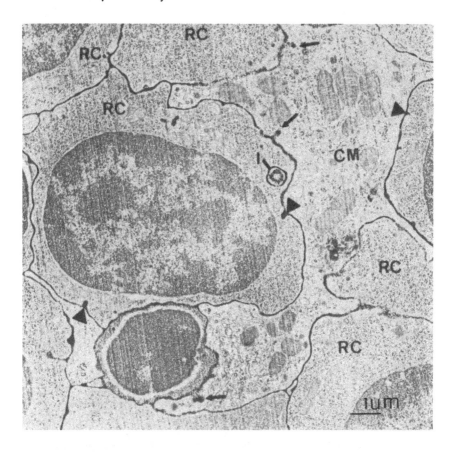

Fig. 9. Lanthanum impregnated, tannic acid-treated thin section of an erythroblastic island. Note the central macrophage (CM) extending from the right upper corner downward and toward the left and interdigitating with developing red cells (RC). Lanthanum tracer has delineated the extracellular space (dark areas). Note in the center of the figure (I) the tracer has identified an area where the central macrophage has invaginated into the developing red cell. Endocytosis is evident in erythroid cells and is well delineated by lanthanum (arrowheads), as well as in the central macrophage (arrows). The cytoplasm of the macrophage contains numerous mitochondria and profiles of endoplasmic reticulum that are delineated by tannic acid (× 8600) (Tavassoli and Shaklai, 1979, courtesy of Blackwell).

macrophage contains numerous micropinocytic and endocytic vesicles, some which contain ferritin.[57,58] When tannic acid is used to enhance the membrane, complementary exocytic ves-

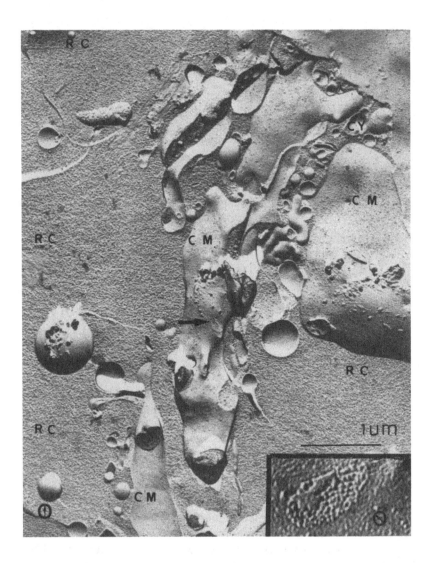

Fig. 10. Freeze-fracture replica of an erythroblastic island. The central macrophage (CM) is seen in the right upper part, extending downward and interdigitating with red cells (RC). The path of the fracture has gone mostly through the cell membrane of the CM displaying its protoplasmic face. Only in a few areas is the cytoplasm revealed (CY). By contrast, the path of fracture through erythroid cells is almost entirely transcytoplasmic. Note the small desmosome-like structure on the membrane of the central macrophage (arrow). This structure is magnified in the inset, displaying a patch of closely packed particles without hexagonal arrangement that is characteristic of gap junctions in this and other freeze fracture figures. The direction of coating is identified by an encircled arrow (× 23,000, inset × 170,000) (Tavassoli and Shaklai, 1979, courtesy of Blackwell).

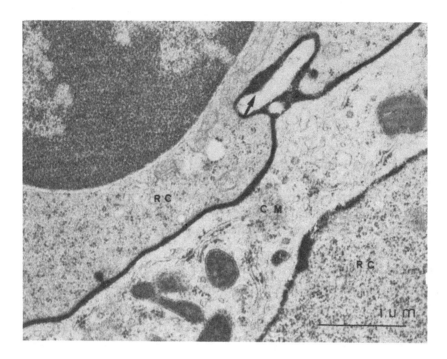

Fig. 11. Lanthanum-impregnated thin section showing part of an erythro-blastic island. Extension of a central macrophage (CM) is seen between two red cells (RC). The extracellular space is well perceived owing to the density of lanthanum. Note the continuity of two endocytic vesicles with the extra-cellular space. Note also within the cytoplasm of the erythroid cell (arrow), that the process of a central macrophage is completely surrounded by the extracellular space, as delineated by lanthanum. This type of cellular inter-digitation is commonly identified when lanthanum is used (× 31,000) (Tavassoli and Shaklai, 1979, courtesy of Blackwell).

icles from developing erythroid cells sometimes may be seen within the endocytic vesicles of the central macrophage (Fig. 12), suggesting that the macrophage may pinch-off part of de-veloping red blood cells. In mouse bone marrow fixed with tannic acid, structures similar to gap junctions have been re-ported between macrophages and between macrophages and the surrounding erythroid cells, as well as between macro-

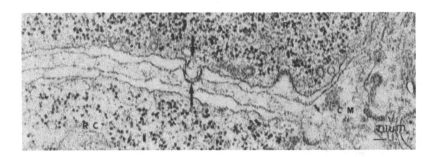

Fig. 12. Cytoplasmic processes of a central macrophage (CM) is running between two developing red cells (RC). In one area (arrows), an exocytic vesicle from a developing red cell appears within a complementary vesicle of the CM, suggesting that the latter cell may "pinch off" a portion of RC cytoplasm (× 57,000) (Tavassoli and Shaklai, 1979, courtesy of Blackwell).

phages and reticular cells.[23] In rat bone marrow, gap junctions are not revealed between macrophages or between macrophages and maturing erythroid cells, even when tannic acid fixation, lanthanum impregnation, or freeze fracture techniques are used. However, in freeze fracture replicas of central macrophages, structures resembling adhering junctions, possibly demosomes, have been seen (Fig. 10). Corresponding structures have also been demonstrated in lanthanum-impregnated preparations (Fig. 13). In freeze fracture specimens of erythroblastic islands, structures resembling intercellular bridges between the membranes of macrophages and erythroid cells have also been reported (Fig. 14).[3,17]

The outstanding morphologic characteristic of the central macrophage is the presence of a large number of inclusions, including breakdown products arising from ingested red cells, extruded nuclei of red cells, lysosomes and phagosomes (Figs. 15 and 16).[2,3,58–61] In the mouse, but not in rat bone marrow, the central macrophages are frequently loaded with paracrystaline inclusions in the cytoplasm that are usually surrounded by a single membrane profile and appear to contain hemoglobin.[58,76] The nucleus of the central macrophage is irregular in shape and

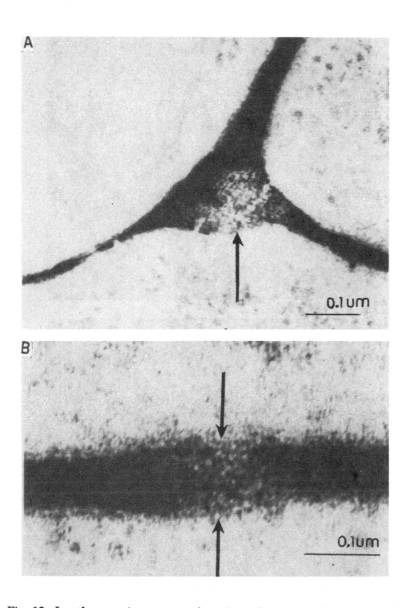

Fig. 13. Lanthanum-impregnated sections showing delineation of desmosomes by the tracer (arrows). The central dense stratum of the intercellular space appears in negative contrast (×158,000 and 220,000) (13a Shaklai and Tavassoli, 1979, courtesy of Academic; 13b Tavassoli and Shaklai, 1979, courtesy of Blackwell).

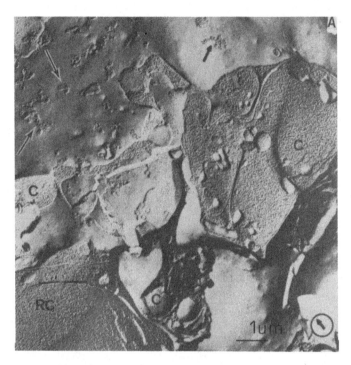

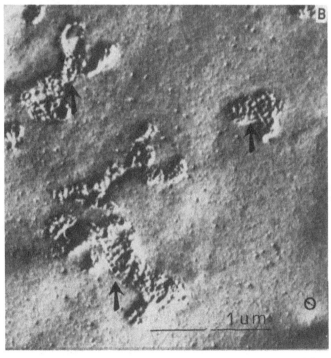

238

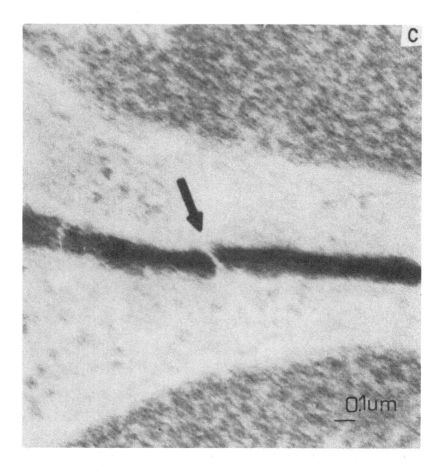

Fig. 14. A central macrophage dominates (a) and, in the left corner, is in contact with a developing red cell (RC) that is fractured transcytoplasmic. The path of the fracture has revealed mostly the protoplasmic face of the cell membrane in the central macrophage but because of its branching characteristics, the cytoplasm has also been revealed in some areas (C). Note on the macrophage membrane that there are patches of depression (arrows), some branching and extending into the cytoplasm. A higher magnification of these patches can be seen (b). In (c), lanthanum is used to trace the extracellular space between the two cells. Note the abrupt interruption of the tracer (arrow), suggesting cytoplasmic continuity between the two cells. This could correspond to areas of depression extending into the cytoplasm as seen by freeze-fracture techniques and could represent an intercellular cytoplasmic bridge (× 11,500, 43,000, and 60,000) (Tavassoli and Shaklai, 1979, courtesy of Blackwell).

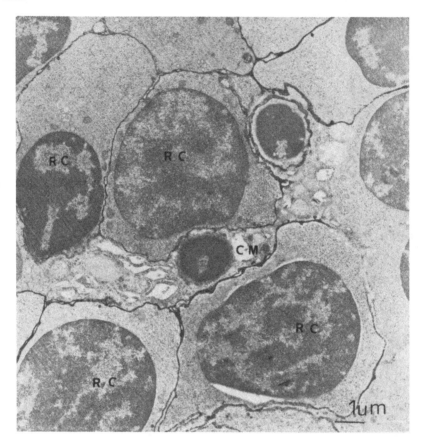

Fig. 15. Lanthanum-treated thin section of an erythroblastic island. The central macrophage (CM), surrounded by several maturing red cells (RC) contains distended profiles of rough endoplasmic reticulum and an ingested nucleus of a red cell (× 8400).

the chromatin condensed in masses of varying sizes, and these are located predominately under the nuclear envelope. Mitoses in the central macrophage is very rare.[74] Iron appears in two forms in the central macrophage. First as hemosiderin, it is derived from the breakdown of red cells and the rim of cytoplasm surrounding extruded red cell nuclei. This iron can be recognized by its diffuse blue color when applying Prussian Blue to smears studied by light microscopy. The second form

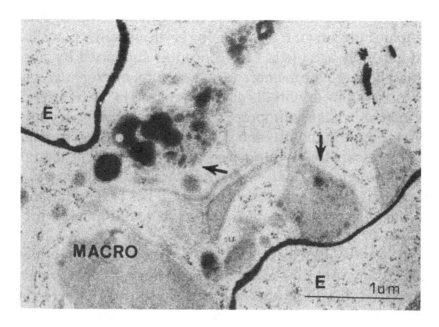

Fig. 16. Thin section of lanthanum-impregnated marrow tissue showing a central macrophage, (MACRO) in an erythroblastic island. The macrophage bordered by two erythroid cells (E), contained many phagosomes inclusions, some of them surrounded by a single membrane (× 39,000) (Tavassoli et al., 1980, courtesy of Springer-Verlag).

is ferritin which is the end product of the digested hemoglobin and can be seen by electron microscopy, either in lysosomes or the cell sap.[57,60]

It is generally accepted that the central macrophage is an important constituent of in vivo erythropoiesis. It is possible that the central macrophage elaborates certain factors that are transferred to the developing erythroid cells. Such a "nursing" function of the central macrophage was first suggested by Bessis, who assumed that ferritin is transported from the macrophage to the erythroblast and is taken up by the latter cell through a process of rhopheocytosis.[57,62,64,68,77,78] Although ferritin transport from the central macrophage to the developing erythroid cell could not be provided by other investigators,[5,8,65,79,80,81] the assumption that the central macrophage has a trophic function for the developing erythroid cell is plausible and generally accepted. This concept is supported by close contact between the membrane of the central macrophage and the surrounding erythroid cells and can lead to the transfer of hormones such as erythropoietin. In culture, however, erythropoiesis occurs without a central macrophage, but erythropoietin is necessary for erythropoiesis to occur in vitro. Although there is no evidence that erythropoietin is released by marrow macrophage in vivo or in cell culture,[81] it has been found that the liver macrophages are involved in erythropoietin production.[83–85]

The possibility exists that macrophages of the erythroblastic island produce or process erythropoietin that is then transferred directly to the erythroid cells through the membrane's channels of communications[3,17,23] and, therefore, cannot be detected even in cultures of marrow macrophages. These channels, formed by appositions of plasma membranes, are better perceived when tracers such as lanthanum and tannic acid are used to define the extracellular space,[17,23,86] or a freeze fracture technique is applied to disclose intramembranous structures (Figs. 11, 12, 14b, 14c, and 15).[3,17]

Further evidence supporting the existence of a functional relationship between the central macrophage and the maturing erythroid cell, derives from experimental work in which erythropoiesis is modified. Hypoxia, which stimulates red cell production, also leads to an increase in the central macrophage's size and enhances of its phagocytic activity.[59,60,74] Similar changes are seen following induction of server hemolysis.[87] On the other hand, when erythroid production is suppressed by hypertransfusion, the central macrophage is destroyed. This is then followed by rapid development of an adipocyte that replaces the macrophage to retain the fixed volume of marrow. The disappearance of central macrophages from the marrow is further followed by lack of erythrophagocytosis and the marrow's inability to respond to stimuli such as hemolytic stress that can be induced by phenylhydrazine.[88]

The importance of the central macrophage to in vivo erythropoiesis is additionally supported by the observation that during erythropoietic stress, ectopic erythropoiesis in liver sinusoids and heterotopic marrow transplants is preceded by migration of monocytes that can develop into central macrophages.[73]

Locomotion of erythroid cells in the erythoblastic island is an additional function that has been attributed to central macrophages. It has been suggested that erythroid cells move along the processes of the central macrophage that can then serve as a guide to give the locomotion a direction.[89] In this fashion, a mechanism for cell egress into the circulation has been attributed to macrophages.[24]

Perisinal Macrophage

A perisinal macrophage has no specific morphologic characteristics that may distinguish it from the central or other macrophages located in other parts of the hematopoietic cord. Its function has been explored predominately in rabbit bone marrow.[90,91] The cell is located preferentially in the vicinity of venous sinuses interspersed with adventitial cells. Similar to the adventitial cell, it covers varying proportions of the sinus endothelium's abluminal surface. Its cytoplasmic protrusions penetrate the endothelium, engulf senescent or defective red cells, and remove them from the circulation. The proportion of red cells removed in this fashion is not exactly known, but the perisinal macrophage is extensively engaged in the removal of senescent erythrocytes in some situations.

Macrophages Dispersed
in the Hematopoietic Cord

Morphologic features of these cells are similar to central and perisinal macrophages. They are distinguished from the fibroblastic reticular cells by large amounts of primary and secondary lysosomes and phagocytized materials. With the use of acid phosphatase staining, they can be easily recognized. They extend their cytoplasmic processes for long distances, making contact with the perisinal and central macrophages. These cells show intimate association with extracellular fibrillar deposits, similar to those described for the fibroblastic reticular cells.[16,92] The functional significance of these cells is not clarified. It has been suggested that they may take part in an interconnecting network of macrophages that are widely dispersed in the granulocytic microenvironment.[86]

Macrophages of Bone Marrow Origin in Long-Term Culture

Macrophages from mouse, human, and canine bone marrow have been grown in long-term bone marrow cultures. [36–8,40,41,45,93–95] Like fibroblastic reticular cells, they are highly adhesive and are necessary for the support of hemopoiesis in vitro.[96] Like other cells in LTMC, their characterization is controversial, and controversy still remains regarding which of the stromal components in culture is of bone marrow macrophage or fibroblast origin. Corresponding to the fibroblastic reticular cells, the characterization of macrophages is based on morphological, cytochemical, ultrastructural, and immunological features.

In light and phase microscopy, the macrophage appears pleomorphic, bipolar,[75] flattened or elongated, and interconnected as network-forming cells.[95] On cytochemical staining, it gives a positive reaction for nonspecific esterases and acid phosphatase.[47,75] It is highly phagocytic,[35,45] and its plasma membrane is negative when stained with polycationized ferritin in transmission electron microscopy. By scanning electron microscopy in human, canine, and mouse marrow cultures, the cell is usually small, 10-15 μm in diameter, exhibits membrane folding and ruffling (Fig. 4), and its surface is covered with microvilli.[35,42,95] By transmission electron microscopy, the cell has a round nucleus with a considerable amount of heterochromatin. Its cytoplasm is vesiculated and contains numerous dense granules. Its cell surface is covered with a variable number of microvilli (Fig. 5). Mouse macrophages in LTMC have recently been defined with the monoclonal antibody F4/80.[75] It has been shown that several cell types in LTMC, previously thought to be of fibroblastic origin, carry antigens that react with the antibody F4/80.[75,86,95,98] Applying this antibody to mouse marrow in vivo, positively-reacting cells have been found to be distributed throughout the hematopoietic compartment.

It is thought that in LTMC, macrophages create an interconnecting network through the granulopoietic regions of the culture.[86] The membrane appositions between neighboring macrophages in this network are impermeable to lanthanum, a finding that suggests a functional unity. Gap junctions have been detected between the progeny of canine macrophage colony-forming cells. These intercellular structures have been detected using the freeze fracture technique and lanthanum as a tracer to delineate the special structure of these junctions. Structures similar to gap junctions have been shown in mouse marrow, *in situ*, when tannic acid has been incorporated into the fixative.[23] However, these findings could not be corroborated with the use of freeze fracture technique, the optimal method for demonstration of a gap junction.

Additional information on morphologic and functional features of marrow macrophages have been obtained by cloning and analysis of various cellular components of the marrow stroma.[52,54,55] Two monocyte cell lines were derived in continuous liquid culture which cells exhibit a high number of cytoplasmic protrusions upon scanning electron microscopy. They have the capacity to degrade and process antigen, are dependent on colony-stimulating factors, and stain positively for acid phosphatase and nonspecific esterase.[99] These monocytic lines have the capacity to suppress adipogenesis in a cloned fibroblastic line that is derived from a marrow adherent cell line.

Other Cellular Components
of the Marrow Stroma

Adipocytes and endothelial cells are the important components of marrow stroma. These are discussed in detail in Chapters 7 and 9.

BRANCHED STROMAL CELLS. This stromal cell is distinctive in its appearance. It is an extensively branched cell that possesses a relatively dense cytoplasm with dilated nuclear cisternae and abundant endoplasmic reticulum. Mitochondria are seen in moderate numbers. The cell has a euchromatic nucleus and large nucleoli. Multinucleation is frequent. The cell is nonphagocytic, does not contain acid phosphatase activity, and is associated with extensive hemopoiesis.[11,88,100] The origin and function of this cell and its relationships to other cell types are not yet clear.

A STROMAL CELL RECOGNIZED BY LANTHANUM UPTAKE. This cell has been described in rat bone marrow. It is widespread in the hematopoietic compartment and is associated with both erythropoietic and granulopoietic areas of marrow parenchyma. This cell displays a light branching cytoplasm with very few cytoplasmic organelles, sparse endoplasmic reticulum, and few mitochondria. This cell can be distinguished from other stromal cells by their preferential uptake of tracer lanthanum in low concentrations (Fig. 17).[101] Its function is not yet known.

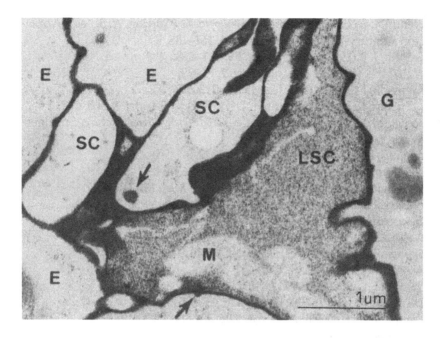

Fig. 17. Thin section of rat marrow tissue impregnated with lanthanum in the concentration of 5 mM. In this concentration, the tracer remained confined to the extracellular space with no uptake in erythroid (E), granulocytic (G), or many stromal cells (SC). The only cell type that took up the tracer in this concentration was the light stromal cell (LSC) that could be readily identified in moderately low power micrographs. The tracer appeared diffusely through the cell sap and organelles such as mitochondria (M), rending the otherwise light cytoplasm dense (× 33,500) (Tavassoli et al., 1980, courtesy of Springer-Verlag).

References

[1]Moore, M. A. S. (1975) *Adv. Bioscience* **16,** 87–96.
[2]Weiss, L. (1976) *Anat. Rec.* **186,** 161–184.
[3]Shaklai, M. and Tavassoli, M. J. (1979) *Ultrastruct. Res.* **69,** 343–361.
[4]Lichtman, J. (1981) *Exp. Hematol.* **9,** 391–410.
[5]Tavassoli, M. and Yoffey, J. M. (1983) *Bone Marrow: Structure and Function,* Liss, New York, pp. 47–64.
[6]Curry, J. L., Trentin, J. J. and Wolf, N. (1967) *J. Exp. Med.* **125,** 703–720.

[7]Trentin, J. J. (1970) *Regulation of Hemopoiesis* (Gordon, A. S., ed.) Apple-ton-Century-Crofts, New York, pp. 161–186.

[8]Trentin, J. J. (1971) *Am. J. Pathol.* **65**, 621–628.

[9]Wolf, N. S. (1974) *Cell Tissue Kinet.* **7**, 89–98.

[10]Tavassoli, M. (1975) *Exp. Hematol.* **3**, 213–226.

[11]LaPushin, R. W. and Trentin, J. J. (1977) *Exp. Hematol.* **5**, 505–522.

[12]Bessis, M. (1973) *Living Blood Cells and Their Ultrastructure*, Springer-Verlag, New York, pp. 477–517.

[13]Kaplow, L. S. (1955) *Blood* **10**, 1023–1029.

[14]Loffler, H. (1961) *Folia Haematol* (Leipzig) **6**, 164.

[15]Trubowitz, S. and Masek, B. (1979) *J. Exp. Med.* **150**, 919–937.

[16]Westen, H. and Bainton, D. F. (1979) *J. Exp. Med.* **150**, 919–937.

[17]Tavassoli, M. and Shaklai, M. (1979) *Br. J. Haematol.* **41**, 303–307.

[18]Weiss, L. (1970) *Blood* **36**, 189–208.

[19]Tavassoli, M. (1977) *Br. J. Haematol.* **35**, 25–32.

[20]Weiss, L. (1965) *J. Morph.* **117**, 467–537.

[21]Campbel, F. R. (1972) *Am. J. Anat.* **135**, 521–536.

[22]Tavassoli, M. (1978) *Exp. Hematol.* **6**, 257–269.

[23]Campbel, F. R. (1980) *Anat. Rec.* **196**, 101–117 .

[24]Campbel, F. R. (1982) *Anat. Rec.* **203**, 365–374.

[25]Tavassoli, M. (1979) *Br. J. Haematol.* **41**, 297–302.

[26]McCusky, R. S., Meinke, H. A., and Towsend, S. F. (1972) *Blood* **39**, 697–712.

[27]McCusky, R. S. and Meink, H. A. (1977) *Kidney Hormones* (Fisher, J. W., ed.) Academic, London, pp. 311–327.

[28]Noordegraaf, E. M., Erken-Versluis, E. A., and Ploemacher, R. E. (1981) *Exp. Hematol.* **9**, 326–331.

[29]Bentley, S. A., Alabaster, O., and Foidart, J. M. (1981) *Br. J. Haematol.* **48**, 287–291.

[30]Bentley, S. A. (1982) *Br. J. Haematol.* **50**, 1–6.

[31]Ploemacher, R. E., Piersma, A. H., and Brockbank, K. G. M. (1984) *Blood Cells* **10**, 341–367.

[32]Piersma, A. H., Brockbank, K. G. M., Ploemacher, R. E., Van Viellt, E., Brakel-van Peer, K. M. J., and Visser, P. J. (1985) *Exp. Hematol.* **13**, 237–243.

[33]Friedenstein, A. J., Chailakhyan, R. K., Latsink, A. N. B., Panasuk, F., and Keiliss-Borok, Z. V. (1974) *Transplantation* **17**, 331–340.

[34]Friedenstein, A. J., Deriglasova, U. F., Kulagina, N. N., Panasuk, A. F., Rudakowa, S. F., Luria, E. A., and Rudakow, I. A. (1974) *Exp. Hematol.* **2**, 83–92.

[35]Wilson, F. D., Grady, L. O., McNeill, C. J., and Munn, S. L. (1974) *Exp. Hematol.* **2**, 343–354.

[36]Dexter, T. M. and Testa, N. G. (1976) *Meth. Cell Biol.* **14**, 387–405.

[37]Dexter, T. M., Allen, T. D., and Lajtha, L. G. (1977) *J. Cell Physiol.* **91**, 335–344.

[38]Wilson, F. D., Tavassoli, M., Greenberg, B. R., Hinds, D., and Klein, A. K. (1981) *Stem Cells* **1**, 15–29.

[40]Farnes, P. and Barker, B. E. (1963) *Exp. Cell Res.* **29**, 278–288.

[41]Tavassoli, M. (1982) *Scan. Elect. Micro.* **1**, 349–357.

[42]Tavassoli, M. and Takahashi, K. (1982) *Am. J. Anat.* **164**, 91–111.

[43]Bentley, S. A. and Foidart, J. M. (1980) *Blood* **56**, 1006–1012.

[44]Bentley, S. A., Tralka, T. S., and Alabaster, O. (1981) *Exp. Hematol.* **9**, 313–318.

[45]Reinchke, U., Hsieh, P. H., Mawch, P., Hellman, S., and Chen, L. B. (1982) *J. Histochem. Cytochem.* **30**, 235–244.

[46]Weiss, L. (1970) *Regulation of Hemopoiesis* (Gordon, A. S., ed.) Appleton-Century-Crofts, New York, pp. 79–92.

[47]Allen, T. D. and Dexter, T. M. (1983) *Scanning Electron Microscopy* (Johari, O., ed.) SEM Inc., Chicago, vol. IV, pp. 1851–1866.

[48]Dexter, T. M. (1979) *Clin. Haematol.* **8**, 453–467.

[49]Dexter, T. M. (1982) *Cellular and Molecular Biology of Hemopoietic Stem Cell Differentiation* (Mak, T. W. and McCulloch, E. A., eds.) Liss, New York, p. 87.

[50]Zucker-Franklin, D., Grusky, G., and Marcus, A. (1978) *Lab. Invest.* **38**, 620–628.

[51]Tavassoli, M. and Friedenstein, A. (1983) *Am. J. Hematol.* **15**, 195–203.

[52]Harigaya, K., Cronkite, E. P., Miller, M. E., and Shadduck, R. K. (1981) *Proc. Natl. Acad. Sci.* **78**, 6963–6966.

[53]Kodoma, H. A., Amagai, Y., Koyama, H., and Kasai, S. (1982) *J. Cell Physiol.* **112**, 89–95.

[54]Lanotte, M., Scott, T. D., Dexter, M., and Allen, T. D. (1982) *J. Cell Physiol.* **111**, 117–186.

[55]Zipori, D., Friedman, A., Tamir, M., Silverberg, D., and Malik, Z. (1984) *J. Cell Physiol.* **118**, 143–152.

[56]Besis, M. (1958) *Rev. Hematol.* **13**, 8–11.

[57]Besis, M. and Breton Gorius, J. (1962) *Blood* **19**, 635–663.

[58]Berman, I. (1967) *J. Ultrastruct. Res.* **17**, 291–313.

[59]Ben Ishay, Z. and Joffey, J. M. (1971) *Isr. J. Med. Sci.* **7**, 948–962.

[60]Ben Ishay, Z. and Joffey, J. M. (1971) *J. Reticuloendothel. Soc.* **10**, 482–500.

[61]Ben Ishay, Z. and Joffey, J. M. (1971) *Lab. Invest.* **26**, 637–647.

[62]Sorensen, G. D. (1962) *Am. J. Path.* **40**, 297–314.

[63]Sorensen, G. D. (1961) *Lab. Invest.* **10**, 178–189.

[64]Grasso, J. A., Swift, H., and Ackerman, G. A. (1962) *J. Cell Biol.* **14**, 235–241.

[65]Zamboni, L. (1965) *J. Ultrastruct. Res.* **12**, 509–517.

[66]Chui, D. H. and Russell, E. S. (1974) *Develop. Biol.* **40,** 256–269.

[67]Fukuda, T. (1974)*Virchows Arch. B.* **16,** 249–270.

[68]Orlich, D., Gordon, A. S., and Rhodin, J. A. (1965) *J. Ultrastruct. Res.* **13,** 516–542 .

[69]Pictet, R., Orci, L., Forssman, W. G., Girardier, L. Z. (1969) *Zellforsch Mikrosk. Anat.* **96,** 372–399.

[70]Djaldeti, M., Bessler, H., and Rifkind, R. H. (1972) *Blood* **39,** 826–841.

[71]Tavassoli, M. and Crosby, H. W. (1968) *Sciences* **161,** 54–56.

[72]Tavassoli, M. and Weiss, L. (1971) *Anat. Rec.* **171,** 477–494.

[73]Ploemacher, R. E. and Van Soest, P. L. (1977) *J. Cell Tissue Res.* **178,** 435–461.

[74]Joffey, J. M. and Yaffe, P. (1980) *J. Reticuloendothel. Soc.* **28,** 37–47.

[75]Dexter, T. M., Spooncer, E., Schofield, R., Lord, B. I., and Simmons, P. (1984) *Blood Cells* **10,** 315–339.

[76]Shaklai, M. and Tavassoli, M. (1977) *Lancet* **2,** 305 (letter).

[77]Policard, M. and Besis, M. (1958) *Acad. Sci.* **246,** 3194–3197.

[78]Tanaka, Y., Bricher, G., and Bull, B. (1966) *Blood* **28,** 758–769.

[79]Jones, O. P. (1964) *Anat. Rec.* **148,** 296.

[80]Jones, O. P. (1965) *J. Natl. Cancer Inst.* **35,** 139–146.

[81]Zamboni, L. (1965) *J. Ultrastruct. Res.* **12,** 525–541.

[82]Gordon, L. I., Miller, W. J., Bronder, R. F., Zanjani, E. D., and Jacob, H. S. (1980) *Blood* **55,** 1047–1050.

[83]Peschle, C., Marone, G., Genovese, A., Magli, I. A., and Condorelli, M. (1976) *Blood* **47,** 325–338.

[84]Peschle, C., Marone, G., Genovese, A., Magli, I. A., and Condorelli, M. (1976) *Br. J. Haematol.* **32,** 105–119.

[85]Gruber, D. F., Zucali, J. R., and Mirand, E. A. (1976) *Exp. Hematol.* **5,** 392–398.

[86]Allen, T. D. and Dexter, T. M. (1984) *Exp. Hematol.* **12,** 517–521.

[87]Tavassoli, M. (1974) *Acta. Anat.* **90,** 608–616.

[88]Brookoff, D. and Weiss, L. (1982) *Blood* **60,** 1337–1344.

[89]Besis, M., Mize, C., and Prenant, M. (1978) *Blood Cells* **4,** 155–174.

[90]Tavassoli, M. (1974) *J. Reticuloendoth. Soc.* **15,** 163–169.

[91]Tavassoli, M. (1977) *Br. J. Haematol.* **36,** 323–326.

[92]Hulme, D. A., Robinson, A. P., MacPherson, G. G., and Gordon, S. (1983) *J. Exp. Med.* **158,** 1522–1536.

[93]Allen, T. D. and Dexter, T. M. (1976) *Differentiation* **6,** 191–194.

[94]Moor, M. A. S., Sheridan, A. P. C., Allen, T. D., and Dexter, T. M. (1979) *Blood* **54,** 775–793.

[95]Harrison, B., Reincke, U. , Smith, M., and Hellman, S. (1984) *Blood Cells* **10,** 451–466.

[96]Allen, T. D. and Dexter, T. M. (1976) *Blood Cells* **2**, 591–606.

[97]Austyn, M. M. and Gordon, S. (1981) *Eur. J. Immunol.* **11**, 805–815.

[98]Simmans, P. J., Allen, T. D., Dexter, T. M., Hirsch, S., and Gordon, S. (1983) *Exp. Hematol.* **11**, 144.

[99]Zipori, D., Duksin, D., Tamir, M., Argaman, A., Toledo, J., and Malik, Z. (1985) *J. Cell Physiol.* **122**, 81–90.

[100]Brookoff, D., Maggio-Price, L., Bernstein, S., and Weiss, L. (1982) *Blood* **59**, 646–651.

[101]Tavassoli, M., Aoki, M., and Shaklai, M. (1980) *Exp. Hematol.* **5**, 68–57.

Chapter 7

Stromal Cells in Long-Term Bone Marrow Cultures

Peter J. Quesenberry

Introduction

The introduction of systems for the growth of long-term liquid culture of murine marrow cells has provided unique opportunities for the study of the role of accessory stromal cells in regulating hemopoiesis.[1-3] A number of in vivo observations (reviewed elsewhere in this volume) including those on the selective anatomical localization of different differentiation pathways after marrow transplant,[4-6] the organ distribution of hemopoiesis under stressed conditions (endotoxin, anemia),[7-8] and the stromal deficit in SL/SLd[9-10] mice all provided evidence for the existence of an hematopoietic inductive microenvironment. But these in vivo systems did not lend themselves to studies on the specific stromal cells involved in such regulation. Bessis and colleagues[11] have provided intriguing morphologic observations indicating that macrophages may act as "nurse cells" for erythroid cells. Weiss and coworkers[12-15] and Chamberlin et al.[16] have described the adventitial reticular cell (ARC) of the marrow as an interesting candidate stromal cell. This "ARC" abutts the abluminal side of sinusoidal endothelial cells[17,18] and sends processes throughout the marrow sinusoid touching many different cells and providing an obvious means of "networking" among the marrow cell populations. Further work has indicated that an alkaline phosphatase positive reticular cell, similar in many respects to the ARC, appears to be selectively associated with granulocytes.[19] These two candidate stromal cells will be of particular interest as we discuss the adherent cells that are critical to in vitro long-term lymphohemopoiesis in culture.

As noted above, the in vitro system first established by Dexter and colleagues for long-term culture of hematopoietic cells[1-3] and later by Whitlock and Witte[20,21] for the long-term culture of lymphoid cells has allowed for the detailed study of adherent stromal cells necessary for growth in these systems. In both murine systems, long-term growth is dependent upon the formation of an adherent layer by the marrow cells. In the Dexter system, progressive adherent layer formation is seen from initiation to 2–4 wk of growth and if an "adequate" adherent layer forms, then growth may continue dependent upon the strain of mouse[22] and the lot of horse serum[23,24] for many months. If an adherent layer does not form, growth rapidly declines. Furthermore, if adherence is prevented by utilization of siliconized flasks, growth rapidly ceases.[25] Other conditions that lead to poor stromal formation also lead to poor growth in the system. This includes the inadequate lots of horse serum or the use of stromal cells from other organs such as the spleen.[26] Further indications that the adherent layer plays a central supporting role in Dexter cultures are the findings that the stem cells with the highest proliferative and self-renewal capacity appear to be resident in the stroma, giving rise to supernatant stem cells with less proliferative and self-renewal capacity.[27] Finally, the stromal deficiency of the SL/SLd mouse has been reproduced in the Dexter culture system[28] once again indicating the critical nature of stromal cell support for maintenance of hemopoiesis in this system.

Many early studies ignored, or did not address, the fact that the stroma is a rich source of stem cells. Thus, studies in which the stroma was refed with marrow or directly manipulated, (i.e., exposed to radiation or drugs) and then the supernatant, stem cell, or differentiated cell production evaluated as a measure of stromal function are, of necessity, difficult to interpret. In many cases, there were no controls for the potential effects of the experimental manipulations on the stromal stem cells. In addition, it is important to emphasize that the lots of horse serum utilized in the Dexter culture may dramatically change the nature of growth in this system.[23,24] The observation that supplementation of hydrocortisone allowed growth with many otherwise "poor" horse serum lots,[29] has, in part, overcome these difficulties, but the marked variability between different serum lots, with regard to the basic nature of both adherent and stem cell growth in these systems, remains an important factor that may explain many discrepancies currently present in the literature.

It is clear that with an appropriate stromal cell formation, a wide variety of hematopoietic stem cells, are supported in the Dexter system. These include CFU-S,[1-3,30] GM-CFU-C,[1-3,30] CFU-Meg,[31] CFU-diffusion chamber,[32] and the high proliferative potential colony forming cell.[33,34] In addition, stem cells selectively responsive to partially purified GM-CSA or pure IL-3 are also supported in this system.[35] Lymphoid cell growth is not supported in the classical Dexter system although cells with the capacity for in vivo B lymphocyte repopulation are present.[36,37]

We will deal with the true B-lymphocyte potential further below.

Cell Types in Adherent Layer

Initial studies on the adherent layer supporting myeloid growth indicated that a mixture of cells was present. The adherent layer, of course, included hemopoietic stem cells, granulocytes, macrophages, and monocytes. In addition to these primary hemopoietic cells, Dexter and colleagues described the presence of phagocytic mononuclear cells, flattened cells forming a confluent monolayer and adipocytes.[1-3,25] In addition, they also referred to endothelial cells in various publications. The basic nature of the cells supporting growth in this system was clarified in work by Tavassoli and Takahashi[38] and Song and Quesenberry.[39] The former group, in careful studies utilizing indices of phagocytosis, scanning electron microscopy, and transmission electron microscopy, described the presence of two basic cell types. One was a large alkaline phosphatase, positive epithelioid type cell with a diameter greater than 100 μm containing numerous thin, elongated mitochondria and adhering strongly to polycationized ferritin, indicating a negatively-charged cell surface. These particular cells "blanketed large areas." This epithelioid cell appeared to exist in two different phases, a synthetic phase in which the cell contained numerous profiles of rough endoplasmic reticulum and a storage phase containing numerous storage granules and lipid inclusions. The macrophage cell types were smaller, 10–15 μm in diameter, phagocytosed latex and carbon particles and contained lysosomes. Their surface did not stain with polycationic ferritin and they were acid phosphatase positive. Both the epithelioid cells and macrophages appeared to have the capacity to accumulate fat under appropriate culture conditions. Tavassoli and Takahashi[38] further speculated, based on work by Weiss and Faucet[40] and Sutton and Weiss,[41] that there may be a common monocytic stem cell for both the macrophage and epithelioid cell types. Work by Song and Quesenberry,[39] and Gualtieri et al.[42] also indicated that these same two cell types were probably the critical components for marrow support in the Dexter culture system. Their studies, utilizing both in vivo irradiation and marrow explant to culture and in vitro irradiation of preformed adherent layers, indicated the existence of two relatively radioresistant cell types, i.e., macrophages and large alkaline phosphatase positive epithelioid cells. In the work by Song et al.,[39] mice were exposed to 1000R in vivo and 24 h later, marrow was harvested and used to establish adherent layers in the Dexter liquid culture system. In this setting, no hemopoiesis occurred, but adherent cells capable of growth and support of stem cells from long-term liquid cultures (out 8–10 wk) were present. If explant cultures were established at relatively low inoculum levels, colonies of adherent cells were seen (Fig. 1) that consisted of the above two noted cell types. Colonies were either mixed (the majority) (Fig. 2), or consisted of pure populations of macrophages or epithelioid cells (Fig. 1). These data further suggested that there might be a common precursor stem cell for macrophage and epithelioid types of adherent stromal cells (Fig. 3). However, in these studies, individual adherent macrophages were scattered throughout the flask bottom so there was never a truly isolated colonial type. If these stromal colonies were overlaid with supernatant cells from long-term murine Dexter culture, which were incapable of forming stromal cells themselves, hemopoiesis as evidenced by peroxidase positive cells occurred directly on the epithelioid, but not the macrophage colonies. These data suggested that the large epithelioid cell may have a role in directly nurturing hemopoietic stem cells. The studies by Gualtieri et al.[42] indicated that after in vitro exposure to 950R irradiation, 95% of the residual stromal cells were either consistent with the macrophage cell

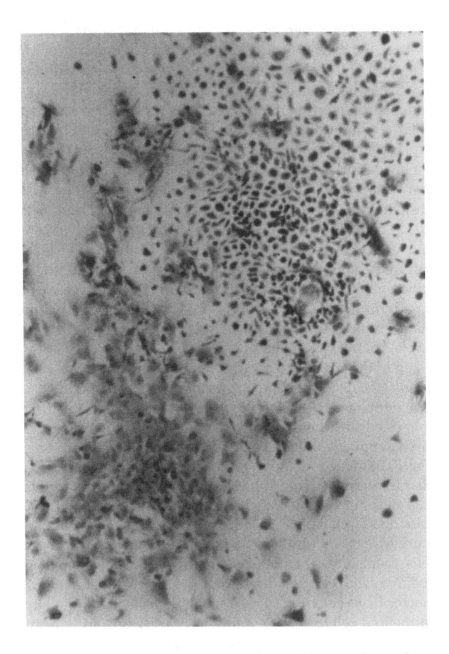

Fig. 1. Stromal cell colonies—a mixed colony and a macrophage colony at 1 wk of growth (reproduced courtesy of Song and Quesenberry (1984) *Exp. Hematol.* **12**, 523 (Fig. 5b).

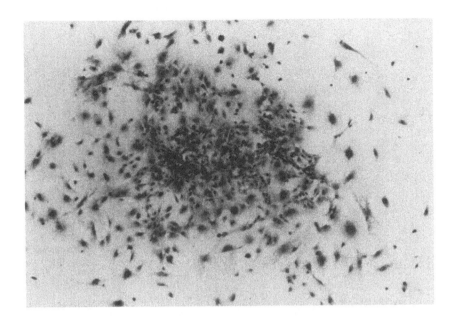

Fig. 2. Stromal cell colonies—a mixed colony at 1 wk of growth (reproduced courtesy of Song and Quesenberry (1984) *Exp. Hematol.* **12,** 523 (Fig. 5a).

type, or the large alkaline phosphatase positive epithelioid cell type; however, a small percentage (less than 3%) of cells could not be accurately categorized. In this setting, it was clear that these stromal cells were potent sources of hemopoietic growth factors (*vide infra*). In addition, in work by Dexter and colleagues, "blanket cells" actually overlying macrophage cell types have been described.[43]

The question of whether endothelial cells are an important component of the Dexter culture stroma has been controversial. Based on morphologic evidence, Dexter and colleagues[1-3,25,43] initially described endothelial cells, whereas Bentley and associates[44,45] presented evidence based upon Factor VIII staining and collagen biosynthesis indicating that the cells in the culture system were basically fibroblastic and not endothelial. Zuckerman and colleagues,[46] however, found

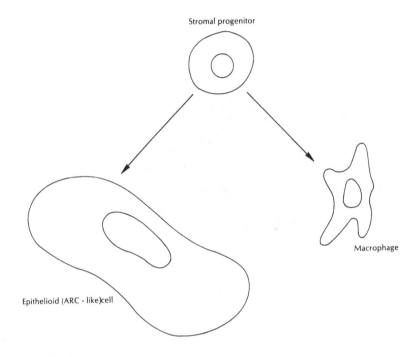

Fig. 3. Model for stromal progenitor cell giving rise to macrophages and epitheliod (ARC-like) cells.

both Factor VIII positive staining cells and type 4 collagen in the stromal cells of their in vitro murine liquid culture system, indicating that at least a percentage of the stromal cells were endothelial in type. Gualtieri et al.,[42] however, were unable to find factor VIII positive cells although the factor VIII antibody preparations clearly cross-reacted with murine factor VIII on both endothelial and megakaryocyte cells. More recently, work by Waterhouse and colleagues[47] has indicated that Dexter stromal cells produce collagens type 1, 3, and 4, along with fibronectin, confirming the work of Zuckerman[46] and once again raising the question of the presence of endothelial cells in these cultures. In these studies, a unique small mol wt collagen was also detected. However, it should be noted that collagen subtypes are not a definitive indication of cell type and, in fact, may change with prolonged cell culture.[48]

The question of the role of adipocytes in supporting long-term marrow growth from different species has concerned a number of investigators, some presenting positive correlations of the presence of adipocytes with hemopoiesis,[1,49,50] and others indicating a lack of correlation with this cell type and hemopoietic support.[51] Work by Tavassoli and Takahashi,[38] as noted above, indicates that both macrophages and the epithelioid cells could become fat cells, but work by Simmons and colleagues,[52] utilizing the monoclonal antibody F4/80 that marks monocyte–macrophages, has indicated that all of the adipocytes in their system were nonmacrophage. In addition, longitudinal observations of culture by Song and Quesenberry[39] indicated that fat cells developed in the large epithelioid cells and not in the macrophage-like cells. Thus, the bulk of evidence seems to indicate that the adipocytes in this culture system may represent the storage phase of these large alkaline, phosphatase-positive epithelioid cells. But whether fat accumulation *per se* is an important component or necessary for the support of hemopoiesis, or possibly an indication that the system is aging and running down is still not established. Possible insights from the derivation of cell lines from these adherent stromal cells are dealt with in a separate chapter in this book.

The question of interactions between these stromal cells or the stromal and hemopoietic cells is also an important one. In studies dealing with junctional structures in hematopoietic tissues, typical gap junctions are generally not found.[53,54] Pits and vesicles, however, are common in hemopoietic tissues probably involving endocytosis and representing a means of direct transfer of vesicles between cells.[53] In Tavassoli and Takahashi's work,[38] widespread cellular interactions were observed in the culture system in the stromal layer. The interactions, however, were mostly between macrophages and epithelioid cells with both cells type extending projections toward each other and epithelioid cells often encompassing macrophages. Dexter and colleagues[43] have noted coated vesicles in regions of membrane contact between macrophages and hemopoietic cells, possibly indicating a mode of short-range message transfer. They utilized the electron dense tracer lanthanum to establish whether occluding or tight junctions existed at the surface of cells. In the cobblestone regions of mouse cultures, they found no evidence of tight junctions between macrophages and granulocytes, but did between macrophages, possibly indicating a means of macrophage–macrophage communication. Overall, present data seem to indicate the presence of two critical stromal cells. The first, a large alkaline, phosphatase-positive epithelioid cell that, in many respects, appears to be similar to the adventitial reticular cell (ARC) described in vivo.[12,13] This cell is also alkaline, phosphatase-positive and appears to be a particularly important cell for nurturing granulocytes.[19] The ARC in vivo appears to extend processes throughout marrow tissue whereas the large epithelioid cell in vitro also appears to have extensive and widespreading processes enabling it to contact a number of different cells. The second basic cell type is a macrophage, and it is particularly interesting that this is the other basic type described in human marrow, possibly representing an analog of the nurse cell of Bessis.[11] Along these lines, Dexter and co-workers have described manipulations that allow the Dexter system to support erythropoiesis, i.e., inclusion of erythropoietin-rich serum. In this situation, erythroid cell maturation takes place in association with macrophages.[43] This appears to be analogous with the in vivo situation. Thus, both of these cell types in vitro appear to recapitulate critical in vivo stromal cells. Characteristics of these two adherent cell types are summarized in Table 1.

The capacity of these cell types to act as stroma was established by Song and Quesenberry.[39] In their studies, cell

Table 1
Adherent Stromal Cell Characteristics

Characteristic	Epitheloid "ARC-like" cell	Macrophage
Size	Large	Smaller
Growth Pattern	Confluent	Individual
Phagocytosis	No	Yes
Acid phosphatase	–	+
Alkaline Phostphatase	+	–
Nonspecific esterase	–	+
Factor VIII	–	–
Directly support growth of hemopoietic cells	+	–

populations explanted from mice exposed to 1000R, which consisted of these two basic cell types, were shown to be able to support CFU-S and CFU-C growth for at least 6 wk of culture. These studies also indicated the stromal cells were relatively radioresistant, in contrast to a number of earlier studies.[55,56] Certainly the CFU-F, which may be a model for the fibroblastic or epithelioid-type adherent cell, was found to have a radiation sensitivity reasonably close to hemopoietic stem cells.[58] However, it is not clear if the CFU-F is in fact an adequate model of hemopoietic stromal cells. A number of studies have presented data indicating that stromal cells were relatively or possibly exquisitely radiosensitive,[56,57] but a major problem with these early studies was a failure to disassociate the effect of this radiation on adherent stromal hemopoietic stem cells from effects on stromal function. In addition, differences in serum supplementation, altering the basic characteristics of growth in these systems, may also have contributed to these divergent results.[23,24] Overall, however, it appears that the stromal cells are relatively radioresistant and capable of supporting liquid culture hemopoiesis.

Growth Factor Production
by Adherent Cells

In addition, these same stromal cells appear to be capable of producing a variety of hemopoietic growth factors that may be adequate to explain all of the aspects of in vitro cell support.[39,42,57] Earlier studies indicated that the system may not produce hemopoietic colony stimulating factors[3,58,59] and, in fact, this data was utilized to propose that these factors may not be important in the regulation of hemopoiesis. However, as we will outline below, the negative results first presented were probably owing to the fact that the colony stimulating factors are rapidly absorbed and utilized in the system,[42,57] as first suggested by Tavassoli and Takahashi.[38] CSA activity had been detected in other studies,[30] but Heard and colleagues[57] were the first to show significant stromal-derived CSA activity utilizing an agar overlay system. Adopting this agar overlay system, Gualtieri et al.[42] demonstrated that adherent layers were capable of producing granulocyte–macrophage–megakaryocyte CSA. They also showed that increasing levels of hemopoietic colony stimulating activities were seen with increasing levels of irradiation from 250 to 950 rads in vitro X-irradiation. Increasing CSA production, as detected in agar overlayers containing target bone marrow cells, correlated inversely with the level of hemopoiesis, particularly the level of granulocyte production. Furthermore, mixture experiments, in which normal stroma replete with granulocytes and megakaryocytes was added back to irradiated stroma, effectively blocked growth factor production.

Finally, the addition of an exogenous source of GM-CSA to normal Dexter cultures resulted in the recovery of only approximately 30% of activity after 7 d. Addition of the same amounts of GM-CSA to irradiated stroma resulted in recovery of more than 70% of activity. These data strongly indicated that: (l) stroma was a potent source of hemopoietic colony stimulating activities and that; and (2) failure to detect activities in this system was probably related to the rapid utilization and/or degradation of these factors by end cell progeny of the hemopoietic system, most likely granulocytes. Further studies with this same system indicated the production of colony stimulating factor–1 under baseline conditions, confirming reports by others,[59] but there were no elevations after irradiation. In addition, at the higher levels of radiation (750 and 950 rads), megakaryocyte colonies, mixed megakaryocyte–macrophage–granulocyte colonies, large granulocyte–macrophage colonies, and colonies of early myeloid or possibly blast cells were seen. This indicated the production of multilineage CSA(s) in this system. An antibody to CSF-l at high titer blocked the majority of granulocyte–macrophage colony formation, but had no effect on, and in several instances appeared to augment, megakaryocyte colony formation. Further results indicated that these stroma were capable of producing growth factors that stimulated the IL-3 dependent cell line, FDC-Pl.[35,60] This was particularly interesting, because IL-3 is the factor identified in WEHI-3 conditioned media (cm) that is responsible for the induction of marrow cell lines from long-term Dexter marrow cultures.[61,62] However, antibody to IL-3 did not block the FDC-Pl stimulatory activity indicating that it was not IL-3.[35] The growth factors stimulating both murine marrow mixed lineage colonies and FDC-Pl cells were markedly increased when the stroma were treated with the lectin, pokeweed mitogen, and studies utilizing a specific antibody to murine GM-CSF and CSF-l have indicated that the activity stimulating the factor dependent cell line is GM-CSF whereas those stimulating marrow colonies are GM-CSF plus CSF-l.[35] However, only GM-CSF (not CSF-l) is increased by exposure of stromal cells to pokeweed mitogen. In addition, recent evidence indicates the presence of a growth factor that synergizes with CSF-l to give

Table 2

Growth Factor Production by Adherent Stromal Cell

Activity	Assay
CSF–1[a]	RIA
GM–CSA[b]	Bioassay and antibody inhibition
Synergistic activity	Synergizes stimulation of colony formation by CSF–1
Factor dependent cell line proliferation	3H–TdR incorporation into FDC–P1 cells (not blocked by anti-IL–3[c] antibody)

[a]CSF–1, colony stimulating factor–1.
[b]GM–CSA, granulocyte–macrophage colony stimulating activity.
[c]IL–3, Interleukin–3.

large macrophage colonies.[63] It is interesting that lithium, which has been demonstrated to stimulate a wide variety of hemopoietic stem cells in the Dexter culture system,[23,30–33] appears to act via a radioresistant adherent marrow cell[23] and that present evidence indicates this action to be mediated by the production of growth factors probably including the synergizing activity and GM-CSF.[63] Others have reported on the presence of bioactivities in Dexter culture that may either stimulate or inhibit DNA synthesis of CFU-S, dependent upon the interval of culture from which the conditioned media is collected,[64] but the relationship of these activities to GM-CSF, synergistic activity, or CSF-l is unclear. Growth factor production by adherent Dexter culture cells is summarized in Table 2. Further insights on stromal growth factor production, derived from the study of the TC-l cell line[39] isolated from adherent stromal cells, will be expanded upon below.

Some additional issues regarding the murine adherent stromal cells in the Dexter culture warrant comment. We have already emphasized the importance of the serum supplementation in this system and this has been well documented in several articles.[23,24] The role of collagen production and extracellular matrix will be dealt with separately in this book. Certainly evidence suggests that collagen production, and possibly mucopolysaccharide production, are important aspects of stromal support of hemopoiesis.[43-46] A number of additional modulating influences undoubtedly exist. The production of prostaglandins,[65] interferon,[66] Interleukin-1,[67] and probably a number of other potential modulators of hemopoietic cell growth and differentiation undoubtedly plays an important role in the regulation of in vitro hemopoiesis by stromal cells. The possible significance and role of the fibroblast colony forming units (CFU-F)[68-71] remains unclear.

CFU-F may, in fact, be a model of the epithelioid component of the stroma described above. If this is so, studies on its growth, differentiation, and factor production may provide important insights into the regulation of hematopoiesis. Piersma and colleagues[72] have indicated that CFU-F may be a noncycling cell that is positive for fibronectin, lipid, alkaline phosphatase, and nonspecific esterase, but nonphagocytic and without desmosomes and negative for Mac-1. Perhaps this cell may represent the progenitor of both the macrophage and epithelioid cell (Fig. 3). Further studies appear warranted regarding the relevance of this cell in microenvironment studies.

Studies in Other Species Including Human

A number of other species have been studied regarding the characteristics of the in vitro liquid culture of bone marrow. Significant species variation has been found to exist,[65] but perhaps studies of greatest note are those of Eastment and Ruscetti[65,73] on the Syrian hamster. In this species, impressive long-term marrow growth and proliferation exists for both erythropoiesis and granulopoiesis in the absence of an adherent monolayer. In fact, growth improves with the removal of an adherent monolayer apparently removing growth inhibitors. Thus, here we have an example of long-term sustained hemopoiesis in the absence of adherent cells.

Eastment and Ruscetti summarized differences between species regarding long-term marrow growth that have been previously reported.[65] Granulocyte production was found in long-term marrow cultures from mouse,[1] hamster,[73] treeshrew,[74] and human,[75] as was blast cell and macrophage production. Megakaryocyte production had not been observed in the treeshrew and human, and lymphoid production was observed only in the human.[65] In addition, erythropoiesis occurred in the presence of erythropoietin with both mouse and hamster,[76,77] but the data was unclear in treeshrew and human. Optimal culture conditions varied between species with murine growth and probably human growth being superior at 33°C, whereas hamster and treeshrew cultures performed better at 37°C.[65] Raising the temperature to 37°C in the murine system, along with the addition of erythropoietin and anemic mouse serum, appeared to facilitate erythroid cell production,[76] whereas other studies indicated that initiating human cultures at 37°C, and then switching to 33°C, might give equally good long-term growth.[78] Important methodologic aspects affecting in vitro long-term marrow culture are summarized in Table 3. A number of important differences exist between these culture systems. In general, human long-term marrow cultures have given suboptimal growth with an apparent steady decline in hemopoiesis with time.

Evidence suggests that the most proliferative stem cells may be present in the adherent layer in human cultures,[78] as with mouse, but as yet it is not clear that an optimum human system has been established. In general, conditions for human

Table 3
Growth Requirements for Long-Term Bone Marrow Cultures[a]

	Murine, 10^6/ML	Hamster, 10^6/ML	Tree shrew, 10^6/ML	Human, 2.5-3.7×10^6/ML
Cell Density				
Culture constituents				
Medium	Fischer's	RPMI-1640	Fischer's	MEM-alpha
Serum type	Horse	Horse	Horse	Horse/FCS
(%)	(20)	(20)	(20)	(12.5) (12.5)
Supplements inositol	10^{-6}M HC	None	None	10^{-6}M HC glutamine, folic acid, 2-mercaptoethanol
Temperature (°C)	33	37	37	33
Special manipulations	None	Removal of stem cells from the adherent layer	None	Separation of mature elements
Maintenance regimen	Half refed weekly	Complete medium change every 5–7 d	Half refed weekly	Half refed vs complete medium change
Stem cell location	Both adherent layer and in suspension	Rapid decline in adherent layer, survival in suspension	Cyclical reestablishment of adherent layer	Preferentially located in adherent layer

[a]Reproduced courtesy of Eastment and Ruscetti (1984) *Long Term Bone Marrow Culture* (Wright, D. G. and Greenberger, J. S., eds.), Liss, New York, NY, p. 99.

growth have involved the addition of hydrocortisone, horse serum, and fetal calf serum included with Fischer's media,[75] McCoys 5A,[79] or MEM alpha.[77] Human multipotent stem cells, as detected by in vitro assay, have been found in the adherent fraction for as long as 12 wk of growth,[77] and CFU-C were able to be recovered for as long as 20 wk.[75] Whether the human system that shows this steady decline also provides an appropriate model for stromal cells, analogous to that seen with the murine culture system, remains an open question. Studies characterizing the adherent cells that form with human stroma have indicated the presence of multiple different cell types, including fibroblastoid cells, endothelial cells, smooth muscle, and macrophages.[75,80–83] These cells clearly appear to be able to support hemopoiesis, and studies by Singer and colleagues[84] have shown that irradiated stroma has the capacity to support an Ia-depleted marrow population for relatively long-term growth in vitro. The human stromal layers also have the capacity to produce multilineage CSAs, as noted for the mouse, and probably do serve as a reasonable model for the human marrow microenvironment.[85,86] In the human system, T-cells and other lymphoid populations have been noted[87,88,95] along with the synthesis of types 1, 3, 4, and 5 collagen.[83] Keating and colleagues[83] studied long-term bone marrow cultures derived from transplant recipients who had received marrow from a donor of the opposite sex. These studies indicated that the stromal cells (or adherent cells) became progressively more donor with time and that 5–25% of these cells stained for Factor VIII, suggesting that they were endothelial cells. The data were interpreted as indicating that stroma could be transplanted and that at least part of the stroma was endothelial. Further work by the same investigators analyzed marrow cultures from individuals heterozygous for G6PD isoenzymes.[80,89] Studies using G6PD isoenzyme determination as a clonal marker indicated that the adherent cells from these individuals were also clonal and that many of these cells might, in fact, be of endothelial or smooth muscle origin. These data suggested that stromal cells, more specifically endothelial cells, might derive from the same progenitor as the hemopoietic cells.

As noted above, Eastment and Ruscetti[65] have studied Syrian hamster bone marrow cultures and reported significant and potentially important differences in these long-term marrow cultures from those of murine, human, or treeshrew systems. These cultures could be established with Fischer's media and a wide variety of horse serum lots.[65] It was found that the development of an adherent layer in these cultures was necessary for the initiation of stem cell replication, but not for long-term maintenance.[65,73,90] In addition, no fat cells were seen. Most interesting was the observation that for sustained proliferation in this system, the cells had to be removed from the stromal layers. After approximately 2 wk of initiation of the culture, blast clumps were seen. If these were not removed from the adherent layer, hemopoiesis usually ceased within 2–5 wk of culture, but if cultured separately from the adherent layer, long-term hemopoiesis was seen and, in the presence of erythropoietin-active, erythropoiesis ensued. This could be augmented by the addition of prostaglandin and was clearly inhibited both in the presence of an adherent layer, or of conditioned media derived from the adherent layer. This erythroid inhibition occurred quite rapidly and appeared to act at early erythroid stem cell levels although with longer incubations, both CFU-GEM and CFU-C were inhibited.[65] If hamster adherent layers after 6 wk or more of growth were evaluated, no erythroid or multipotent stem cells were seen, but they did contain CFU-C with the capacity to make macrophages. Thus, in the hamster long-term marrow system, there is evidence that stroma actually produced substances that inhibited cell growth, raising questions regarding the need for stromal cells or their equivalent in long-term marrow culture. One possibility was that regulator cells were present, but simply not adherent. However, when Eastment and Ruscetti[65] evaluated bursts or clusters in these cultures, neither macrophages, fat cells, endothelial cells, nor fibroblasts, as determined by standard morphologic and cytochemical criteria, were observed. Thus, at least one system appears to be able to grow in long-term liquid culture without an apparent adherent layer or other regulator cells. Whether as yet unidentified regulator cells are present, or whether an autocrine type mechanism may be involved, remain open questions at the present time.

Lymphoid Growth and Long-Term Culture

The predominant differentiated cells produced in murine long-term Dexter cultures are granulocytes, macrophages, and megakaryocytes. A similar spectrum of cells are seen in most of the other long-term culture systems from different species. Erythropoiesis can be induced in murine and hamster species by the addition of erythropoietin with or without other manipulations, as noted above. Lymphocyte production, however, ceases very quickly in murine Dexter cultures. B-cells are virtually undetectable after a week or so,[37,91,92] as are T-cells.[93,94] This is in contrast to the situation in humans in which long-term cultures have terminal transferase positive cells, cells responsive to PHA, mature T-cells, and T-lymphocyte colony forming units.[37,87,88,95] However, despite a failure to produce cells in the differentiated B lineage, including B-cells or differentiated T-cells, the long-term murine Dexter cultures have stem cells that are capable of repopulating not only myelopoiesis in vivo after transplantation, but also T- and B-lymphopoiesis.[36-37,96] These data indicated that early stem cells, for both lymphopoiesis and myelopoiesis, are supported in the classical Dexter culture system although the system is only permissive for myeloid differentiation in vitro. A modification of the Dexter system, however, allowed for proliferation of murine marrow B-lymphocyte precursors and B-cell differentiation.

In the Whitlock-Witte system,[20-21] growth was also dependent on the presence of adherent cells. This system differed from the Dexter culture systems in that fetal calf serum was substituted for horse serum, no hydrocortisone was included, 2-mercaptoethanol was included, and the temperature at which cells are cultured was raised to 37°C (Table 4). The adherent cells appeared similar to those noted in the Dexter system and long-term lymphocyte proliferation was found to be absolutely dependent on the presence of such adherent cells. Two predominant adherent cell types have been noted in these long-term cultures on the basis of morphology, cytochemical staining pattern, receptor expression for the Fc portion of IgG, and phagocytosis.[97] These two cell types are similar to those noted in Dexter cultures: macrophages along with large nonphagocytic cells, many of which stained with alkaline phosphatase. In lymphoid cultures, it was observed that lymphocytes seemed to occur around these large cells with macrophages surrounding the periphery of the lymphocyte-laden large cells. Other studies have indicated that macrophages may be necessary for late stages of B-cell differentiation in vitro,[98,99] and this may well be their role in the long-term culture system. As noted above, lymphocytes from the long-term Whitlock-Witte system can reconstitute immunity in vivo. Phillips et al.[100] reported B lineage cell reconstitution in peripheral lymphoid tissues, whereas Kurland et al.[101] found bone marrow reconstitution. It appears from the extant data that progenitor cells early in the B lineage can be established in long-term cultures with appropriate stromal support. Several factors, acting on relatively differentiated B-cells, have been described including BSF-1[102] and BCGF-2.[103] More recently, a pre-B inducing factor has been described from the urine of cyclical neutropenics.[104,105] It was noted that, when the neutrophil numbers were lowest, there

Table 4
Differences between Dexter and Whitlock-Witte
Long-Term Marrow Cultures

Characteristics	Dexter	Whitlock-Witte
Serum additive	Horse	Fetal calf
Hydrocortisone	+	−
2-mercaptoethanol	−	+
Media	Fischers	RPMI-1640
Temperature	33°C	37°C

was a marked increase in numbers of pre-B-cells in the marrow of a patient with cyclical neutropenia.[106] A pre-B inducing activity was found in this patient's urine. Both human and murine cells were responsive to this factor which is capable of inducing cells with cytoplasmic mu-chain and the 14.8 antigen.[107–110] There appeared to be two activities in the urinary preparations; one of 44,000–46,000 mol wt that induced pre-B-cell formation directly, and another lower mol wt fraction that appeared to act via a second accessory cell. These data are pertinent to our discussions of stromal cell regulation of myelo- and lymphopoiesis in that recently, a pre-B activity has been detected in conditioned media from the adherent marrow cell line TC-1.[111] Cell lines isolated from these cultures are dealt with in more detail in a separate chapter, but we will discuss this particular cell line since it appears to provide insights into the basic manner in which stromal cells may regulate both lymphoid and myeloid differentiation.

TC-1 Cell Line

The TC-1 cell line was isolated from murine C57/black marrow cells utilizing Fischer's media supplemented with fetal calf serum and no hydrocortisone.[39] These latter conditions were used to enhance the ability to establish cell lines, but it is now realized that these were, in essence, lymphoid permissive conditions approaching those seen with Whitlock-Witte cultures. The TC-1 cells were large alkaline phosphatase positive cells that produced high levels of colony-stimulating factor-1 and a "synergistic" activity that augmented the effect of CSF-1 and produced giant macrophage colonies in short-term in vitro agar culture. This synergistic activity appears to be a molecule distinct from the synergistic activities reported by Bradley et al.[112] as demonstrated by differing physiochemical and immunological properties.[113,114] This synergistic activity was clearly separate from CSF-1 and was not IL-3.[115] This activity was also capable of synergizing with IL-3 to give giant multilineage colonies including granulocytes, macrophages, and megakaryocytes and with GM-CSA to give giant granulocyte–macrophage colonies.[115] In addition, supernates from this cell line contained a potent pre-B inducing activity similar to that described in cyclical neutropenic urines.[111] Synergizing activity and the pre-B inducing activity thus far have copurified through a series of biochemical purifications and would appear to be the same factor.[111] In addition, conditioned media from this line also appears to contain a B-cell differentiating factor analogous to BCGF-2,[116] although different from this described activity in that B-cell proliferation is stimulated without concomitant IgM secretion. Thus, the cell line appears to produce an activity acting on the early stages of B-lymphopoiesis and myelopoiesis plus terminal differentiating hormones acting on the later stages of B-lymphocyte differentiation (Table 5). Finally, recent data from Johnson and Dorshkind[117] has indicated that when Dexter cultures are switched to lymphoid permissive conditions, i.e., fetal calf serum is substituted for horse serum, the hydrocortisone omitted, 2-mercaptoethanol added, and the temperature raised to 37°C, B-lymphocyte pro-

Table 5
Biologic Activities from TC–1 Cells

Activity	Assay
CSF–1	RIA
Synergistic activity	Bioassay synegizing IL–3, GM–CSA, CSF–1, and erythropoietin
Pre-B-Cell activity	Induction of pre-B-cells in liquid culture
Proliferation of factor dependent cell lines (GM–CSF)	3HtdR incorporation into FDC–P1 and DA–1 cell lines, but not 32D blocked by anti-GM–CSF
B-cell mitogenic activity	Stimulation of proliferation of isolated B-cells without concomitant IgM secretion

duction will ensue. This occurs without any obvious alterations in the basic nature of the stromal supporting cells and suggests that the same cells are capable of supporting both myeloid and lymphoid proliferation and differentiation and that local conditions of these cells may determine whether one pathway or another is supported. In an in vitro situation, the local conditions relate to serum additives, temperature, and hydrocortisone; however, one can envision alterations in local conditions in vivo being related to oxygen tension, local pH, and so on, and being equally potent in altering the stromal support function.

To summarize these points, the concept that there are two basic cell types supporting both Dexter myeloid and Whitlock-Witte lymphoid cultures, can be derived from a number of the observations cited above. Basic observations of Tavassoli and Takahashi[38] and Song and Quesenberry[39] indicate that there are two basic radioresistant cell types that are sufficient to provide the appropriate microenvironment for hemopoietic stem cell support. These cells are an alkaline phosphatase positive, large epithelioid preadipocyte and a macrophage. Similar cell types have been postulated to represent the essential microenvironment for the Whitlock-Witte B-lymphoid system.[97] The observations of a number of workers indicate that myeloid cultures, although not containing cells that can be recognized as phenotypic B-cells or B-cell precursors in vitro, do contain cells capable of in vivo B-cell reconstitution[36-37] and that by switching myeloid cultures to lymphoid conditions, these cultures begin to actively produce B-cells.[117] The switched conditions involve omitting hydrocortisone, increasing the temperature to 37°C, and substituting fetal calf serum for horse serum plus the addition of 2-mercaptoethanol. Under these conditions, the cultures switch from the support of myelopoiesis to that of lymphopoiesis. In addition, preliminary observations suggest that the production of myeloid growth factors is shut off under these switched conditions.

Morphologic analysis of the cell types involved indicates no basic change in the adherent supportive cells. These data show that the basic stromal cell populations may support either myelopoiesis or lymphopoiesis, dependent upon the particular culture conditions employed. Further observations on the TC-1 cell line isolated from normal stroma, indicate the capacity of at least one cell type to produce an early acting growth factor capable of inducing pre-B-cells in liquid culture and synergizing with virtually all known myeloid growth hormones. Initial data suggests that these activities reside in one molecule. This particular cell line also appears to be capable of producing CSF-1 and GM-CSF. In addition, factors produced by Dexter stromal cells can account for all the phenotypic end cells in the Dexter myeloid system, i.e., CSF-1 nurturing macrophages and GM-CSA supporting the growth of macrophages, monocytes, granulocytes, and megakaryocytes.[118] Ongoing work also indicates the presence of a BCGF-2-like molecule capable of stimulating differentiated B-cell proliferation. Finally, observations of Weiss and Faucet[40] and Sutton and Weiss[41] indicated that monocytes may be able to transform into macrophages, epithelioid, and multinucleated giant cells. In their in vitro studies, monocytes apparently transform through various stages to become large epithelioid cells. These data, as summarized by Tavassoli and Takahashi,[38] suggest that a single stromal stem cell exists that may give rise to both the epithelioid and macrophage type cells. If the TC-1 cell line in fact represents this particular common stromal progenitor cell, or the lymphoid permissive ARC-like cells, then a general hypothesis to explain stromal regulation of both B-lymphopoiesis and myelopoiesis may be proposed.

Hypothesis

The factors produced by the TC-1 cell line and the isolated Dexter stromal cells in in vitro culture may represent the range of factors capable of being produced by the derived macrophages and epithelioid cells seen in the stromal layers of both Dexter and Whitlock-Witte cultures. One may then envision that the large alkaline, phosphatase positive epithelioid cell produces CSF-1 that is known to be an absolute prerequisite for macrophage proliferation and survival. The macrophage in turn, which has been shown to produce messenger RNA for GM-CSA, is the source of GM-CSA, a molecule capable of stimulating the macrophage, granulocyte, and megakaryocyte lineages seen in Dexter culture.[118] One of these two cell types presumably is capable of producing a permissive growth factor that supports early stem cell proliferation and survival and expands these populations that may then respond to the appropriate terminal differentiating hormones. Thus, under the

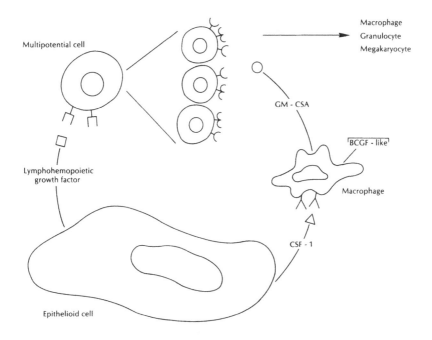

Fig. 4. Model for Dexter myeloid cultures.

appropriate conditions for myelopoiesis, i.e., hydrocortisone, horse serum, and a 33°C temperature in the classical Dexter system, this early acting growth factor stimulates early multipotent lymphohemopoietic stem cells that can then respond to GM-CSF and CSF-l (Fig. 4). When conditions are altered in the culture system, i.e., switching to fetal calf serum, raising the temperature to 37°C, omitting hydrocortisone, and adding 2-mercaptoethanol, the GM-CSF production is diminished or ceases altogether and the production of B-cell differentiating factor is induced. This would constitute the basic system for the Whitlock-Witte cultures in which the same early acting growth factor supports the population of multilineage stem cells that then could respond to the terminal B-cell differentiating hormones and produce B-lymphocytes (Fig. 5). This hypothesis would explain both the switching phenomenon and the range

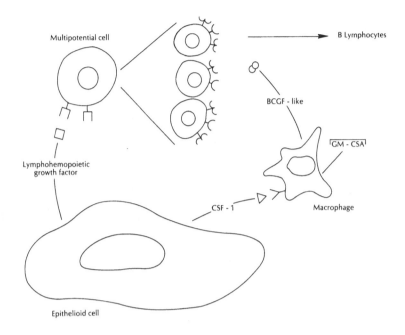

Fig. 5. Model for Whitlock-Witt lymphoid cultures.

of bioactivities observed from cell lines derived from adherent Dexter cells. The current rapid progress in this area of research should soon either definitively confirm or reject this hypothesis.

References

[1]Dexter, T. M., Allen, T. D., and Lajtha L. G. (1977) *J. Cell. Physiol.* **91,** 335–344.
[2]Dexter, T. M. and Lajtha, L. G. (1974) *Br. J. Haematol.* **28,** 525–530.
[3]Dexter, T. M. (1979) *Clinical Haematology* **8,** 453–468 (Lajtha, L., ed.), W. B. Saunders, Philadelphia, PA.
[4]Wolf, N. S. and Trentin, J. J. (1968) *J. Exp. Med.* **127,** 205–214.
[5]Curry, J. L. and Trentin, J. J. (1967) *Dev. Biol.* **15,** 395–413.
[6]Curry, J. L., Trentin, J. J., and Wolf, N. (1967) *J. Exp. Med.* **125,** 703–719.
[7]Quesenberry, P., Halperin, J., Ryan, M., and Stohlman, Jr., F. (1975) *Blood* **45,** 789–800.
[8]Quesenberry, P. J., Levin, J., Zuckerman, K., Rencricca, N., Sullivan, R., and Tyler, W. (1979) *Br. J. Haematol.* **41,** 253–269.

[9]McCulloch, E. A., Siminovitch, L., Till, J. E., Russell, E. S., and Bernstein, S. E. (1965) *Blood* **26**, 399–410.

[10]Bernstein, S. E. (1970) *Am. J. Surg.* **119**, 448–451

[11]Bessis, M., Miye, C., and Prenant, M. (1978) *Blood Cells* **4**, 155–174.

[12]Lichtman, M. A. (1981) *Exp. Hematol.* **9**, 391–410.

[13]Weiss, L. (1976) *Anat. Rec.* **186**, 161–184.

[14]Weiss, L. and Che, L.-T. (1975) *Blood Cells* **1**, 617–638.

[15]Weiss, L. (1970) *Blood* **36**, 189–207.

[16]Chamberlain, J. K., Leblond, P. F., and Weed, R. I. (1975) *Blood Cells* **1**, 655–674.

[17]Ito, J. (1965) *Bull. Tokyo Med. Dent. Univ.* **12**, 1–28.

[18]Zamboni, L., and Pease, D. C. (1961) *J. Ultrastruct. Res.* **5**, 65–85.

[19]Westen, H. and Bainton, D. F. (1979) *J. Exp. Med.* **150**, 919–937.

[20]Whitlock, C. A. and Witte, O. N. (1982) *Proc. Natl. Acad. Sci.* **79**, 3608–3612.

[21]Whitlock, C. A., Robertson, D., and Witte, O. N. (1984) *J. Immunol. Method* **67**, 353–369.

[22]Sakakeeny, M. A. and Greenberger, J. S. (1982) *J. Natl. Can. Inst.* **68**, 305–317.

[23]Quesenberry, P. J., Coppola, M. A., Gualtieri, R. J., Wade, P. J., Song, Z. X., Doukas, M. A., Shideler, C. E., Baker, D. G., and McGrath, H. E. (1984) *Blood* **63**, 121–127.

[24]Eliason, J. F. (1984) *Exp. Hematol.* **12**, 559–567.

[25]Dexter, T. M. (1982) *J. Cell. Physiol.* **1**, 87–94.

[26]Reimann, J. and Burger, H. (1979) *Exp. Hematol.* **7**, 52–58.

[27]Mauch, P., Greenberger, J. S., Hannon, E. C., and Hellman, S. (1980) *Proc. Natl. Acad. Sci.* **77**, 2927–2930.

[28]Dexter, T. M. and Moore, M. A. S. (1977) *Nature* **269**, 412–414.

[29]Greenberger, J. S. (1978) *Nature* **275**, 752–754.

[30]Levitt, L. J. and Quesenberry, P. J. (1980) *N. Eng. J. Med.* **302**, 713–719.

[31]McGrath, E., Liang, C., Alberico, T., and Quesenberry, P. (1987) *Blood* **70**, 1136–1142.

[32]Doukas, M., Niskanen, E., and Quesenberry, P. J. (1986) *Exp. Hematol.* **14**, 215–221.

[33]Wade, P. and Quesenberry, P. J. (1983) *J. Cell. Biochem.* (Suppl. 7B) (Fox, C. F., ed.), Liss, New York, NY, p. 30.

[34]Hodgson, G. S. and Bradley, T. R. (1979) *Cancer Treat. Rep.* **63**, 1761–1769.

[35]Alberico, T., Ihle, J., and Quesenberry, P. (1987) *Blood* **69**, 1120–1127.

[36]Dorshkind, K. and Phillips, R. A. (1982) *J. Immunol.* **129**, 2444–2450.

[37]Schrader, J. W. and Schrader, S. (1978) *J. Exp. Med.* **148**, 823–828.

[38]Tavassoli, M. and Takahashi, K. (1982) *Am. J. Anat.* **164**, 91–111.

[39]Song, Z. X. and Quesenberry, P. J. (1984) *Exp. Hematol.* **12**, 523–533.

[40]Weiss, L. and Fawcett, D. W. (1953) *J. Histochem. Cytochem.* **1**, 47–65.

[41]Sutton, J. S. and Weiss, L. (1966) *J. Cell Biol.* **28**, 303–332.

[42]Gualtieri, R. J., Shadduck, R. K., and Quesenberry, P. J. (1984) *Blood* **64,** 516–525 .

[43]Dexter, T. M., Spooncer, E., Simmons, P., and Allen, T. D. (1984) *Long-Term Marrow Cultures* (Wright, D. C. and Greenberger, J. S., eds.), Liss, New York, pp. 57–96.

[44]Bentley, S. A. and Foidart, J. M. (1980) *Blood* **56,** 1006–1012.

[45]Bentley, S. A. and Tralka, T. S. (1982) *Scand. J. Haematol.* **28,** 381–388.

[46]Zuckerman, K. S. and Wicha, M. S. (1983) *Blood* **61,** 540–547.

[47]Waterhouse, E. J., Quesenberry, P. J., and Balian, G. (1986) *J. Cell. Physiol.* **127,** 397–402.

[48]Benya, P. D., Padilla, S. R., and Nimni, M. E. (1978) *Cell* **15,** 1313–1321.

[49]Allen, T. D. and Dexter, T. M. (1976) *Differentiation* **6,** 191–194.

[50]Gordon, M. Y., Goldman, J. M., and Gordon-Smith, E. C. (1983) *Int. J. Cell Cloning* **1,** 429–439.

[51]Touw, I. and Lowenberg, B. (1983) *Blood* **61,** 770–774.

[52]Simmons, P. J., Allen, T. D., Dexter, T. M., Hirsh, S., and Gordon, S. (1983) *Exp. Hematol.* **14,** 144.

[53]Tavassoli, M. and Shaklai, M. (1979) *Br. J. Haematol.* **43,** 235–241.

[54]Campbell, F. R. (1980) *Anat. Rec.* **196,** 101–117.

[55]Tavassoli, M. (1982) *Exp. Hematol.* **10,** 435–443.

[56]Crouse, D. A., Mann, S. L., Anderson, R. W., and Grazulewicz, S. (1980) *Exp. Hematol.* **8,** 94.

[57]Heard, J. M., Fichelson, S., and Varet, B. (1982) *Blood* **59,** 761–767.

[58]Williams, N., Jackson, H., Sheridan, A. P. C., Murphy, M. J., Elste, A., and Moore, M. A. S. (1978) *Blood* **51,** 245–255.

[59]Dexter, T. M. and Shadduck, R. K. (1980) *J. Cell. Physiol.* **102,** 279,280.

[60]Ihle, J. N., Keller, J., Henderson, L., Klein, F., and Palaszynski, E. (1982) *J. Immunol.* **129,** 2431–2436.

[61]Greenberger, J. S., Sakakeeny, M. A., Krensky, A., Burakoff, S., Reid, D., Novak, T., and Boggs, S. (1984) *Long Term Bone Marrow Culture,* (Wright, D. G. and Greenberger, J. S., eds.), Liss, New York, pp. 255–269.

[62]Ihle, J. N., Keller, J., Greenberger, J. S., Henderson, L., Yetter, R. A., and Morse, H. C., III (1982) *J. Immunol.* **129,** 1377.

[63]McGrath, H. E., Quesenberry, P. J., and Alberico, T., unpublished data.

[64]Toksoz, D., Dexter, T. M., Lord, B. I., Wright, E. C., and Lajtha, L. G. (1980) *Blood* **55,** 931–936.

[65]Eastment, C. E. and Ruscetti, F. W. (1984) *Long Term Bone Marrow Culture* (Wright, D. G. and Greenberger, J. S., eds.) Liss, New York, pp. 97–118.

[66]Shah, G., Dexter, T. M., and Lanotte, M. (1983) *Br. J. Haematol.* **54,** 362–372.

[67]Lomedico, P. T., Gubler, U., Hellman, C. P., Dukovich, M., Giri, J. G., Pan, Y. E., Collier, K., Semionow, R., Chua, A. O., and Mizel, S. B. (1984) *Nature* **312,** 458–462.

[68]Zipori, D., Reichman, N., Arravi, L., Shtalrid, M., Berrebi, A., and Resnitzky, P. (1985) *Exp. Hematol.* **13,** 603–609.

[69]Lauer, J., Ebell, W., and Castro-Malaspina, H. (1986) *Blood* **67,** 1090–1097.

[70]Castro-Malaspina, H., Gay, R. E., Jhanwar, S. C., Hamilton, J. A., Chiarieri, D. R., Meyers, P. A., Gay, S., and Moore, M. A. S. (1982) *Blood* **59,** 1046–1054.

[71]Castro-Malaspina, H., Gay, R. E., Resnick, G., Kapoor, N., Meyers, P., Chiareri, D., McKenzie, S., Broxmeyer, H. E., and Moore, M. A. S. (1980) *Blood* **56,** 289–301.

[72]Piersma, A. H., Brockbank, K. G. M., Ploemacher, R. E., Uliet, E., Brakel Van Peer, K. M., and Visser, P. J. (1985) *Exp. Hematol.* **13,** 237–243.

[73]Eastment, C. E., Denholm, E., Katznelson, I., Arnold, E., T'so, P. (1982) *Blood* **60,** 130–135.

[74]Moore, M. A. S., Sheridan, A. P. C., Allen, T. D., and Dexter, T. M. (1979) *Blood* **54,** 775–793.

[75]Gartner, S. and Kaplan, H. (1980) *Proc. Natl. Acad. Sci.* **77,** 4756–4759.

[76]Dexter, T. M., Testa, N. G., Allen, T. D., Rutherford, T., and Scolnick, E. (1981) *Blood* **58,** 699–707.

[77]Eastment, C. E. and Ruscetti, F. W. (1982) *Blood* **60,** 999–1006.

[78]Coulombel, L., Eaves, A. C., and Eaves, C. J. (1983) *Blood* **62,** 291–297.

[79]Greenberg, H. M., Newburger, P. E., Parker, L. M., Novak, T., and Greenberger, J. S. (1981) *Blood* **58,** 724–732.

[80]Singer, J. W. (1984) *Long Term Bone Marrow Culture,* (Wright, D. G. and Greenberger, J. S., eds.), Liss, New York, pp. 235–242.

[81]Golde, D. W., Hocking, W. G., Quan, S. G., Sparkes, R. S., and Gale, R. P. (1980) *Br. J. Haematol.* **53,** 183–187.

[82]Wilson, F. D., Greenberg, B. R., Konrad, P. N., Klein, A. K., and Walling, P. A. (1978) *Transplantation* **25,** 87,88.

[83]Keating, A., Singer, J. W., Killen, P. D., Striker, G. E., Salo, A. C., Sanders, J., Thomas, E. D., Thorning, D., and Fialkow, P. J. (1982) *Nature* **298,** 280–283.

[84]Keating, A., Powell, J., Takahashi, M., and Singer, J. W. *Blood* (in press).

[85]Gordon, M. Y. (1982) *Stem Cells* **1,** 80.

[86]Brockbank, K. G. M. and Van Peer, C. M. J. (1983) *Acta Hematol.* **69,** 309.

[87]Shibata, T. and Inoue, S. (1986) *Exp.Hematol.* **14,** 234–240.

[88]Touw, I. and Lowenberg, B. (1984) *Blood* **64,** 656.

[89]Singer, J. W., Keating, A., Cattner, J., Gown, A. M., Jacobson, R., Killen, P. D., Moohr, J. W., Najfeld, V., Powell, J., Sanders, J., Striker, G. E., and Fialkow, P. J. (1984) *Leuk. Res.* **8,** 535.

[90]Eastment, C. E., Ruscetti, F. W., Denholm, E., Katznelson, I., Arnold, E., and T'so, P. (1982) *Blood* **60,** 495–502.

[91]Aspinall, R. and Owen, J. J. T. (1983) *Immunology* **48,** 9–15.

[92]Jones-Villeneuve, E. and Phillips, R. A. (1980) *Exp. Hematol.* **8,** 65–76.

[93]Schrader, J. W., Goldschneider, I., Bollum, F. J., and Schrader, S. (1979) *J. Immunol.* **122,** 2337–2339.

[94]Schrader, J. W., Schrader, S., Clark-Lewis, I., and Crapper, R. (1984) *Long Term Bone Marrow Culture,* (Wright, D. G. and Greenberger, J. S., eds.), Liss, New York, pp. 293–307.

[95]Hocking, W. G. and Golde, D. W. (1980) *Blood* **56,** 118–124.

[96]Dorshkind, K. (1983) *J. Immunol.* **131,** 2240–2245.

[97]Kincade, P. W., Witte, P. L., and Landreth, K. S. (1986) *Current Topics in Microbiology and Immunology* (Gisler, R. and Paige, C., eds.), Springer (in press).

[98]Kincade, P. W., Lee, G., Paige, C. F., and Scheid, M. P. (1981) *J. Immunol.* **127,** 255–260.

[99]Gisler, R. H., Paige, J., and Hollander, G. (1984) *Immunobiol.* **1114** (in press).

[100]Phillips, R. A., Bosma, M., and Dorshkind, K. (1984) *Long Term Bone Marrow Culture,* (Wright, D. G. and Greenberger, J. S., eds.), Liss, New York, pp. 309–321.

[101]Kurland, J. I., Ziegler, S. F., and Witte, O. N. (1984) *Proc. Natl. Acad. Sci.* **81,** 7554–7558.

[102]Noelle, R., Krammer, P. H., O'Hara, J., Uhr, J. W., and Vitetta, E. S. (1984) *Proc. Natl. Acad. Sci.* **81,** 6149–6153.

[103]Swain, S. L. and Dutton, R. W. (1982) *J. Exp. Med.* **156,** 1821–1834.

[104]Landreth, K. S., Engelhard, D., Beare, M. H., Kincade, P. W., and Good, R. A. (1984) *Fed.Proc.* **43,** 1485 (abstract).

[105]Landreth, K. S., Engelhard, D., Beare, M. H., Kincade, P. W., Kapoor, N., and Good, R. A. (1985) *J. Immunol.* **1134,** 2305–2309.

[106]Engelhard, D., Landreth, K. S., Kapoor, N., Kincade, P. W., DeBault, L. E., Theodore, A., and Good, R. A. (1983) *Proc. Natl. Acad. Sci.* **80,** 5734–5738.

[107]Landreth, K. S., Kincade, P. W., Lee, G., and Medlock, E. S. (1983) *J. Immunol.* **131,** 572–580.

[108]Landreth, K. S., Kincade, P. W., Lee, G., and Harrison, D. (1984) *J. Immunol.* **132,** 2724–2729.

[109]Medlock, E. S., Landreth, K. S., and Kincade, P. W. (1984) *Dev. Comp. Immunol.* **8,** 887.

[110]Landreth, K. S. and Kincade, P. W. (1984) *Dev. Comp. Immunol.* **8,** 773.

[111]Quesenberry, P. J., and Landreth, K. S., unpublished data.

[112]Bradley, T. R. and Hodgson, G. S. (1979) *Blood* **54,** 1446–1450.

[113]Bradley, T. R., Kriegler, A. B., McNiece, I. K., and Hodgson, G. S. (1982) *Exp. Hematol.* **10,** 10.

[114]Quesenberry, P. J., Song, Z. X., Gualtieri, R. J., Wade, Jr., P. M., Alberico, T. A., Stewart, F. M., Doukas, M. A., Levitt, L., McGrath, H. E., Rexrode,

L. A., and Innes, D. J. (1984) *Long Term Bone Marrow Culture*, (Wright, D. G. and Greenberger, J. S., eds.), Liss, New York, pp. 171–193.

[115]Quesenberry, P. J., Song, Z., McGrath, E., Shadduck, R., Waheed, A., Baber, G., Kleeman, E., and Kaiser, D. (1987) *Blood* **69,** 827–835.

[116]Quesenberry, P. J. and Isakson, P. C., unpublished data.

[117]Johnson, A. and Dorshkind, K. (1986) *Blood* (in press).

[118]Quesenberry, P. J., Ihle, J. N., and McGrath, H. E. (1985) *Blood* **65,** 214–217.

Chapter 8

Cultured Stromal Cell Lines from Hemopoietic Tissues

Dov Zipori

The Hemopoietic Microenvironment

Putative Functions

Hemopoietic tissues are highly active in terms of cell proliferation, differentiation, and migration. Their microorganization into discrete regions of cells from defined lineages or a given differentiation stage implies the existence of an instructing mechanism that acts locally.

Cell organization during organ formation in the embryo and regenerating tissues indicates that connective tissue elements carry instructive information that defines pattern formation.[1,2] Thus, the first stage of organization is the accumulation of a connective tissue network that serves as a template for the forming tissue. Connective tissue-like cells, referred to by the collective name stromal cells, form tridimensional networks of supportive tissue, in various blood-forming organs, that embed hemopoietic cells.[3,4] In view of the above mentioned functions of connective tissue cells, it appeared logical to assume that the stromal cells control hemopoiesis. Trentin suggested the term hemopoietic inductive microenvironment (HIM), implying that the stromal tissue serves to instruct the direction of differentiation rather than act as a substrate for hemopoietic cell proliferation.[5] Bone marrow transplantation experiments, coupled with microhistology, supported this notion. Additional suggestive evidence for the instructive role of the hemopoietic stroma came from the study of genetically-determined anemias as well as from a variety of disorders of the blood system in rodents and humans (this area of research has been reviewed extensively).[6]

In vitro models constructed during the late 60's suggested a humoral model for the regulation of hemopoiesis. Schematically, glycoprotein inducers of proliferation and differentiation have been identified.[7-9] Those were able to effectively induce a complete differentiation cascade in vitro. A single isolated stem cell, exposed to a specific factor purified to homogeneity, gave rise to mature and functional progeny.[10] It appeared that the whole spectrum of events in the hemopoietic system involved only the action of lineage-specific differentiation factors. Each of the factors would induce the differentiation of other types of progeny. The relative proportion of the different mature cells could simply be determined by the number of committed stem cells and the relative proliferative potential of each of the intermediate differentiating progeny of the committed cell. Moreover, the relative proportion of the committed stem cells would be stochastically determined[11,12] during the proliferation and first stage of differentiation of multipotential stem cells (Fig. 1).

This simplistic mechanism, with minor modifications, may account for a variety of events occurring in blood-forming

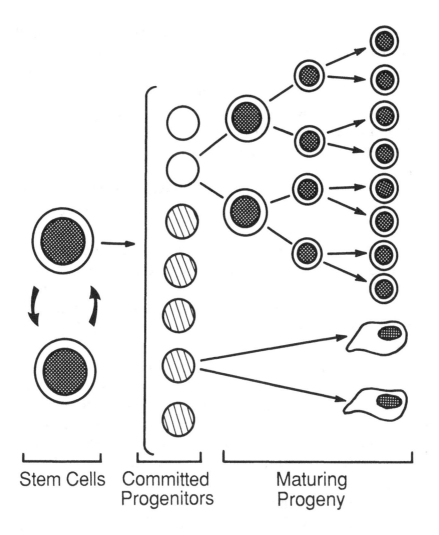

Fig. 1. A schematic representation of cell proliferation and differentiation in the hemopoietic system. Stochastic models suggest a preprogrammed continuum of events in which both the probability for production of a given progenitor cell and stem cell self-renewal are intrinsic properties of the given cell. The scheme indicates self-renewal (thick arrows) and differentiation (line arrows). It further shows that committed stem cells are produced at different incidences and the production of mature cells in a given time period is a result of the incidence of progenitor cells and the degree of proliferation of their descendants.

organs. Nevertheless, there are many observations that cannot be accounted for by the above. Primarily, hemopoietic organs are highly ordered. The pattern formation seen in those tissues would have to be determined by local factors rather than circulating hormone-like substances. Such local factors may create conditions preferential to particular cell lineages. Alternatively, they may inhibit differentiation or growth of certain cell types.

Self-renewal of stem cells is an obligatory step in hemopoiesis. Without strict control over this process, the whole stem cell pool may be swept into terminal differentiation. Thus far, none of the hemopoietic factors isolated has the capacity to induce long-term self-renewal of stem cells.[7-9] It could be argued that self-renewal is intrinsically imposed on the stem cell by the same stochastic mechanism that determines the probability for production of committed stem cells. However, a variety of experimental systems indicate that the degree of stem cell renewal can be modulated and that stem cells totally lose their ability to self-renew upon their in vitro culture. Therefore, it appears that a major function of the microenvironment is to protect the stem cell pool from excess differentiation by creating conditions that favor self-renewal. Hemopoietic stromal tissues may thus control the organization of blood-forming organs by directing differentiation, by restricting the growth or the differentiation of particular cell types and by inducing self-renewal of stem cells (Figs. 2 and 3).

Nature of Stromal Cells

An unequivocal definition of cells from the hemopoietic stroma cannot be provided to date in view of the lack of specific markers that would discriminate these cells from others. Alternatively, they may be described in terms of their tissue localization and morphology in vivo (*see* Shaklai's chapter, this

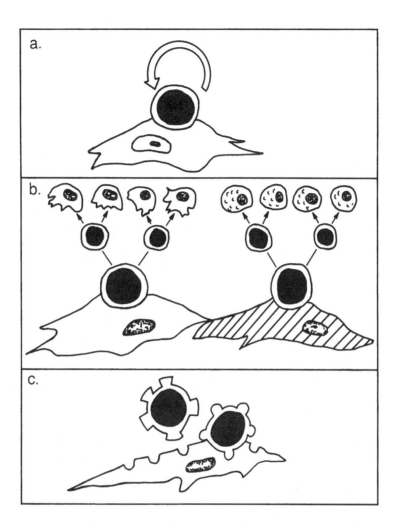

Fig. 2. Schematic view of some hypothetical functions of hemopoietic stromal cells. Section A demonstrates the capacity of particular stromal cells to control self-renewal (arrow) of stem cells. This function may be the same as the capacity of the stroma to restrain differentiation (*see* also p. 321). Section B represents the hemopoietic inductive microenvironment (HIM) that determines the differentiation pathway "taken" by the stem cell. The striated cell would drive stem cells to produce one type of progeny, whereas a similar stem cell in contact with a different stromal cell will give rise to another type of progeny. In Section C, it is shown that stromal cells may be nonpermissive to particular cell types, a phenomenon termed "restrictive stroma." An example for a possible mechanism is displayed. It assumes that stromal cells have receptors to ligands on particular hemopoietic cells, but not others. Some receptor molecules may be homing receptors or growth stimulating signals, whereas a different set of receptors may be inhibitory. An inhibitor that may represent the latter mentioned class, LCIA, is discussed on p. 321–322.

291

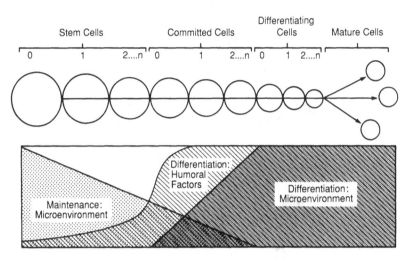

Fig. 3. Hierarchy of cell populations in the hemopoietic system and a hypothetical view of the involvement of stroma in various stages of hemopoietic differentiation. The lower part of the figure schematically demonstrates that early stages of the hemopoietic cell cascade, i.e., stem cells, are under the influence of microenvironmental factors that maintain the integrity of the stem cell pool (maintenance:microenvironment). The sensitivity of hemopoietic cells to this activity diminishes as they differentiate. In turn, these cells become responsive to differentiation-inducing signals provided by humoral factors, such as lymphokines (differentiation:humoral factors). Finally, at late stages of differentiation, the involvement of the stroma in differentiation increases again in terms of provision of the right milieu for the homing of each cell type, consequently determining the end stage of maturation and cell organization within tissues (differentiation:microenvironment).

volume). Here, the properties of cultured stromal cells will be discussed. All of those cells, originating from hemopoietic tissues that are adherent in culture, are included for the sake of this discussion under the collective name "stromal cells." This terminology should however be regarded as tentative and requires further verification.

Adherent cell types, most frequent in primary bone marrow cultures, are fibroblast-like cells and macrophages. It has been recognized by many investigators that this population may be very heterogeneous, as evidenced by the presence of several morphologically distinct cell types within the fibroblastoid population.[13–19] These include fibroblasts, fat cells, epithelial, reticulum, and endothelial cells. It was not clear, though, whether this heterogeneity represented phenotypic flexibility of one cell population or stromal cell subpopulations that have different origins and a variety of distinct functions.

Primary Cultures of Bone Marrow Stromal Cells

In Dexter's long-term bone marrow cultures, hemopoiesis strictly depends upon an adherent layer of stromal cells.[16] Stem cell maintenance occurs in these cultures continuously for up to several months. This is the best in vitro approximation of self-renewal processes that occur in vivo and clearly indicates that stromal cells are involved in the formation of suitable conditions for stem cell proliferation. Substances stimulating and suppressing DNA synthesis in stem cells were detected in regenerating and resting bone marrow, respectively.[20] Similar activities were observed in long-term bone marrow cultures and were suggested to account for the control of stem cell proliferation.[21] However, it has not been shown that these factors support stem cell proliferation in the absence of the stroma.

One piece of evidence from Dexter's long-term cultures supports the putative HIM. When these cultures are treated with anemic mouse serum, specific areas in the adherent cell layer that otherwise were myeloid become erythropoietic. This is accompanied by retraction of adipocytes that are suspected to support myelopoiesis in culture.[22] Additional support for the capacity of stromal cells to direct differentiation may be derived from studies on a modified culture system in which B-cells are continuously produced.[23,24]

Indications that stromal cells may be involved in restriction of hemopoietic growth and differentiation emerge from an experimental system designed by Zipori et al. that examined the clonal growth of myeloid progenitor cells in the presence of an excess number of stromal cells (Fig. 4).[25-30] Sparse bone marrow cell suspensions were seeded onto confluent layers of stromal cells. The interactions between almost isolated progenitors and the stroma can be assessed, at least during the first few days of culture. The contribution of interactions between stem cells and mature progeny, which occur in long-term bone marrow cultures, are minimized. Under these conditions, stromal cells from the bone marrow interfere with the capacity of colony-stimulating factor-1 (CSF-1, M-CSF) to induce the formation of myeloid colonies. Concomitantly, the stromal cells cause the accumulation of myeloid progenitors that, under control conditions, are eliminated through terminal differentiation. Therefore, the presence of stroma appears to block the capacity of the progenitors to respond to this differentiation factor. The alternative pathway is continued proliferation, resulting in an accumulation of progenitors. It was proposed that stromal cells allow stem cell self-renewal by restraining the differentiation flow.[28]

Most quantitative studies on interactions between hemopoietic cells and the stroma deal with stem cells and precursors, rather than with mature cells, owing to the absence of a suitable experimental system for study of the latter. Little is known, therefore, about the influence of the stroma on functions of maturing or mature cells. To circumvent this difficulty, leukemia cell lines were used as a model for hemopoietic cells at various stages of maturation. Primary stromal cells were found to affect the in vitro growth of hemopoietic tumors; the growth of leukemia cell lines with an immature phenotype (such as pre-B-lymphomas) was stimulated by the stroma, whereas the growth of cell lines with a mature phenotype (such as plasma-

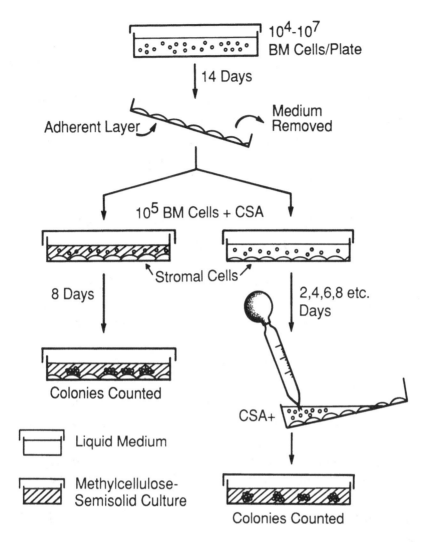

Fig. 4. A modified CFU-C assay used to investigate the effects of adherent stromal cells on the proliferation and differentiation of hemopoietic progenitor cells. The scheme is based on experiments in which the growth of bone marrow (BM) cells, stimulated with a source of colony stimulating factor (CSA), was studied. The effect of the stroma (adherent layer) on the formation of hemopoietic colonies in semisolid medium (left side of figure) and the production of colony forming cells monitored by subcloning of cells grown in liquid medium (right side of figure) may be studied. In the methylcellulose cultures, the hemopoietic cells sediment to the bottom of the plate shortly after seeding and come in close contact with the stroma. The use of methylcellulose allows further examination of the progenitor cell content in individual colonies by the subculture of single colonies.[29] In addition, such cultures are used to determine whether the activity of the stroma is mediated by cell–cell interactions or secreted factors. This is done by the addition of a separating agar layer between the stromal cells and the methylcellulose containing the target hemopoietic cells.[25-30]

295

cytomas) was inhibited. This was interpreted as reflecting the capacity of the marrow stroma to serve as an accumulation site for immature rather than mature lymphoid cells.[31,32] A detailed review of the mode of action of the hemopoietic stroma is presented elsewhere.[33]

The Requirement for Permanent Stromal Cell Lines

The study of the nature and functions of cells from the hemopoietic stroma has suffered from two major deficiencies. One is the heterogeneity of the cell population involved. This made it impractical to precisely define the role of each cell type (or phenotype) in the regulation of hemopoiesis in culture. Attempts were made to separate precursors of stromal cells from those of macrophages, which are very common in primary bone marrow cultures, using density gradient centrifugation.[14] This approach yielded results suggesting that the fibroblastoid cells, rather than macrophages, were responsible for the stimulation of growth of pre-B-lymphoma cells. Data derived from this kind of experiment cannot exclude the involvement of minor cell populations that copurify with the major cell of interest.

A second major difficulty for the use of primary stroma became evident when the abovementioned functions of the stroma were reported. The molecules mediating the stromal cell activities attracted much interest, but appeared to be rare or unstable. The activities mediating stem cell renewal in long-term cultures could not be found in conditioned media. Similarly, differentiation restraining activities were not detected in media conditioned by primary stromal cells, and CSF could be induced in stromal cells by glucose, but was found in an exceedingly low titer.[25-30] Any progress in biochemical characterization of stromal cell factors requires a source for large numbers of cells constituting uniform populations. Inevitably, attempts to derive continuous cell lines began.

Hemopoietic Stromal Cell Lines

Derivation

In contrast to embryonic or skin fibroblasts, which proliferate readily and can be propagated as primary cell strains, bone marrow cultures tend to give rise to layers of adherent cells that remain quiescent for prolonged periods of time.[26,27] The culture conditions used for the in vitro growth of stromal cells in a number of different laboratories is summarized in Tables 1 and 2 (*see* pp. 298–301). In several attempts, the incubation temperature, as well as the medium and type of serum used, were selected to match the conditions of the Dexter culture. However, these conditions were not essential.

Different methods were employed; long-term bone marrow cultures were established in which active hematopoiesis occurred. Following a period of continuous culture, particular areas showing accumulation of fibroblasts or adipocytes were removed and subcultured.[37] Using similar cultures, other investigators found that during routine harvesting of the nonadherent population, some cells in the inoculum gave rise to adherent stromal cells.[51] This phenomenon also occurs in nonhemopoietic stromal cell cultures.[14] Probably, it results from removal of mitotic cells that tend to round up and detach from the adherent layer. This was the basis of the method used to clone the MBA-1 stromal cell line (Fig. 5). Additional methods involved the establishment of nonhemopoietic cultures containing only the stromal component of the bone marrow or other hemopoietic tissues.[46]

The methodology established by Todaro and Green[54] for the derivation of fibroblast cell lines was the basis of many attempts to derive cell lines from mouse stroma. Contrary to

Table 1
Stromal Cell Lines from Hemopoietic Tissues of Mouse and Humans

| | Origin[a] | | | Culture conditions | | | | | | |
Designation	Strain	Age, wk	Status	Initial inoculum, cells $\times 10^6$	Use of proteolytic enzyme for passaging	Pre-passage period, d	Temp., °C	CO_2, %	Serum type (%)	Medium
RCN-BM 5	C57BL/6	6–8	Tumor-bearing	100	Yes	6–7	NM	NM	NM	Weymouth's
MC₁	C57BL/6	NM	Normal	NM[b]	Yes	NM	33	5	Horse (20)	Fischer's
MC₃	C57BL/6	NM	Normal	NM[b]	Yes	NM	33	5	Horse (20)	Fischer's
MC₄	C57BL/6	NM	Normal	NM[b]	Yes	NM	33	5	Horse (20)	Fischer's
H-1	C57BL/6	7	Normal	NM[c]	Yes	98	33	5	Horse (10)	Fischer's
LP20, HP1, LP20a LP4 (human origin)	—	NM	Normal	0.1–1[b]	Yes	14	37	5	Horse (20) or FCS (20)	Fischer's
MC3T3-G2/PA6	C57BL/6	Newborn	Normal	0.3	Yes	3	37	5	NBCS (10)	αMEM
MS3-2A	DBA/2 (C57 BLx)	6–10	Normal	10	Yes	28–42	33	NM	Horse or FCS (15)	Fischer's
MS2-2A	DBA) F1	6–10	Normal	10	Yes	28–42	33	NM	Horse or FCS (15)	Fischer's
MS1	Swiss	6–10	Normal	10	Yes	28–42	33	NM	Horse or FCS (15)	Fischer's
MS4	Swiss	6–10	Normal	10[d]	Yes	28–42	33	NM	Horse or FCS (15)	Fischer's
266AD	Balb/c	6–20	Normal	0.2[b,e]	Yes	14	37	5	Horse (15) FCS (10)	RPMI
V209, V213	AKR/rho Ico	8–12	Normal[f]	NM[c]	No	42–82	37	5	Horse (25)	α-Medium
BMA1	DDY	NM	Normal	15[g]	NM	42	37	5	Horse (20)	Fischer's
MBA-1	SJL/J	4	Normal	42	No	30	37	10	FCS (10)	DMEM
MBA-15	SJL/J	4	Normal	42	No	30	37	10	FCS (10)	DMEM
MBA-13	nude-ICR	4	Normal	42	No	90	37	10	FCS (10)	DMEM

MBA-2	RF/J	4	Normal	42	No	~300	37	10	FCS (10)	DMEM
14M1	Balb/c	4	Normal	42	No	120	37	10	FCS (10)	DMEM
14F	Balb/c	4	Normal	42	No	120	37	10	FCS (10)	DMEM
AP63[A]	(CBA/Rij × C57BL/Rij)	NM	Normal	NM	Yes	90	37	NM	FCS (20)	α-Medium
D2X R II c17	C3H/Hej	NM	Normal	NM	NM	154[i]	37	7	FCS (10)	DMEM
KM-101 KM-102, KM-103 Km-104, KM-105 [human origin][j]	—	[48yr]	[Lung surgery]	10	Yes	60[k]	37	NM	FCS (20)	McCoy's
B.Ad	Balb/c	NM	Normal	NM	Yes	270[l]	37	5	FCS (20)	DMEM
TC-1	C57BL/6J	NM	Normal	NM	Yes	7	33	5	FCS (20)	Fischer's
K-1	(C57 BL/6 × DBA/2)	8–12	Normal	NM	Yes	161	33	5	Horse (25)	Fischer's

[a]Most cell lines are of femural or tibial bone marrow origin. The human cell lines, and the human lines are from sternum marrow[39] or from rib marrow.[50] Cell line AP63 was derived from mouse spleen. Cell line MC3T3-G2/PA6 is from mouse calvaria.

[b]Cell lines were derived from stromal colonies removed from original cultures.

[c]Cell line obtained from the adherent population in long- term bone marrow cultures.

[d]Cultures infected with F-MuLV.

[e]Cell line derived from collagen gel cultures.

[f]This mouse strain has a high incidence of leukemias at about 8 mo of age.

[g]Bone marrow cultures were transfected with adenovirus 5 DNA.

[h]A spleen derived cell line.

[i]At the indicated time following seeding, nonadherent cells were removed from long-term cultures. The adherent cell line was derived from this nonadherent population.

[j]These cell lines were derived from adherent cell populations transfected in vitro with recombinant plasmid pSV3 gpt DNA containing the coding sequence of the early region of simian virus 40 (SV40).

[k]Time following transfection.

[l]Nine months after initiation of culture by seeding of nonadherent cells from long term cultures of mast cells in WEHI-3B conditioned medium. FCS = fetal calf serum; FBS = fetal bovine serum; NBCS = new born calf serum; DMEM = Dulbecco's modified Eagle medium; and NM = not mentioned in publication.

Note: References are cited in Table 2.

Table 2
Stromal Cell Lines from Hemopietic Tissues of Mouse and Humans

Designation	Number of passages	Single-cell cloned	Main criteria used for characterization	Cell Type	Reference
RCN-BM 5	>18	Yes	Morphology	Epithelial	34,35
MC$_1$	NM	No	Response to insulin In vivo transplantation	Preadipose	36
MC$_3$	NM	No	Response to insulin In vivo transplantation	(?) Preadipose	36
MC$_4$	NM	No	Response to insulin In vivo transplantation	(?) Preadipose	36
H 1	40	Yes	Morphology Cytochemical analysis	Fibroblast or fibroblast-type reticulum cell	37,38
LP20, HP1, LP20a, LP4 [human origin]	>30	No	Morphology Cytochemical analysis	Fibroblast or fibroblast-type reticulum cell	39
MC3T3-G2/PA6	>40	Yes	Hydrocortisone vs insulin responsiveness	Preadipose	40,41
MS3-2A	>64	Yes	Hydrocortisone vs insulin responsiveness	Preadipose	42
MS2-2A	>64	Yes	Hydrocortisone vs insulin responsiveness	Preadipose	42
MS1	>64	Yes	Hydrocortisone vs insulin responsiveness	Preadipose	42
MS4	>64	Yes	Hydrocortisone vs insulin responsiveness	Preadipose	42
266AD	>30	Yes	Morphology	Preadipose	42
V209, V213	>18	No	Morphology	Preadipose	43
BMA1	>80	No	Morphology	Fibroblastoid or epitheloid	44
MBA-1	>50[a]	Yes	Analysis of extracellular matrix (ECM) constituents Cytochemistry	Fibroblastoid	45
			Presence of junctional complexes (EM) Macrophage function tests	Fibroblasts	46,47

Cell line	Passage	Cloned	Characterization	Cell type	Ref.
MBA-15	>20[a]	Yes	Analysis of extracellular matrix (ECM) constituents; Cytochemistry; Presence of junctional complexes (EM); Macrophage function tests	Fibroblasts	46,47
MBA-13	>70[a]	Yes	Analysis of extracellular matrix (ECM) constituents; Cytochemistry; Presence of junctional complexes (EM)	Fibroendo-thelial; Endothelial-like	46,47; 46,47
MBA-2	>20[a]	Yes	Analysis of extracellular matrix (ECM) constituents; Cytochemistry; Presence of junctional complexes (EM); Macrophage function tests		
14M1	>20[a]	Yes	Analysis of extracellular matrix (ECM) constituents; Cytochemistry; Presence of junctional complexes (EM)	Macrophage	46,47
14F	>20[a]	Yes	Analysis of extracellular matrix (ECM) constituents; Cytochemistry; Presence of junctional complexes (EM); Macrophage function tests	Preadipocyte	46,47
AP63[a]	13	No	Cytochemistry; Surface antigens	Fibroblastic	48
D2x R II c17	>12	Yes	Cytochemistry; Surface antigens; Analysis of ECM	Fibroblast or Preadipocyte	49
KM-101, KM-102, KM-103 KM-104, KM-105 [human origin]	>40	Yes	Morphology	Fibrocytic	50
B-Ad	NM	Yes	Cytochemistry; Cell surface markers	Preadipose (?)	51
TC-1	>76	Yes	Cytochemistry; EM (for junctional complexes)	Epitheloid	52
K-1	>35	Yes	Morphology	Preadipose	53

[a]The passage number given refers to the cloned lines. Prior to cloning, each of the cell lines had been passaged between 20 and 30 times.

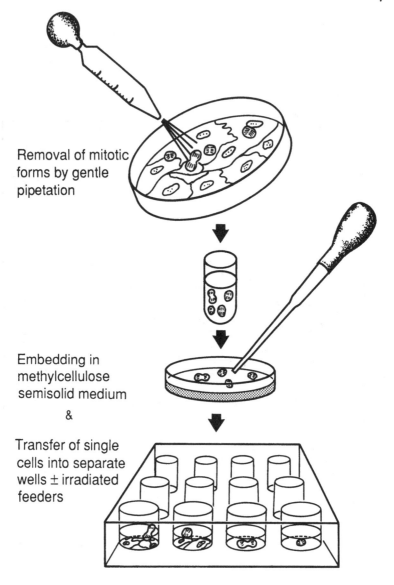

Removal of mitotic
forms by gentle
pipetation

Embedding in
methylcellulose
semisolid medium

&

Transfer of single
cells into separate
wells ± irradiated
feeders

Fig. 5. Cloning of MBA-1[46] stromal cells by selective transfer of mitotic forms.

the classical method for derivation of fibroblast cell strains, care was taken not to create strong selective pressures while deriving MBA cell lines. Cells were maintained in the original plates for up to 10 mo of incubation. Passaging was performed only when all of the cell populations, observed in the primary cultures, had the opportunity to increase in number and consequently survive passage.[46,55] Furthermore, this method excluded the use of proteolytic enzymes for the transfer of cells from one plate to another in order to maintain the contacts between cells and limit selection of cells that do not require contact with their neighbors (Fig. 6). Finally, in two separate attempts, changes were introduced in the bone marrow population, by transfection with either adenovirus-5 DNA[45] or a recombinant plasmid DNA,[50] apparently with the aim of increasing the probability of emergence of the desired cell line. As can be seen in Table 1, all these methods yielded continuous cell lines. It appears though that the method used to derive the cell lines influences the type of cell that emerges (*see* below). The MBA cell line series, derived in the author's laboratory, will be discussed in some detail along with cell lines obtained in other laboratories.

Growth

Substantial variability exists among stromal cell lines in their rate of in vitro proliferation. The MBA-1 cell line, derived from the bone marrow of SJL/J mice, had an initial rapid growth pattern. Following a number of passages, the cells established a population doubling time of about 17 h.[47] The MBA-14 cell line, which was the origin for sublines 14F and 14M1 (Table's 1 and 2), retained a long and variable doubling time for over a year of continuous culture. Additional variability existed in the maximal density that the various cell lines could reach in vitro. The adipogenic cell line 14F could not crowd over 1.5×10^2 cells/mm^2. At the other extreme, the MBA-2 cell line reached a maximal density of about 3×10^3/mm^2.[47] These properties may relate to the cell performance in the support of in vitro hemopoiesis discussed below.

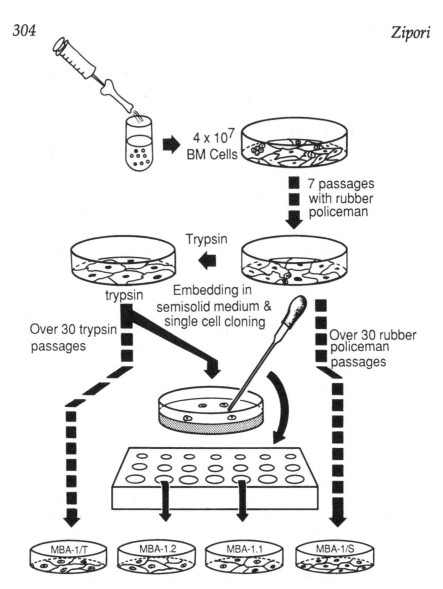

Fig. 6. Derivation of MBA cell lines (for further details, *see* text).[46,47]

Morphology

Morphological studies are limited in the lack of objective and quantitative tools for a clear definition of what a "fibroblast" or an endothelial-like cell would be. Consequently, there is no guarantee that cells designated "fibroblastoid" in one laboratory would be regarded as such by other investigators. Nevertheless, there was a remarkable correlation between initial description of cell lines in the MBA series, based solely on their appearance in phase contrast microscopy[46] and subsequent classification, based upon the examination of extracellular matrix composition.[47,56] Thus, the MBA-1 cell line was fibroblast-like. The 14F cells were extremely flattened, each covering a surface area that would occupy over 10 fibroblast-like cells. In addition, these cells had long cytoplasmic protrusions. Upon confluence, the cells formed monolayers and adipogenesis was triggered. A completely different phenotype was exhibited by MBA-2 cells. These were spindle-shaped and grew in bundles. Upon confluence, they formed highly dense and compact layers. The MBA-13 cell line was yet another morphologically-distinct type in that the cells were polygonal and tended to form epithelioid layers with distinct boundaries between adjacent cells. This feature was not observed in fibroblast-like cells for which upon confluence, cell boundaries tended to disappear. Finally, the 14M1 cell line had a characteristic macrophage/monocyte morphology. This was supported by scanning and transmission electron microscope observations. The latter technique also revealed the presence of junctional complexes in the MBA-2 cell line and implied that it is endothelial or epithelial.[47]

RCN-BM 5[34,35] is a representative of 31 cell lines derived from hemopoietic tissues of mice bearing reticulum cell neoplasms (RCN). Their morphology was epithelial or fibroblastoid. The cell lines were primarily used to produce RCN-inducing virus and were not characterized in detail or reported to have hemopoietic functions. Fibroblast-like morphology was common to a variety of cell lines.[37-39,44,45,48,50] Anderson and Sharp[57] identified a number of cell shapes in stromal cell cultures during initial passages. The cell lines that emerged were eventually found to be preadipocytes, as indicated by their fat conversion in response to insulin.[36] Harigaya et al.[37] derived the fibroblastoid cell line H-1 from mouse bone marrow long-term cultures. The latter and the cell lines obtained by Kodama et al. (MC3T3-G2/GA6)[40,41] and Lanotte et al. (MS series),[42] as well as cell lines from human bone marrow,[39] were all capable of undergoing fat conversion. This property was found to be common to additional stromal cell lines derived in other laboratories.[49,51,53]

Adipogenesis

The induction of fat accumulation in the MC_1 stromal cell line occurred in medium containing horse serum. Transfer of the cells to FCS reversed the process. Adipogenesis could also be induced by insulin. The MC_1 cell line responded to 10^{-9} insulin. Other cell lines of this series responded to much higher and nonphysiologic concentrations.[36] The MC3T3-G2/PA6[40,41] and cells in the MS series[42] accumulated fat when grown with hydrocortisone, but not insulin (about $10^{-6}M$). In MS cells, adipogenesis depended on the use of horse serum rather than FCS.[42] Dexamethasone at $10^{-7}M$ was the most potent inducer of fat conversion in the MC3T3-G2/PA6 cell line. The steroid, however, was not required for progression of adipogenesis, and in this system, newborn calf serum rather than horse serum was used.[41] About 90% of the lipids accumulated by these cells were triglycerides. Hydrocortisone also induced fat accumulation in human stromal cell lines.[39] Similarly, fat accumulated in the H-1 cell line derived by Harigaya et al.[37,38] and the 266AD line derived by Hines et al.,[43] grown in horse serum. Spontaneous fat accumulation was observed by Zipori et al. in the cell line 14F1.1 This occurred in FCS.[46]

The results from various laboratories concerning hormone responsiveness of adipocytes are contradictory. It is possible that a number of adipose cell populations exist in the bone marrow that differ in their hormonal responses. Whether the cell population that responded to hydrocortisone is specific to the marrow stroma, as suggested by Kodama et al.,[41] requires further examination.

Cytoplasmic Enzymes

The cell lines of the MBA and MS series, and the H-1, B.Ad, TC-1, and K-1 mouse cell lines as well as some human cell lines have been assayed for the expression of cytoplasmic enzymes by standard cytochemical reactions.[38,47,51–53,58] Results from most laboratories confirm that marrow stromal cell lines are α-naphtyl acetate esterase and periodic acid Schiff (PAS) positive and peroxidase negative. In addition, the various cell lines were oil red-O positive to various degrees irrespective of whether they were capable of making large fat droplets. On the other hand, there is obvious disagreement in the reports on alkaline and acid phosphatase enzymes. Acid phosphatase was detected in all cell lines of the MBA series, in the human stromal cell lines of Lanotte et al., and the H-1, B.Ad, TC-1, and K-1 cell lines. Cell lines in the MS series (preadipocytes) were negative, as was the AP63 cell line derived from mouse spleen.

The MBA cell line series exhibited high heterogeneity in terms of expression of alkaline phosphatase. The macrophage-like cell line 14M1 was negative, and in the preadipose cell line 14F, only occasional cells were weakly positive. Similarly, the MBA-2 cell line was negative. In contrast, the fibroblast-like cells MBA-1, MBA-15, and MBA-13 were positive. K-1 and the cell lines from human bone marrow of Lanotte et al. were also negative. TC-1, AP63, H-1, and cells of the MS series were positive to alkaline phosphatase. Twenty α-hydroxysteroid dehydrogenase was detected in stromal cell lines of the MS series,[59] but it has not been examined in other stromal lines.

Extracellular Matrix

Connective tissue cells produce an extracellular matrix that serves primarily as a substrate for their growth. It is also involved in the formation of boundaries between tissues, in cell–cell interactions, and in the control of cell morphology and tissue pattern formation.[60] The extracellular matrix is an extremely complex structure and its precise organization has not been totally resolved. Nevertheless, many components of this matrix have been identified and purified. There are differences among cell populations in the composition of the matrix they produce. Therefore, it was anticipated that the heterogeneity in morphological appearance of stromal cell lines would also be reflected in the composition of their extracellular matrix.

The MBA cell line series has been studied in great detail using both biochemical analysis of proline-labeled proteins[47] and immunofluorescence, using antibodies specific to a variety of matrix components.[56] The MBA-1 cell line produced type I and III collagens that confirm its fibroblast morphology. The MBA-2.1 cell line produced mainly collagen type IV and V, whereas the MBA-13 cell line made all four types of collagens. Accordingly, these cell lines were termed endothelial-like and fibroendothelial, respectively. The adipose cell line 14F1.1 was positive for collagens I, IV, and V. All of the cell lines made fibronectin and laminin. Whereas most cell lines made a loose network of matrix fibers, the 14F1.1 cells made a prominent basal lamina-like matrix that seemed to engulf the cells. The macrophage cell line 14M1 was devoid of matrix proteins. Cronkite et al. reported that the H-1 fibroblast cell line made collagen types I and III[38] and the D2XRII was found to produce collagens I, II, and III.[61]

Thus far, cells producing basal lamina collagens were reported only in the MBA series. It is possible that this is owing to the method used for the derivation of these cell lines, i.e., the lack of proteolytic enzymes and passage of cells at high densities.[55] These conditions may allow maintenance of a phenotype that otherwise is lost in culture.

Cell Surface Markers

Fc receptors assayed by binding of protein A-(SRBC) or aggregated IgG and factor VIII associated antigen, assayed by immunofluorescence, were not detected on the human stromal cell lines.[39] These markers could not also be detected on the H-1[38,62] and AP63[48] cell lines. The latter were Mac-1 negative. The B.Ad cell line was positive to H-2, but negative to Ia, Ig, Ly1, and Ly2.[51]

Classification

In order to introduce some starting point for future efforts to characterize stromal cell types, the author suggests the following classification that seems to account for the majority of the available cell lines.

Endothelial–Adipose Cell

Many of the cell lines derived from mouse and human bone marrow have been termed adipocytes (adipose cells, preadipocytes, and fat cells), but appear to differ in a variety of functions. Heterogeneity in adipocyte populations, in terms of response to hormones, was discussed above. Does this variability represent the existence of subpopulations of adipogenic cells within the bone marrow? Indeed, fibroblast-like cell lines that can be maintained for prolonged periods of time in vitro, without passage, tend to accumulate moderate amounts of fat. These clearly differ in morphology, growth properties, and collagen production from the 14F1.1 adipocytes that make an extracellular matrix reminiscent of endothelial cells. In contrast to all other cells in the MBA cell series, this cell line forms large fat droplets that occupy most of the cytoplasm.

It is therefore proposed that this type of stromal cell be termed marrow endothelial–adipose cell, to account for its additional properties that distinguish it from cells such as the H-1 cell line, that are adipogenic but make collagen types I and III characteristic of fibroblasts.[62,63] Unfortunately, the adipogenic cell line MC3T3-G2/PA6[64] and the TC-1-C-11 clone[52] have not been examined for their ECM composition. They may, however, belong to the endothelial–adipose cell category, as indicated by their ability to support stem cell growth, a feature they share with 14F1.1 cells (*see* below).

Fibroblast or Adventitial Reticulum Cell

This cell type is collagen types I and III positive. It may (as H-1 cells) or may not (as MBA-1 cells) be adipogenic. It is both acid and alkaline phosphatase positive and does not exhibit any of the endothelial–epithelial features discussed above.

Endothelial-Like Cell

The MBA-2 cell line and its clones MBA-2.1 and MBA-2.4 are unique among the MBA cell line series. Their derivation was the most difficult, both in terms of preincubation time that was needed before the cells could be passaged (10 mo) and in their failure to grow at low concentrations. Cloning of these cells was consequently more tedious than of all the others. It is possible that this cell subtype is unable to normally grow in culture. This would also explain the fact that other cell lines, with properties reminiscent of the above, have not been reported. MBA-2 cells mainly make collagen types IV and V. They form junctional complexes with adjacent cells. In contrast with fibroblast cell lines from the marrow, these cells are negative to alkaline phosphatase, a feature common with the endothelial–adipose cells described above.

Fibroendothelial Cell

The main features of these cells are their cuboidal-epitheli-oid morphology in confluent cultures, and more importantly, their capacity to produce both interstitial and basal lamina collagens. The enzymatic profile of these cells is identical to the fibroblasts described above.

Macrophage

The classification of this cell type is not controversial. The 14M1 cells that represent this group of cell lines are dependent upon CSF-1, the macrophage differentiation and growth factor for their survival and proliferation. They are phagocytic and can degrade and present antigen to primed lymphocytes. Thus far, not one function of these cells was found to be unique, compared to macrophages from other sources. These cells, though, may play a major role in the regulation of hemopoiesis, in view of the known functions of macrophages in erythropoi-esis, as well as their effects on preadipocytes. This latter subject is discussed below.

Long-Term In Vitro Hemopoiesis

It is well established that primary stromal cells are essen-tial for the maintenance of hemopoietic activity in culture. The role of each of the various cell types observed in these cultures is unclear, however. It was anticipated that the availability of cloned stromal cell lines would reveal the type of stroma cell required for stem cell proliferation in vitro. Fibroblast stroma cell lines, such as H-1[63] and MBA-1,[46] were incapable of suppor-ting hemopoiesis, whereas the MC3T3-G2/PA6 preadipose cell line maintained colony-forming units spleen (CFU-S) for 3 wk of culture.[40,64] A direct contact between the stroma and the hemopoietic cells was required. Hydrocortisone did not im-prove the performance of this cell line, and the cells supported

CFU-S more effectively in the preadipose rather than the fully adipogenic state. Conversely, in Dexter long-term cultures, hydrocortisone enhanced the recovery of CFU-S, and fat accumulation correlated with active hemopoiesis. The uncloned cell line MBA-14, derived by Zipori et al., consisted of a mixture of preadipocytes and macrophages. This cell line supported the proliferation of granulocyte/macrophage colony-forming cells (GM-CFC or CFU-C) in short-term bone marrow cultures[46] and up to 8 wk (Fig. 7) under conditions that do not favor hemopoiesis (i.e., 37°C, FCS, and no hydrocortisone added). Cloned cell lines prepared from MBA-14, designated 14F1.1 (adipocytes), and 14M1 (macrophages) were each tested for its ability to support stem cells. The macrophage cell line was devoid of such activity. On the other hand, the 14F1.1 clone induced accumulation of GM-CFC and allowed the maintenance of CFU-S in short-term bone marrow cultures.[56] Other stromal cell types, including endothelial-like and fibroblastoid cells, were unable to perform similarly.

It is concluded that the only stromal cell type that supports stem cell proliferation in vitro is the endothelial–adipose cell. The activity of these cells does not seem to account for all the events occurring in long-term cultures, and the participation of other stromal cell types must be examined. Among the various stromal cells, preadipocytes exhibit the lowest cell density at confluence. It is not clear to what extent this property contributes nonspecifically to their effects on hemopoietic cells.

It is conceivable that endothelial–adipose cells play a major role in the induction of stem cell self-renewal in long-term bone marrow cultures. The interpretation of the above experiments is complicated, however, by the fact that they were performed using heterogeneous bone marrow cell populations that include stroma cell precursors. To minimize the contribution of the latter, small numbers of bone marrow cells were seeded onto the stroma.[64] Further experiments should in-

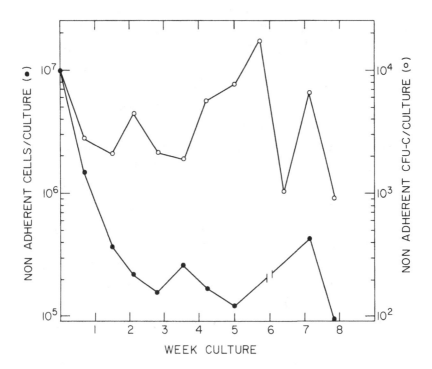

Fig. 7. Long-term proliferation of myeloid progenitor cells, induced by an uncloned cell line from the bone marrow (MBA-14). The total number of cells in these cultures was reduced to about 2%, compared to the seeding inoculum. In contrast, the number of the CFU-C fluctuated around 10% of the input. This resulted in a significant enrichment of CFU-C at various time points.[46]

clude the use of cloned stromal cell lines in coculture with purified stem cells.

Colony Stimulating Factors (CSF)

Stromal cells from mouse bone marrow stimulated the formation of myeloid colonies in methylcellulose cultures and were therefore suggested to produce CSF.[15,26-29] It is noteworthy, though, that a lot of discrepancies exist in the literature in relation to CSF production by stromal cells. Chan and Metcalf reported local production of colony stimulating activity (CSA) by nonhemopoietic cells in the bone marrow.[65] In long-term Dexter cultures, CSA was not initially detected.[16] Experiments performed by Zipori et al. have shown that the stroma CSA is inducible, whereas cultures of primary stroma cells had poor CSA, and significant activity was observed when the growth medium was supplemented with high concentrations of glucose.[26,27] This sugar activity appeared to be distinct from its primary role as an energy supply. Various reports indicated that the stroma CSA stimulated differentiation of target bone marrow cells into granulocytes and macrophages. In some of its bioactivities, the stroma CSA differed from CSF of other sources. Primary stromal cells antagonized CSF-1 or GM-CSF in the formation of myeloid colonies. On the other hand, CSA produced by the stroma was capable of overcoming this inhibition.[27] Moreover, dose response analysis of colony formation, induced by the stroma CSA, implied that the population of colony forming cells responding to this factor is more closely related to stem cells than committed progenitors.[27] Therefore, it is possible that stromal cells produce a "resident-CSF" that is limited to the marrow microenvironment. However, no characterization of stromal cell specific CSFs on either the protein or the mRNA level have been reported thus far.

The question concerning production of CSFs was reapproached when stroma cell lines became available. During early passages, adherent cell populations from the bone marrow produced CSA. In marrow cultures from SJL/J, Balb/c, and nude-ICR mice, CSA in conditioned media obtained from cells during the first passages and of the emerging cell lines, was of a higher titer than that observed in primary cultures.[47] Adherent cell layers of the H-1 cell line stimulated the formation of myeloid colonies in a double-layer agar system, under conditions where there was no direct contact between the interacting cells.

Media conditioned by these cells contained CSA that stimulated differentiation into macrophages and neutrophils and was neutralized by antibodies raised against L-cell conditioned medium.[37] A number of studies reported production of CSF-1-like activity by preadipocyte cell lines. Antibodies specific to CSF-1 eliminated the stimulating activity in media conditioned by these cells.[47,66] A cell line dependent upon CSF-1 for its growth in culture was developed (designated 14M1).[46] One clone of this cell line, 14M1.4, was highly dependent on this factor, but did not respond to human and mouse recombinant GM-CSF (rGM-CSF), γ-interferon (γ-IF), or mouse rIL-3 (Zipori and Lee, unpublished). 14M1 cells were used to screen the MBA stroma cell line series. All those, including preadipocytes, endothelial-like cells, fibroblasts, and fibroendothelial cells, were found to produce CSF-1 like activity by this criterion. This observation was substantiated by the finding that anti-CSF-1 antiserum neutralized CSA from the various cell lines. However, in the endothelial-like cell line MBA-2.1, as well as in the fibroendothelial cell clone MBA-13, the antibody did not totally eliminate the stimulating activity. The remaining CSA induced the formation of GM colonies. It was consequently proposed that particular stromal cells may produce CSF other than M-CSF.[47]

The secretion of GM-CSA (i.e., induction of the formation of colonies containing granulocytes and macrophages) by stromal cell lines was reported by several laboratories.[44,45,48] It was not clarified, though, whether this CSA represented the genuine GM-CSF or alternatively a mixture of GM, G, and M-CSF in the various possible combinations. It also must be kept in mind that a small proportion of cells induced by CSF-1 are granulocytes. Godard et al.[44] compared CSA produced by the V209 and V213 stromal cell lines to mouse lung conditioned medium. The cell populations responding to factors from these sources coincided. Recent experiments[67] indicated that particular stromal cell lines produce GM-CSF. Others make G-CSF and both types also make M-CSF. These findings were based upon the use of factor dependent cell lines. Further analysis of poly A^+ RNA from the stromal cell lines substantiated the finding that one of the cell lines had messenger RNA for GM-CSF. The MBA cell line series was similarly studied. None of the cell lines of this series produced a significant titer of GM-CSF nor had mRNA for GM-CSF detectable by Northern analysis and *in situ* hybridization.[68] The possibility that stroma cells make minute amounts of colony stimulating factors that are detectable only in bioassays in which the producer and target cells are cocultured, seems unlikely. It cannot be excluded, though, that stromal cells make some colony stimulating factors other than the species characterized thus far.

One implication of the findings discussed above is that there may be no direct correlation between the titer of CSF produced by a particular cell line and its ability to support the in vitro proliferation of myeloid progenitor cells. 14F1.1 stromal adipocytes were found to support both GM-CFC and CFU-S in culture, but did not show detectable titers of CSF apart from some CSF-1 like activity. The latter, in its purified form, does not induce in vitro accumulation of progenitor cells and, therefore, may not account for the activity of the stromal cells. IL-3 has often been suggested to support stem cell proliferation. This factor was not, however, reported to be produced either in long-term bone marrow cultures or in stromal cell lines.

Differentiation-Restraining Activities

Under conditions that allow direct contact between hemopoietic and primary stromal cells (i.e., in methylcellulose cultures), the response of CFU-C to CSF is diminished. The differentiation-restraining factor(s) produced by the stromal cells can be demonstrated only under conditions where the stromal cells are cocultured with the target hemopoietic stem cells. Conditioned media are devoid of inhibitory activity.[25-30] Zipori et al. found that some of the restraining activity diffuses through agar.[27] It appears, therefore, that the factor(s) is cell bound and shedded in low amounts. At least part of this differentiation-restraining activity operates across species barriers.[69] Although prostaglandins were detected using a radioimmunoassay in primary stromal cell cultures, they did not account for the inhibition of GM-colony formation by the stroma.[28] The H-1 cell line was also found to produce inhibitory substances that crossed agar barriers. Some, but not all, of this activity was ascribed to prostaglandins.[70] In addition, conditioned medium from this cell line inhibited erythroid colony formation.[71] Prostaglandin-like activity was also detected in a cell line, designated AP63, obtained from mouse spleen.[48]

Other Regulators of Hemopoiesis

Human stromal cell lines secreted β-interferon (β-IF), but not γ-interferon.[72] β-IF appears to be involved in the regulation of differentiation of hemopoietic cells.[73] Its importance in the mediation of stromal cell functions was not studied in detail. Quesenberry et al.[74,75] reported that the TC-1 stromal cell produced activities that synergize with CSF-1 and IL-3.

Leukemia Cell Inhibitory Activity (LCIA)

A number of cell lines from the MBA series were capable of modulating the growth of leukemia cells in a manner similar to primary stromal cells.[31,32,47,56] This activity of the primary stroma crossed allogeneic barriers and was not determined by the H-2 haplotype (Fig. 8). Attempts were made to isolate the

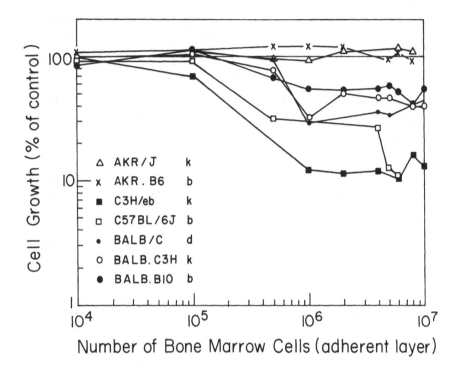

Fig. 8. Inhibition of growth of the MPC-11 plasmacytoma cell by primary stromal cells from congenic mouse strains. The capacity of stromal cells of different origins varies considerably. It is shown that the specific activity of each mouse strain is not dictated by the H-2 haplotype.[76]

active component from stromal cells. Conditioned media prepared from these cell lines did not affect the growth of the MPC-11 plasmacytoma that was found to be most sensitive to inhibition by both primary stroma and stromal cell lines. It was therefore assumed that stromal cells carry some cell surface associated factor(s) that account for this inhibition. Cell surface proteins were released from stromal cells by either enzymatic digestion[76] (Fig. 9) or spontaneous shedding under serum-free conditions (Fig. 10) and were examined for their effects on leukemia cells. Only the endothelial-like cell line MBA-2.1 was

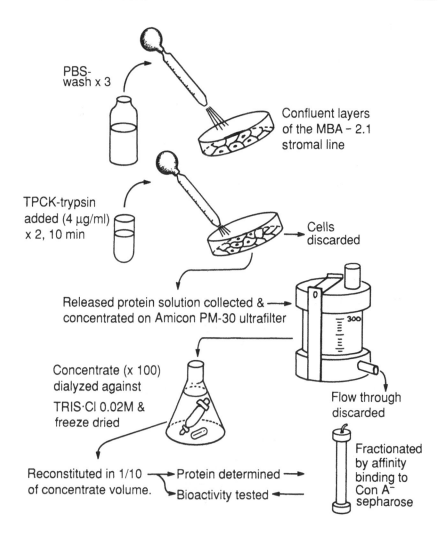

PBS-
wash x 3

Confluent layers
of the MBA – 2.1
stromal line

TPCK-trypsin
added (4 μg/ml)
x 2, 10 min

Cells
discarded

Released protein solution collected &
concentrated on Amicon PM-30 ultrafilter

Concentrate (x 100)
dialyzed against

TRIS·Cl 0.02M &
freeze dried

Flow through
discarded

Fractionated
by affinity
binding to
Con A⁻
sepharose

Reconstituted in 1/10
of concentrate volume.

Protein determined

Bioactivity tested

Fig. 9. Preparation of cell surface release proteins by TPCK-trypsin digestion. Enzymatic digestion is performed at room temperature, although 37°C was also used and found to yield essentially similar results. A standard preparation involved either 100 90-mm tissue culture plates, or alternatively, 10 roller bottles. This procedure was slightly modified for cells grown on cytodex microcarriers. Such a preparation contains 500 LCIA U (1 U is defined as amount of factor that reduces the growth of MPC-11 myeloma by 50% under the given assay conditions, i.e., 150 μL of MPC-11 cell suspension [1000 cells/mL] incubated for 5 d).[76]

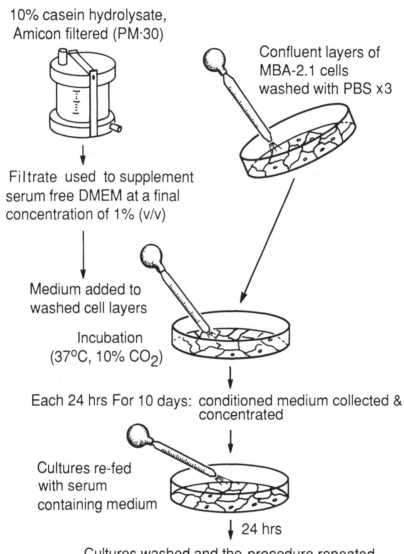

10% casein hydrolysate,
Amicon filtered (PM·30)

Confluent layers of
MBA-2.1 cells
washed with PBS x3

Filtrate used to supplement
serum free DMEM at a final
concentration of 1% (v/v)

Medium added to
washed cell layers

Incubation
(37°C, 10% CO_2)

Each 24 hrs For 10 days: conditioned medium collected &
concentrated

Cultures re-fed
with serum
containing medium

24 hrs

Cultures washed and the procedure repeated

Fig. 10. Spontaneous release of LCIA under serum free conditions. The figure schematically demonstrates the procedure as previously reported by Kadouri and Bohak.[77] Casein hydrolysate is fractionated to contain molecules and aggregates that flow through Amicon PM-30. This is done to ensure the removal of small peptides during the concentration of LCIA. The hydrolysate fraction is then added at 1% to DMEM. This conditioned medium, collected from such cultures, is then treated as in Fig. 6 (i.e., concentrated and fractionated on Con A-Sepharose). The advantage of this method over the one employing TPCK-trypsin is discussed in the pertaining text.[76]

consistently found to release a high molecular weight activity that specifically inhibited the MPC-11 plasmacytoma[76] (Fig. 11). The inhibitor bound to Concanavalin A-sepharose columns was trypsin resistant and proteinase K sensitive and is thus, most likely, a glycoprotein.[76] It was designated, tentatively, as leukemia cell inhibitory activity (LCIA).

In contrast to all plasmacytomas tested and to a few B- and T-lymphomas, other leukemia cell lines, including myeloid, macrophage, and erythroid tumors, were resistant to LCIA. Similarly, LCIA did not affect mitogen stimulation of normal spleen cells, formation of GM colonies induced by CSF, and proliferation of CFU-S in long-term bone marrow cultures.[76] This selective inhibitory activity of LCIA that excludes normal stem cells may be of use in eliminating plasma cell tumors from bone marrow inocula without harming the CFU-S population. Furthermore, LCIA seems to have differentiation and cell lineage specificity. Whereas tumor cells at a relatively early stage of the B-cell lineage, i.e., pre-B-cell lymphomas, were almost unaffected by the factor, 3 out of 10 B-cell tumors and all the plasmacytomas tested thus far were sensitive to its presence in culture.[76] It is possible, therefore, that LCIA reacts with a differentiation-related ligand in the target lymphoma cell. Whether this activity of LCIA also affects normal plasma cells and restricts the accumulation of plasma cells in vivo, remains to be determined.

Promotion of Leukemia Cell Growth

As discussed above, stromal cells from the bone marrow inhibit the growth of B-lineage lymphoma cells with a mature phenotype. Conversely, pre-B tumors required stromal cells for their initial growth in culture and retained a considerable dependence upon the stroma, even following adaptation to in vitro growth and development of cell line characteristics.[14,31,32]

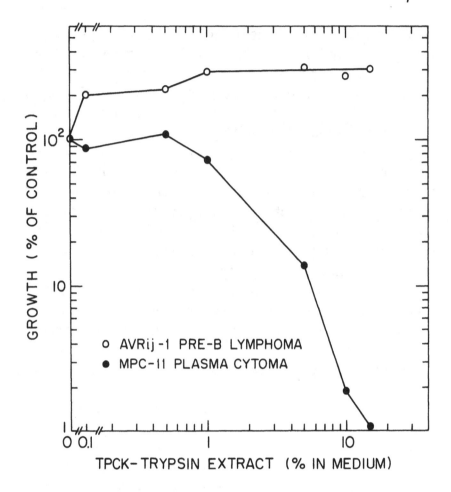

Fig. 11. Effect of cell surface-associated glycoproteins extracted by TPCK-trypsin digestion from MBA-2.1 stromal cells on the growth of lymphoma cells of the B-lineage.

This was interpreted as indicating the supportive role of the stroma regarding growth of the early stages of hemopoietic differentiation.[31] This activity may be related to the capacity of the stroma to support stem cell maintenance.

In a recent study, infant leukemia cells with a mixed pre-B/myeloid phenotype and a capacity to differentiate into two distinct pathways were grown in culture. This stem cell-like leukemia exhibited a strict dependence on stromal cells from the donor.[78] Upon removal from the stromal cells, the leukemia cells died. The autologous stroma could be replaced only by the 14F1.1 endothelial–adipose cell line that is also capable of supporting the in vitro growth of mouse stem cells.

Promoters of Leukemia Cell Differentiation

Media conditioned by the 266AD cell line contained both CSA and an activity that induced the differentiation of a promonocytic cell line.[43] Cells of the MBA series did not induce differentiation of the Friend erythroleukemia, but were found to enhance the differentiation of the tumor cells in synergy with Me_2SO.[56] This promoting activity was first detected only in the fibroendothelial cell line MBA-13.[56] Recently, nondialyzable activity could be concentrated from conditioned media of the MBA-2.1 endothelial cell line (Zipori and Ben-Hur, unpublished). In addition to the promotion of Friend cell differentiation, stromal cells from the MBA series were found to antagonize Me_2SO-induced differentiation. This activity could be observed when Friend cells that had been induced to differentiate were washed from the inducer and seeded in the presence of stromal cells. This activity was not, however, specific to marrow stromal cell lines.[56]

Transplantation and Tumorigenesis

The study of in vivo effects of stromal cells may contribute to the understanding of their functions. Unfortunately, many of these cells are tumorigenic. This considerably complicates the interpretation of their effects on hemopoiesis.

Cells of the MC series were grown in culture, collected as a thick slurry, and placed onto filters. The latter were cultured, floating on liquid medium for 24 h, and then transplanted under the kidney capsule. Histological examination of the transplanted stroma following 30 d indicated that adipogenesis occurred mainly in the MC_1 cell line. This correlated with in vitro findings. Transplantation of the cell lines did not result in development of hemopoietic activity, with the exception of the MC_1 cell line in which hemopoietic foci containing granulocytes and mononuclear and erythroid cells were observed.[79] However, cell lines of the MC series were tumorigenic in syngeneic mice and killed their hosts within 3 mo following transplantation.

Cronkite et al. found that H-1 cells became tumorigenic at the 40th passage and formed fibrosarcomas upon subcutaneous (sc) or intraperitoneal (ip) inoculation into syngeneic mice.[38] The BMA1 cell line induced fibrosarcomas with focal areas of bone formation in nude mice.[80] These tumors induced granulocytosis in nude mice. This was ascribed to the production of CSA by tumor cell lines. It has been shown, however, that production of CSA by these cell lines and the development of granulocytosis may not correlate.[81,82] Cells of the MBA series have been inoculated to syngeneic and allogeneic mice. Most of the cell lines did not produce tumors, with the exception of MBA-2.1 cells, following about 100 passages.[55]

Modulation of In Vitro Functions

In vivo, stromal cells are organized in discrete patterns and interact among themselves. These fine structures are destroyed when the marrow is cultured, and presumably only partial reconstitution occurs in long-term bone marrow cultures. Therefore, it is important to study the interactions between components of the organ stroma.

The MBA-14 presents an interesting model for the study of such phenomena. It emerged from a culture of bone marrow cells from Balb/c mice and maintained a heterogeneous cellular composition and slow growth rate for a prolonged period of in vitro maintenance. It was eventually cloned, as discussed above. The resulting cell lines were either preadipocytes or macrophages.[46] The preadipocyte clones retained the slow growth pattern characteristic of the parent cell line. The association between those two cell types could result from mutual dependence. The macrophages in those cultures apparently obtained the CSF required for their proliferation from the adipocytes. The latter reverted to a preadipose phenotype upon contact with the macrophages. In fact, the MBA-14 parent cell line did not show fat accumulation before cloning.[46] It was further found that the adipocytes are better stimulators of stem cell maintenance in vitro than preadipocytes.[56] Macrophage incidence *in situ* may therefore determine the functional properties of the stroma. In cocultures of 14F1.1 cell and bone marrow cells, a relatively low proportion of mature cells was beneficial for long-term maintenance of stem cells. The artificial addition of macrophages to these cultures reduced the recovery of stem cells and often terminated the culture.

The mechanism by which macrophages affect adipogenesis and colony stimulating activity of preadipocytes is unknown. It is possible, though, that IL-1 is involved in view of the latter's capacity to induce GM-CSF expression in mouse stromal cells.[67]

Tissue and Cell-Lineage Specificity

It is conceivable that many of the specific functions of hemopoietic organs are mediated by stromal cells from a respective microenvironment. The bone marrow stromal cell population may therefore include cells that control stem cell self-renewal, whereas in the thymus stroma, a frequent cell type may be a product of thymic hormones. This possibility has not been conclusively verified either by study of primary stromal cultures from various hemopoietic tissue or examination of stromal cell lines.

A few cell lines from the thymic epithelium are available. Itoh et al. derived a rat thymic epithelial cell line (IT-45R1). A fraction of cells, obtained by density gradient fractionation of bone marrow cells became sensitive to killing by anti-Thy 1.1 antibodies following incubation with media conditioned by the thymic stromal cell. Incubation of the marrow cell fraction in contact with the stromal line, but not conditioned media, induced the appearance of cells forming rosettes with guinea pig erythrocytes.[83,84] Additional cell lines were derived from human thymic stroma by Hays and Beardsley (HT series).[85] These cell lines were transplanted to nude mice. The consequences were that the mice survived in conventional conditions and developed the capacity to mediate mixed lymphocyte reactions and cell-mediated lysis.[85]

Whitlock and Witte[23,24] designed a long-term culture in which pre-B cells are maintained and their differentiation can be followed. Stromal cell lines were derived from those cultures (AC series) and were also found to support pre-B cell growth.[86,87] The mode of derivation and detailed properties of these and other cell lines, as well as a detailed comparison between stem cells supporting stromal cells and those affecting B-cell growth, were recently published.[88–90] The results seem to indicate that the same stromal cell clone can induce both myelopoiesis and pre-B lymphopoiesis. It is possible that a particular stromal cell subtype would exhibit different functions under various culture conditions.

Summary

Stromal cell lines have been derived from the bone marrow of various mouse strains and characterized by morphological, biochemical, and functional assays. An outline for the classification of bone marrow stromal cells is proposed. Five distinct cell types were identified: endothelial–adipose cells, fibroblast or fibroblast-type adventitial reticulum cells, endothelial-like cells, fibroendothelial cells, and macrophages. The endothelial–adipose cell can support stem cells and myeloid progenitors in vitro. This function is not mediated by other stromal cell subtypes. Some of the latter produce colony stimulating activity for granulocytes and macrophages. These activities, as well as a variety of other hemopoiesis modulators that the stroma cells appear to produce, have not been reported thus far to be biochemically purified and no cDNA clones of these activities are available. Nevertheless, it has been shown that stromal cells secrete CSF-1-like activity, synergistic activities, inhibitors of differentiation of normal hemopoietic cells, and factors that modulate leukemia cell growth and differentiation. Apparently, the mouse fibroblast stromal cell produce prostaglandins, and the human counterpart makes β-IF. This cell subtype may also produce soluble inhibitors of granulopoiesis and erythropoiesis. The endothelial-like cells bear cell surface-associated glycoproteins(s) (designated LCIA) that specifically inhibit the growth of lymphoma cells. Both the endothelial-like and the fibroendothelial cells secrete activities that promote the differentiation of leukemia cell lines.

Cells differentiate in vivo while in contact with each other. The in vitro culture procedures involving hemopoietic colony formation are essential in order to allow a quantitative approach to the study of stem cell differentiation. These assay systems, however, do present basic conceptual difficulties since they do not reproduce the high density of hemopoietic cells *in situ*, the interactions with the stroma that surrounds hemopoietic cells, and the possible "cocktails" of factors that each cell encounters within the hemopoietic tissue. Therefore, it is the future task of hematological research to try and reconstruct in vitro systems from isolated, basic cellular components in order to approach, as closely as possible, the structure of hemopoietic tissues in vivo. The derivation of cell lines of stromal cells is one step in this direction.

The availability of permanent stromal cell lines, and techniques designed to obtain additional ones, will be helpful in the study of a variety of open questions regarding the structure and function of the microenvironment. Stromal cells in long-term bone marrow cultures and stromal cell lines were found to control hemopoietic activities in culture. It has not been shown thus far, however, that the cell lines described above correspond to specific cell populations present in the bone marrow in vivo. This may be approached, for example, by the use of antibodies that recognize stromal cells and discriminate them from cells of other origin. Some functions of the stroma appear to be deficient or absent in certain mouse strains (Fig. 8). This has not been demonstrated to date, however, using stromal cell lines. Are there mouse strains that give rise to cell lines with defective hematological functions? Would this be the case in certain human hematological disorders? Some of the data discussed above suggest that stromal cell activities affect stem cell growth, cross allogeneic barriers, and may even cross xenogeneic barriers.

The nature of factors mediating these activities is still unknown. Furthermore, it is not clear whether the stromal factors that affect leukemia cell growth (such as LCIA) or differentiation are also affecting normal cell functions. These problems are, however, rather difficult to study in cell coculture systems and should await the purification of stromal cell factors. A related question is the production of cytokines by stromal cell lines. What type of colony stimulating factors are produced? Are there factors specific to the stroma? It is similarly unclear whether there are cell lineage-specific stromal cells. It is possible that stromal cell functions are modulated either by the hemopoietic cells themselves or by hemopoietic cell products (lymphokines?). The experimental tools are available. The rest is a matter of time and effort.

Acknowledgments

The author wishes to thank Ken-ichi Arai, Frank Lee, J. Allan Waitz, and Pnina Zipori for critically reviewing the chapter and their constructive advice, and Bonda Lewis, Jill Zahner, and Gary Burget for their invaluable help in preparing the manuscript. The author is an incumbent of the Delta Career Development Chair at the Weizmann Institute of Science. This chapter was prepared during the author's sabbatical leave at the DNAX Research Institute of Molecular and Cellular Biology.

References

[1]Rubin, L. and Saunders, J. W., Jr. (1972) *Dev. Biol.* **28,** 94–112.

[2]Erickson, C. A., Tosney, K. W., and Weston, J. A. (1980) *Dev. Biol.* **77,** 142–156.

[3]Weiss, L. (1980) *Regulation of Hematopoiesis*, vol. 1 (Gordon, A. S., ed.), Appleton-Century-Crofts, New York, pp. 79–92.

[4]Weiss, L. (1980) *Blood Cell and Vessel Wall: Functional Interactions* (Ciba Foundation series 71), Elsevier, North Holland, pp. 3–19.

[5]Trentin, J. J. (1970) *Regulation of Hematopoiesis*, vol. 1 (Gordon, A. S., ed.), Appleton-Century-Crofts, New York, pp. 161–186.

[6]Tavassoli, M. (1975) *Exp. Hematol.* **3,** 213–226.

[7]Metcalf, D. (1984) *The Hemopoietic Colony Stimulatory Factors*, Elsevier, Amsterdam.

[8]Metcalf, D. (1985) *Cell* **43,** 5,6.

[9]Metcalf, D. (1986) *Blood* **67,** 257–267.

[10]Metcalf, D. (1980) *Proc. Natl. Acad. Sci. USA* **77,** 5327–5330.

[11]Ogawa, M. Porter, P. N., and Nakahara, T. (1983) *Blood* **61,** 823–829.

[12]Grossman, Z. (1986) *Leuk. Res.* **10,** 937–950.

[13]Friedenstein, A. J., Chailakhjan, R. K., Latsink, N. V., Panasyuk, A. F., and Keilis-Borok, I. V. (1974) *Transplantation* **17,** 331–340.

[14]Zipori, D. and Bol, S. (1979) *Exp. Hematol.* **7,** 206–218.

[15]Wilson, F. D., O'Grady, L. McNeil, C. J., and Munn, S. L. (1974) *Exp. Hematol.* **2**, 343–354.

[16]Dexter, T. M., Allen, T. D., and Lajtha, L. G. (1977) *J. Cell. Physiol.* **91**, 335–344.

[17]Allen, T. D. and Dexter, T. M. (1983) *Scan. Electron. Microsc.* **4**, 1851–1866.

[18]Allen, T. D. and Dexter, T. M. (1982) *Differentiation* **21**, 86–94.

[19]Wilson, F. D., Tavassoli, M., Greenberg, B. R., Hinds, D., and Klein, A. K. (1981) *Stem Cells* **1**, 15–29.

[20]Lord, B. I. and Wright. E. G. (1980) *Blood Cells* **6**, 581–593.

[21]Toksoz, D., Dexter, T. M., Lord, B. I., Wright, E. G., and Lajtha, L. G. (1980) *Blood* **55**, 931–936.

[22]Dexter, T. M., Testa, N. G., Allen, T. D., Rutherford, T., and Scolnick, E. (1981) *Blood* **58**, 699–707.

[23]Whitlock, C. A. and Witte, O. N. (1982) *Proc. Natl. Acad. Sci. USA* **79**, 3608–3612.

[24]Whitlock, C. A., Robertson, D., and Witte, O. N. (1984) *J. Immunol. Methods* **67**, 353–369.

[25]Zipori, D. and Sasson, T. (1980) *Exp. Hematol.* **8**, 816, 817.

[26]Zipori, D., Sasson, T., and Frenkel, A. (1981) *Exp. Hematol.* **9**, 656–662.

[27]Zipori, D. and Sasson, T. (1981) *Exp. Hematol.* **9**, 663–673.

[28]Zipori, D. (1981) *J. Supramol. Struct. Cell. Biochem.* **17**, 347–357.

[29]Zipori, D., Sasson, T., and Friedman, S. (1982) *Experimental Hematology Today* (Baum, S. J., Ledney, G. D., and Thierfelder, S., eds.), Karger, Basel, pp. 19–26.

[30]Tamir, M., Rozenszajn, L. A., Malik, Z., and Zipori, D. (1987) *Int. J. Cell Cloning* **5**, 289–301.

[31]Zipori, D. (1980) *Cell Tissue Kinet.* **13**, 287–298.

[32]Zipori, D. (1981) *Cell Tissue Kinet.* **14**, 479–488.

[33]Zipori, D. (1988)*Long Term Effects of Chemotherapy and Radiation* (Testa, N. E. G. and Gale, R. P., eds.), Marcel Dekker, New York, pp. 27–62.

[34]Haas, M. and Meshorer, A. (1979) *J. Natl. Cancer Inst.* **63**, 427–436.

[35]Haas, M. and Reshef, T. (1980) *Europ. J. Cancer* **16**, 909–917.

[36]Anderson, R. W., Mann, S. L., Crouse, D. A., and Sharp, J. G. (1981) *J. Supramol. Struct. Cell Biochem.* **16**, 377–384.

[37]Harigaya, K., Cronkite, E. P., Miller, M. E., and Shadduck, R. K. (1981) *Proc. Natl. Acad. Sci. USA* **78**, 6963–6966.

[38]Cronkite, E. P., Harigaya, K., Garnett, H., Miller, M. E., Honikel, L., and Shadduck, R. K. (1982) *Experimental Hematology Today* (Baum, S. J., Ledney, G. D., and Thierfelder, S., eds.) Karger, Basel, pp. 11–18.

[39]Lanotte, M., Allen, T. D., and Dexter, T. M. (1981) *J. Cell. Sci.* **50**, 281–297.

[40]Kodama, H., Amagai, Y., Koyama, H., and Kasai, S. (1982) *J. Cell. Physiol.* **112**, 89–95.

[41]Kodama, H., Amagai, Y., Koyama, H., and Kasai, S. (1982) *J. Cell. Physiol.* **112,** 83–88.

[42]Lanotte, M., Scott, D., Dexter, T. M., and Allen, T. D. (1982) *J. Cell. Physiol.* **111,** 177–186.

[43]Hines, D. (1983) *Blood* **61,** 397–402.

[44]Godard, C. M., Augery, Y. L., Ginsbourg, M., and Jasmin, C. (1983) *In Vitro* **19,** 897–902.

[45]Fujita, J., Yoshida, O., Miyanomae, T., and Mori, K. J. (1983) *Gann* **74,** 334–337.

[46]Zipori, D., Friedman, A., Tamir, M., Silverberg, D., and Malik, Z. (1984) *J. Cell. Physiol.* **118,** 143–152.

[47]Zipori, D., Duksin, D., Tamir, M., Argaman, A., Toledo, J., and Malik, Z. (1985) *J. Cell. Physiol.* **122,** 81–90.

[48]Piersma, A. H., Brockbank, K. G. M., and Ploemacher, R. E. (1984) *Exp. Hematol.* **12,** 617–623.

[49]Greenberger, J. S., Sakakeeny, M. A., Davis, L. M., Moloney, W. C., and Reid, D. (1984) *Leuk. Res.* **8,** 363–374.

[50]Harigaya, K. and Hiroshi, H. (1985) *Proc. Natl. Acad. Sci. USA* **82,** 3477–3480.

[51]Li, C. L. and Johnson, G. R. (1985) *Nature* **316,** 633–636.

[52]Song, Z. X., Shadduck, R. K., Innes, D. J. Jr., Waheed, A., and Quesenberry, P. J. (1985) *Blood* **66,** 273–281.

[53]Katsuno, M., Motomura, S., Kaneko, S., Sakai, H., and Ibayashi, H. (1985) *Int. J. Cell Clon.* **3,** 81–90.

[54]Todaro, G. and Green, H. (1963) *J. Cell. Biol.* **17,** 299–313.

[55]Zipori, D. (1985) *Experimental Hematology Today* (Baum, S. J., Pluznik, D. H., and Rozenszajn, A., eds.), Springer-Verlag, New York, pp. 55–63.

[56]Zipori, D., Toledo, J., and von der Mark, K. (1985) *Blood* **66,** 447–455.

[57]Anderson, R. W. and Sharp, J. G. (1980) *J. Supramol. Struct.* **14,** 107–120.

[58]Dexter, T. M., Spooncer, E., Varga, J., Allen, T. D., and Lanotte, M. (1983) *Haemopoietic Stem Cells*, Alfred Benzon Symposium 18 (Killmann, Sv.-Aa., Cronkite, E. P., and Muller-Berat, C. N., eds.), Munksgaard, Copenhagen, pp. 303–318.

[59]Garland, J. M., Lanotte, M., and Dexter, T. M. (1982) *Eur. J. Immunol.* **12,** 332–336.

[60]Hay, E. D.(1982) *Cell Biology of Extracellular Matrix*, Plenum, New York.

[61]Naparstek, E., Donnelly, T., Shadduck, R. K., Wagner, K., Kase, K. R., and Greenberger, J. S. *J. Cell. Physiol.* (1986) **126,** 407–413.

[62]Garnett, H. M., Harigaya, K., and Cronkite, E. P. (1982) *Stem Cells* **2,** 11–23.

[63]Garnett, H. M., Harigaya, K., and Cronkite, E. P. (1984) *Proc. Soc. Exp. Biol. Med.* **175,** 70–73.

[64]Kodama, H., Sudo, H., Koyama, H., Kasai, S., and Yamamoto, S. (1984) *J. Cell. Physiol.* **118,** 233–240.

[65]Chan, S. H. and Metcalf, D. (1972) *Blood* **40**, 646–653.

[66]Lanotte, M., Metcalf, D., and Dexter, T. M. (1982) *J. Cell. Physiol.* **112**, 123–127.

[67]Rennick, D., Yang, G., Gemmell, L., and Lee, F. (1987) *Blood* **69**, 682–691.

[68]Zipori, D., Moulds, C., and Lee, F. (1986) *Exp. Hematol.* **14**, 499 (abstract).

[69]Zipori, D., Reichman, N., Arcavi, L., Shtalrid, M., Berrebi, A., and Resnitzky (1985) *Exp. Hematol.* **13**, 603–609.

[70]Garnett, H. M., Cronkite, E. P., and Harigaya, K. (1982) *Proc. Natl. Acad. Sci. USA* **79**, 1545–1548.

[71]Cronkite, E. P., Miller, M. E., Garnett, H., and Harigaya, K. (1983) *Haemopoietic Stem Cells, Alfred Benzon Symposium 18* (Killmann, Sv.-Aa., Cronkite, E. P., and Muller-Berat, C. N., eds.), Munksgaard, Copenhagen, pp. 266–284.

[72]Shah, G., Dexter, T. M., and Lanotte, M. (1983) *Br. J. Haematol.* **54**, 365–372.

[73]Resnitzky, D., Yarden, A., Zipori, D., and Kimchi, A. (1986) *Cell* **46**, 31–40.

[74]Quesenberry, P. J., Thomas, C., Alberico, T. A., Landreth, K., Witte, P., He, Y., Song, Z. X., Gualtieri, R., Stewart, F. M., McGrath, H. E., Kleeman, E., Baber, G., and Innes, D. (1988) *Proceedings of the Symposium on Humoral and Cellular Regulation of Erythropoiesis* (Zanjani, E. D., Tavassoli, M., and Ascensao, J., eds.), PMA Publishing Group, New York.

[75]Quesenberry, P., Song, Z. X., McGrath, E., McNiece, I., Shadduck, R.K., Waheed, A., Baber, G., Kleeman, E., and Kaiser, D. (1987) *Blood* **69**, 827–835.

[76]Zipori, D., Tamir, M., Toledo, J., and Oren, T. (1986) *Proc. Natl. Acad. Sci. USA* **83**, 4547–4551.

[77]Kadouri, A. and Bohak, Z. (1985) *Develop. Biol. Stand.* **60**, 431–437.

[78]Umiel, T., Friedman, S., Zaizov, R., Choen, I. J., Gozes, Y., Epstein, N., Kobiler, D., and Zipori, D. (1986) *Leuk. Res.* **10**, 1007–1013.

[79]Crouse, D. A., Mann, S. L., Sharp, J. G. (1984) *Long Term Bone Marrow Culture*, KROC Found. Serv. (USA), Liss, New York, pp. 211–231.

[80]Fujita, K., Shimomura, Y., Fujita, J., and Mori, K. J. (1985) *Experientia* **41**, 504, 505.

[81]Burlington, H., Cronkite, E. P., Heldman, B., Pappas, N., and Shadduck, R. K. (1983) *Blood* **62**, 693–696.

[82]Burlington, H., Cronkite, E. P., Laissue, J.A., Reincke, U., and Shadduck, R. K. (1977) *Proc. Soc. Exp. Biol. Med.* **154**, 86–92.

[83]Itoh, T., Kasahara, S., and Mori, T. (1982) *Thymus* **4**, 69–75.

[84]Itoh, T. (1979) *Am. J. Anat.* **156**, 99–104.

[85]Hays, E. F. and Beardsley, T. R. (1984) *Clin. Immunol. Immunopathol.* **33**, 381–390.

[86]Tidmarsh, G. F., Dailey, M. O., Whitlock, C. A., Pillemer, E., and Weissman, I. L. (1985) *J. Exp. Med.* **162**, 1421–1434.

[87]Muller-Sieburg, C. E., Whitlock, C. A., and Weissman, I. L. (1986) *Cell* **44,** 653–662.

[88]Zipori, D. and Lee, F. (1988) *Blood* **71,** 586–596.

[89]Hunt, P., Robertson, D., Weiss, D., Rennick, D., Lee, F., and Witte, O. N. (1987) *Cell* **48,** 997–1007.

[90]Whitlock, C., Tidmarsh, G. F., Muller-Seiburg, C., and Weissman, I. L. (1987) *Cell* **48,** 1009–1021.

Chapter 9

Cellular Interactions in the Regulation of Human Hemopoiesis In Vitro

Joao L. Ascensao and Esmail D. Zanjani

Normal Hemopoiesis

Role of T-Cells

The complex series of steps leading to the production of adequate numbers of blood cells in animals and humans involve the orderly proliferation and differentiation of the pluripotent and committed hemopoietic progenitors in response to the positive and negative feedback influences of regulatory signals. Both humoral and cell-mediated events play a role in this process. The role of cell–cell interaction in the regulation of hemopoiesis, elegantly demonstrated by the in vivo observations of Trentin,[1] has been firmly established as the result of studies utilizing the in vitro clonal assays for hemopoietic progenitors.[2-6] These studies have shown that accessory cell populations (T-cells, monocyte–macrophages, endothelial cells, stromal cells, and so on) that comprise the normal hemopoietic microenvironment, can play a significant role in the regulation many aspects of blood cell production. Although the mechanism(s) by which these accessory cells affect hemopoiesis is not understood, both helper and suppressive roles have been ascribed to these cells. It is generally accepted that the helper influences of these environmental cells are, for the most part, exercised at the earliest stages of progenitor cell growth, preparing the cells for action by "terminal differentiation" hormones and factors.[5,7] By contrast, the inhibitory effects of accessory cells can be demonstrated at nearly all levels of progenitor development.[5,8] This is illustrated by the following example. The stimulatory effects of T-lymphocytes, considered to be an important accessory cell in the regulation of hemopoiesis[9] via the production of BPA (burst-promoting activity), are primarily exercised at the level of the early erythroid progenitor BFU-E.[9] The resultant late erythroid progenitors (CFU-E) are then acted upon by the hormone erythropoietin (Ep) to undergo terminal proliferation/differentiation into mature red cells.[10]

The production of BPA by normal T-cells is increased when these cells are activated by mitogens, such as PHA (phytohemagglutinin), to undergo rapid proliferation.[11] However, it has been clearly shown that mitogen-activated T-cells can also profoundly suppress erythropoiesis at both BFU-E and CFU-E levels in vitro.[12] The suppressive influence of activated T-cells frequently extends to other progenitor types as well.[13-17] This broad spectrum of target cell reactivity, by in vitro activated normal T-cells, is similar to the effect produced by T-cells from some pancytopenic patients (e.g., aplastic anemia, AA) that target more than one type of hemopoietic progenitor.[18] The mechanism(s) by which these two opposing functions of accessory cells, one progenitor-restricted and the other exhibiting no definitive limitations, come about is not understood, since they are seemingly triggered by the same signal.

The delineation of the role of normal T-cells in hemopoiesis, in general, and erythropoiesis, in particular, has been hampered by the absence of pure populations of precursor cells, as well as defined culture conditions. As a result, some controversy exists regarding the effect these cells exert on hemopoietic progenitors. For example, Nathan et al.[19] showed that human blood CFU-E lacks membrane characteristics of B- or T-lymphocytes and are isolated with the null cell fraction, but they would not grow in the absence of T-cells. We confirmed the null cell antigenic characteristics of blood BFU-E; we were unable to demonstrate an obligatory role of T-cells for the BFU-E growth in vitro.[20] Similarly, Zuckerman[21] reported that T-cells were not required for optimal growth of BFU-E in vitro. By contrast, Mangan et al.[22] and Haq et al.[23] presented evidence supporting the T-cell need for optimal BFU-E development in vitro. In our initial studies, we employed two procedures for removing T-lymphocytes, SRBC rosetting, and OKT3 anti-T-cell antibody. However, in the former case, significant numbers of T-cells, recognized by different monoclonal antibodies, present in the depleted fraction, that may have accounted for our inability to demonstrate a significant effect of T-cells in blood BFU-E development.[20] The use of OKT3 proved to be more effective in removing a greater percentage of T-cells and, in this case, we were unable to detect significant BFU-E growth in the T-cell depleted fraction. However, the addition of autologous T-cells to these cultures did not result in the stimulation of BFU-E growth. We found that this inability of T-cells to promote BFU-E growth was related to the mitogenic influence of OKT3. When isolated T-cells, pretreated with OKT3, were cocultured with autologous bone marrow or with blood mononuclear cells, significant inhibition

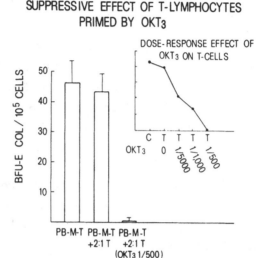

Fig. 1. Effect of incubation of peripheral blood mononuclear cells (PBM) with various concentrations of OKT₃ on BFU-E growth in vitro. Values represent mean ±SD of quadruplicate determinations of one (of three) representative experiment. Insert represents similar data using the 9.6 anti-T-cell antibody.

of erythroid colony formation occurred. This suppressive activity correlated directly with the number of OKT3-treated T-cells added to the culture. This was similar to the suppressive effects produced by PHA-stimulated autologous T-cells (Figs. 1 and 2).[12]

This effect was also dependent on the concentration of OKT3 in culture and was not seen with other anti-T-cell monoclonal antibodies, 9.6 and 7.28 (kindly provided by Dr. John Hansen), (Figs. 1 and 3) that did not stimulate T-cells. The effect of OKT3 was likely owing to its mitogenic effect on T-cells, as seen in Fig. 4. This effect was not blocked by the antibody 38.1 that recognized an epitope in the T3 receptor (Fig. 5). The mechanism leading to erythropoietic suppression is possibly owing to the production of γ-interferon by the activated T-lymphocytes, but other factors may account for this toxicity of

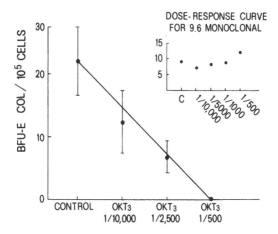

Fig. 2. T-cell requirement for inhibition of circulating BFU-E by incubation with OKT_3; the antibody was added directly to the culture in these experiments, but similar results could be seen with short-term priming of T-cells by OKT_3. Values represent mean ±SD of quadruplicate determinations of a standard experiment. Insert shows concentration of OKT_3 required for induction of suppressive T-cells.

autologous T-cells against the circulating erythroid progenitors. These results and other data are relevant to the analysis of studies that used T-cell depletion with antibodies and that subsequently cultured the cells in the presence of PHA-LCM. We noted that we could deplete T-cells from bone marrow to a remaining 3–4% (Fig. 6). T-cells were enumerated by: rosetting with AET-treated SRBC or by fluorescence with the monoclonal antibodies 9.6 and OKT3. The first two methods are strongly in agreement, but the values obtained with OKT3 were far more variable (Table 1). When T-cell depleted marrow cells were cultured in methylcellulose in the presence of PHA-LCM and Ep, there was a tremendous increase in the number of T-cells found at d 15 of culture (Fig. 7). Blood and bone marrow BFU-E have different requirements for T-cells (24) which may be explained by the continued production of T-lympho-

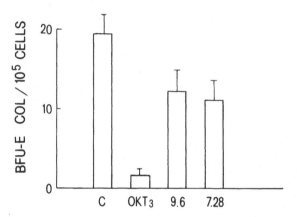

Fig. 3. Effect of long-term incubation of anti-T-cell antibodies with peripheral blood mononuclear cells. Results seen with 9.6 and 7.28 are not statistically significant; those seen with OKT$_3$ were significant. Again, short-term incubation with OKT$_3$ provided suppressor T-cells that were not seen with the other antibodies.

cytes by marrow cells. Whether the continued production of T-lymphocytes by marrow cells may explain the reported difference for T-cell requirements of blood and marrow BFU-E[24] is not known.

More recently, we employed a mixture of three monoclonal anti-T-cell antibodies (TA1, UCHT1, and T101) conjugated to the toxin ricin[25] to achieve total T-cell depletion and were able to demonstrate a significant role of T-cells in the optimal growth of blood BFU-E in vitro. These antibodies, either singly or in combination, did not exhibit significant T-cell mitogenic effect, but they abolished T-cell response to mitogens (Fig. 8). The use of ricin-bound antibodies also permits the delineation of the role of endogenously produced T-cells in BFU-E growth since no T-cells remain after 72 h.

The cells were prepared as shown in Fig. 9; T-cells (SRBC$^+$ cells) were examined for purity and were always >98% pure.

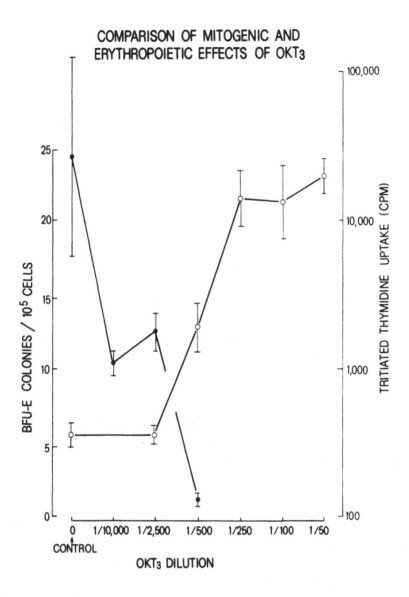

Fig. 4. The hemopoietic inhibitory activity of OKT$_3$ is seen in (o) and appears to correlate somewhat with the degree of proliferative activity—as measured by ^{3}H-thymidine incorporation (•).

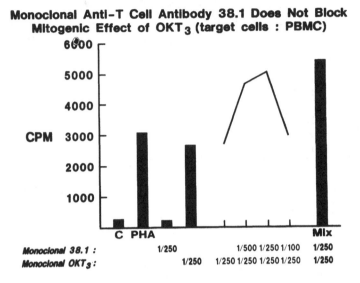

Fig. 5. Preincubation of peripheral blood mononuclear cells with monoclonal antibody 38.1—which was not mitogenic, as seen in the 3rd column
from the left—failed to inhibit OKT_3 driven proliferation (shown in the
linear graph and last bar graph).

Monocyte depletion and repletion was done by adherence and
subsequent removal from plastic surfaces; monocytes were
added back to reconstitute their original numbers, determined
by esterase (NSE) staining and OKM_1 antibody fluorescence.
The results shown in Tables 2 and 3 demonstrate that T-
lymphocytes, even at low concentrations, permit a near optimal growth of blood BFU-E derived colonies; the total T-cell
depletion did result in a significant decrease in blood BFU-E
colony formation. The readdition of T-lymphocytes to T-
depleted blood cells was effective only when such T-cells
remained viable throughout the culture period. The slight
increase in colony growth, seen with the addition of antibody-
treated T-cells suggests that T-lymphocytes are particularly
needed for the early stages of development of the erythroid
progenitors.

NO. OF T-LYMPHOCYTES IN BONE MARROW
BEFORE AND AFTER T-DEPLETION

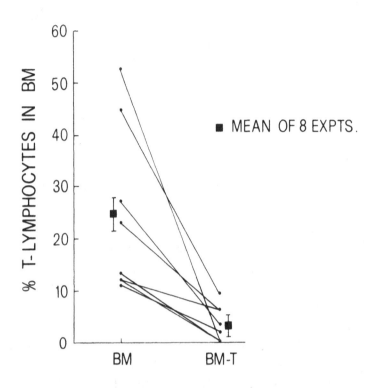

Fig. 6. Effect of separation of T-lymphocytes from bone marrow using a single AET-SRBC rosetting. Results represent the mean ±SD of 8 experiments.

Under these conditions (in a culture system low in BPA) T-cells were required for optimal, but not absolute growth of BFU-E.[25] More recently, there is evidence to suggest that under conditions of maximally stimulated growth (using purified, recombinant-derived growth factors), there is no absolute requirement for T-cells.[26] In fact, this suggests that T-cells play an amplifying role and may also modify the responsiveness of the erythroid progenitors to lineage-specific growth factors, such

Table 1
Identification of Bone Marrow T-Lymphocytes Using
Different T-Cell Markers

Marker	Intact BM,		T-depletedBM,	
	% T-cells	Range	% T cells	Range
9.6[a]	24.5 ± 5.8	11–53%	3.2 ± 1.2	0–9%
OKT$_3$[a]	13 ± 4.3	3–28%	10.8 ± 5.7	2–31%
AET-SRBC	28.7 ± 6.1	11–39%	4.2 ± 1.5	1–8%

[a]Fluorescence with these monoclonal anti-T-cell antibodies.

as erythropoietin. There are substantial amounts of data that strongly suggest that T-cell monocyte cooperation is needed for the production of hemopoietic growth factors,[27–29] whereas the inhibitory effects of T-cells did not depend on monocytes.[30]

The mechanism(s) by which normal cells are "activated" to suppress hemopoiesis is not known. Similarly, the mechanism(s) underlying the inhibitory effects of "activated" accessory cells is not understood. In vivo "activated" T-cells, from patients with aplasias restricted to a specific blood cell type, exhibit a remarkable degree of specificity not usually seen with in vitro "activated" T-cells. Thus, T-cells from patients with T-cell CLL, associated with pure red cell aplasia, inhibit the formation of erythroid colonies by patients' bone marrow, but have no effect on the growth of white cell progenitors in vitro.[31,32]

Similarly, T-cells from some patients with pure white aplasias primarily suppress CFU-GM in vitro.[33] By contrast, normal T-cells activated by exposure to PHA or IF inhibit colonies derived from erythroid (BFU-E, CFU-E), myeloid (CFU-GM), and multipotent (CFU-MIX) hemopoietic progenitors in vitro.[12,34] Although some of these effects can be reproduced by

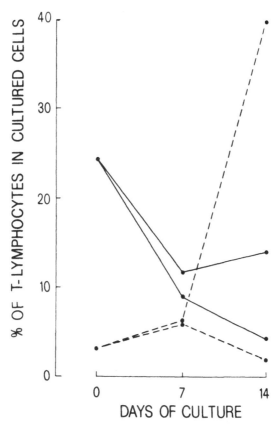

NO. OF T-CELLS IN INTACT AND T-DEPLETED
BONE MARROW THROUGHOUT CULTURE PERIOD
(MEAN OF 8 EXPERIMENT)

Fig. 7. Effect of PHA-LCM (2 top lines of each group) on expansion of T-cell clones in cultures of human marrow. The solid lines represent BMNC, whereas the broken lines represent T-cell depleted BM-T cells. The two bottom lines represent cells cultured with Ep only.

IF, there is recent work to support the notion of nonspecific inhibition by mitogen-activated T-cells[12] or specific inhibition by alloantigen (MLC, mixed lymphocyte culture) stimulated cells.[35] In recent studies, two types of MLC generated cells can be demonstrated. A nonspecific, large "blast" T-cell that has

ANTIBODY-RICIN CONJUGATE "COCKTAIL" INHIBITS MITOGENIC RESPONSE OF T CELLS

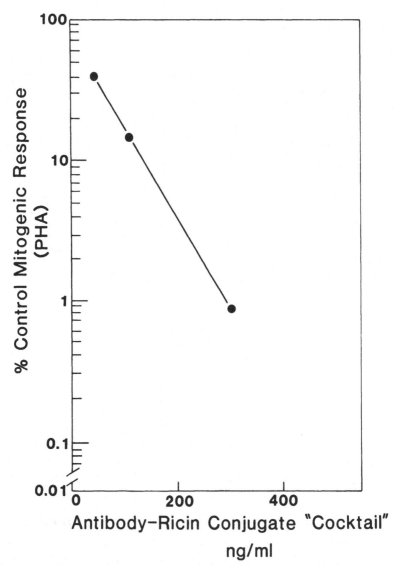

Fig. 8. Although ricin-antibody conjugates fail to kill cells immediately, they curtail their functional properties so that, by 3 d, virtually no mitogenic response was seen to a standard mitogen (PHA).

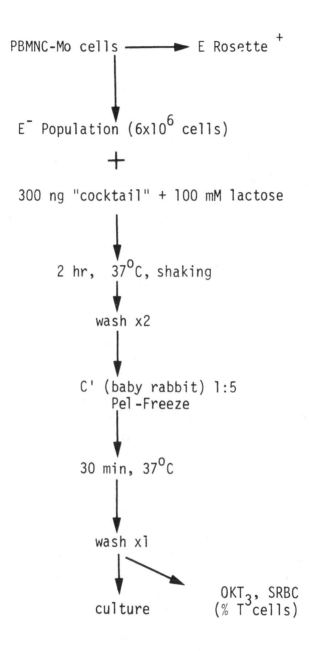

Fig. 9. Sequential steps used for elimination of all T-cells from the target populations. Since ricin A + B chains were used, lactose was needed to prevent nonspecific binding.

suppressive ability is not genetically (HLA) restricted; this cell is seen early (d 6) of mixed lymphocyte cultures and produce γ-IF, which is responsible for their suppressive activity. The d 12, MLC generated small lymphocytes are HLA-DR restricted and do not appear to produce γ-IF. Suppressor cells (T8+) are more common than helper cells (T4+) in the bone marrow. It is not known whether they reside in the marrow for functional reasons (regulating blood cell production) or simply that the traffic patterns brings them through the bone marrow.

Recent studies indicate that the inhibitory effects of activated T-cells of some AA patients may be mediated via interferons (IF).[36,37] Activated T-lymphocytes are known to produce a number of factors, including IF, that inhibit the proliferation of a variety of cell types, including hemopoietic progenitors in vitro.[34,37-39] We found that the inhibitory effects of γ-IF on normal human hemopoiesis in vitro was mediated in part through monocytes (MO) and T-cells.[34] Thus, the removal of MO and/or T-cells significantly reduced the inhibitory effects of γ-IF.[34] Moreover, when MO or T-cells, activated by brief exposure to γ-IF, were cocultured with autologous marrow this resulted in suppression of hemopoiesis.[34] By contrast, α-IF, which also profoundly inhibits human hemopoiesis in vitro, does not require MO and/or T-cells for its effect, and fails to render isolated T-cells/MO inhibitory toward autologous hemopoietic progenitors.[40]

Although both α-IF and γ-IF possess a number of common biological properties, they have different mechanisms of action with respect to their antiviral, immunoregulatory, and antiproliferative properties,[41-44] including their ability to arm accessory cells for tumor cell killing.[41] Thus, although γ-IF can both prime and trigger MO for tumor cytotoxic function, α-IF is capable of only the triggering function.[44] The failure of α-, but not γ-IF to activate T-cells and MO may thus reflect mechanistic differences in the biological functions of the two IFs and, as

Table 2

T-Lymphocyte Depletion and Its Influence on Blood
BFU-E Growth In Vitro

Cells cultured (n = 3)	BFU-E/10^5, non-T	% Monocytes[a]	% T-cells[b]
PBMC	69 ± 21	18 ± 6	74 ± 12
PBMC-T (E+)[c]	51 ± 6	23 ± 3	5 ± 2
PBMC-T (E+Mab-R+C')[d]	19 ± 3	21 ± 4	0
PBMC-T + Mab-R[e]	12 ± 6	19 ± 3	0

[a]Percent monocytes determined by OKM_1 and NSE.
[b]Percent T-cells determined by OKT_3 and SRBC.
[c](E+) T-cells depleted by SRBC rosetting only.
[d]C' complement (baby rabbit, Pel-Freeze prescreened for antistem cell activity).
[e]Mab-R Ricin-linked 'cocktail' of anti-T-cell antibodies (UCHT 1, T101, and TA1).

Table 3

T-Lymphocyte Reconstitution and the Requirement
for Continued Presence of T-Cells Throughout Culture

Cells Cultured (n = 3)	BFU-E/10^5 non-T	% Monocytes[a]	% T-Cells[b]
PBMC-T	19 ± 3	21 ± 4	0
PBMC- T + T (Mab-R)[c]	29 ± 6	24 ± 6	72 ± 9
PBMC-T + T	74 ± 13	21 ± 4	70 ± 7

[a]Percent monocytes determined by OKM_1 and NSE.
[b]Percent T-cells determined by OKT_3 and SRBC.
[c]Mab-R Ricin-linked cocktail of anti-T-cell antibodies (UCHT 1, T101, and TA1).

such, may provide a unique tool for the study of mechanism(s) that render accessory cells inhibitory to the hemopoietic process.

The role of T-lymphocytes in granulopoiesis is somewhat different from their role in erythropoiesis and may be owing to several factors: (1) decreased sensitivity to inhibitors (such as IF); (2) difficulty in growing circulating progenitors (CFU-GM); and (3) less dependence on hemopoietic growth factors other than CSF.

The T-lymphocytes produce and, in part, regulate the production of CSF. This occurs in expanding clones[45] and activated T-cells.[46] Some investigators suggest that only a subset (T4+) for T-cells is capable of producing CSF, whereas (T8+) cells can directly inhibit the CFU-GM colony cells,[47] or CSF production.[48] Mitogen- or antigen-activated T-cells seem able to produce, in addition to CSF, hemopoietic inhibitors that, in certain cases, may mask the CSF effect.[49] T-lymphocytes are not required for CFU-GM colony growth,[13,14] although some authors have found a dual role for T-cells stimulating, circulating CFU-GM and inhibiting marrow CFU-GM.[50] Lymphocytes capable of hemopoietic inhibition can be generated in vitro by mitogen activation.[13,14] Some of these effects can be reproduced by soluble factors present in media conditioned by these cells and it has been shown that γ-IF and, to a certain extent, α-IF modulate some of these effects.[37,40] In some studies, inhibition was only seen in coculture studies;[13] this discrepancy may be owing to concomitant CSF production by the stimulated lymphocytes. The phenotypes of the inhibitory lymphocytes found in MLC reactions were radioresistant T8+ and Ia+;[15] the mitogen-stimulated T-cells were radiosensitive T4+[16] or of the T8+, Ia– phenotype.[17] It is interesting that both helper and suppressor/cytotoxic phenotypes produce γ-IF when activated.[37] Furthermore, it has been suggested that, whereas T-cells from bone marrow of patients with aplasia suppressed autologous or allogeneic hemopoietic progenitors, circulating

T-lymphocytes had no such effect.[50] Standardization of methods, serial determinations, and use of purified cell populations will hopefully clarify the differences in the results reported by various laboratories.

Role of Monocytes

Monocytes are capable of producing factors that stimulate (CSF, IL-1, BPA, and prostaglandins of the F series) and inhibit (IF, PGE_2, IL-1, and TNF) granulopoiesis and erythropoiesis. As such, monocytes may regulate the rate of production of blood cells. The effects are predominantly seen on monocyte/macrophage progenitors (CFU-M) and less on the CFU-GM, and both 7 and 14 d progenitors are equally sensitive.[51,52] The inhibitory effect of PGE_2 is mediated via increases in intracellular cAMP.[53]

Early studies by Kurland and Moore[54,55] elegantly demonstrated the important role of prostaglandins produced by monocyte–macrophages. The prostaglandins appear to act directly on the progenitors and their production was stimulated by increasing levels of CSF.[54,55] The prostaglandins also interfere with IL-1 synthesis by the monocytes[56] that may, in turn, lead to a decrease in CSF production.[29] Another inhibitor produced by mature cells (granulocytes) is lactoferrin,[29,57] which shuts off production of CSF either directly[57] or by decreasing monocyte recruiting activity (MRA) production by monocytes.[29] MRA is a monokine, now thought to be IL-1, that stimulates T-cells, endothelial cells, and fibroblasts to produce CSF.[58] The current hypothesis is that IL-1 (aka MRA) functions as an overall regulator determining the levels of growth factors produced by the various cell types. IL-1 synthesis is stimulated by endotoxin, interferon,[59] and CSF.[60]

Interferon-activated monocytes can inhibit CFU-GM growth but this effect requires high concentrations of γ-IF and is reversed by increasing CSF concentrations.[37,39] Clearly, both the resting or activated macrophages interact with other accessory cells and play a pivotal role in granulopoiesis.

The presence of erythroid islands in the bone marrow suggests that monocytes have a central, nutritive role in erythropoiesis.[61] They provide iron to the progenitors and precursors, produce BPA that acts on early precursors (BFU-E), and is important for cell maintenance in vitro and likely in vivo.[62] Their role in erythropoiesis in vitro has been disputed and is likely dependent on their source, number in erythroid cultures, and activation state. Some studies showed that bone marrow monocyte–macrophages stimulated BFU-E and CFU-E, but only at low monocyte concentrations.[63-65] Peripheral blood monocytes were inhibitory at all concentrations used.[65] Some investigators claim the opposite behavior for circulating monocytes.[21,66] Some of these effects are likely to be artificial and depend on the method used for collecting these cells. Our own studies demonstrated that malignant monocytes (U937 cell line) could produce hemopoietic growth factors (BPA), but that coculture with hemopoietic progenitor cells was generally inhibitory.[67] These cells did not produce CSF constitutively, but could be induced to do so if activated by phorbol esters or lymphokines (likely γ-IF).[68] Contrary to the negative effect of prostaglandins on the granulomonocytopoietic system, PGE_1 and PGA_2 are quite active in stimulating CFU-E and BFU-E growth in vitro.[69] This also appears to be mediated by increasing the intracellular concentrations of cAMP.[69]

Activated monocytes produce more BPA, but they also produce IL-1, TNF, and IF, all of which appear to have a negative effect on erythropoiesis.[70] The production of these factors is bolstered by CSF; these clinical conditions are often associated with anemia and leukocytosis. It is still debated whether CSF and Ep can target early progenitors; competition for cellular receptors at this level could lead to a specific path of differentiation. A controversy still exists whether direct competition exists between CSF and Ep at the level of the early progenitors and whether this may favor a specific path for differentiation.[71] Proponents of the stochastic model believe that the effect of CSF or Ep is exerted only at the level of the committed progenitor or precursor and is an amplifying, rather than a directional signal.[72,73]

Role of NK Cells

The natural killer (NK) cells, habitually known as the large granular lymphocytes (LGL), are radioresistant, can be recruited and activated by lymphokines, and are defined by their ability to lyze tumor cells at high effector:target ratios (50:1 to 20:1).[74] These cells appear to produce BPA[75] and enhance the growth of BFU-E in cultures of blood null cells.[75] Other investigators have demonstrated an inhibitory effect on different types of hemopoietic colonies in vitro.[76,77] This effect may vary with the maturation stage of the progenitor cells. Early CFU-GM colony growth determined at d 7, was enhanced by NK cells, whereas late (d 14) CFU-GM formation was decreased by about 50%.[78] This inhibitory effect is mediated by a factor, NK cell-derived colony inhibiting activity (NK-CIA).[79] Biochemical and immunological studies indicate that NK-CIA is likely TNF; it acts synergistically with γ-IF to augment the sensitivity of the late CFU-GM to the inhibitory effects of NK-CIA.[79]

The hypothesis that NK cells mediate graft rejection in bone marrow transplantation, in particular the phenomenon of hybrid resistance,[80,81] makes it important to understand their biology. With the recent use of T-cell depleted marrow grafts, there has been a rather large increase in the numbers of graft failures, confirming that: NK cells are radioresistant and suggesting that donor T-cells can dampen the negative effects of the hosts' NK cells.

Another area of interest is with the prolonged in vivo use of IL-2 activated cells—LAK (lymphokine activated killer cells)—that results in anemia, thrombocytopenia, and eosino-philia. We have begun a major study to determine the in vitro effects of the LAK cells (mostly NK cells defined as by the monoclonal antibody, Leu 11[+]) in an autologous setting and correlate the results with blood counts, cell surface markers, and interferon levels, in an attempt to understand the effects of these cells in vivo.

Abnormal Hemopoiesis

Aplastic Anemia

Severe aplastic anemia is the most devastating form of hemopoietic failure with a high mortality rate and little re-sponse to conventional hemopoietic stimulatory therapy.[82] Aplastic anemia is in some ways similar to immunodeficiency syndromes and, as such, comparisons between the pathogen-etic mechanisms can be drawn (Table 4). The absolute and rela-tive numbers of detectable hemopoietic progenitors are greatly reduced,[83,84] and remain low during the early remission pe-riod.[85] This decrease in blood cell progenitors was felt to be owing to immunologic suppression of hemopoiesis in some patients.[83] The early studies utilized several methods to dem-onstrate this phenomenon: (1) incubation of the patient's cells with ATG;[86] (2) removal of T-lymphocytes by physical separa-tion (elutriation);[87] and (3) incubation of the patient's lympho-cytes with normal marrow cells.[83,88] These studies were later criticized because of the detection of suppressor lymphocytes in transfusion recipients,[89] but other investigators did not find evidence of transfusion-induced suppression activities.[88] Fur-thermore, coculture studies of untransfused patients, using HLA-matched target cells, did show a percentage (20%) of patients with lymphocyte-mediated aplasia.[90]

The majority of studies done have been able to demon-strate the presence of these inhibitory cells. We studied 32

Table 4
Pathogenetic Mechanism in AA
and Comparison with Immunodeficiencies

Aplastic anemia	Immunodeficiencies
Stem Cell Defect	SCID[a]
quantitative	
qualitative	
Defective microenvironment	DiGeorge syndrome
Suppressor mechanism	CVI[b] (hypo γ)

[a]Severe combined immunodeficiency.
[b]Common variable immunodeficiency.

consecutive patients diagnosed with aplastic anemia. The characteristics of the patient population is shown in Table 5 and is similar to other reported series. As seen in Table 6, 9 of the 32 patients (29%) were felt to have a demonstrable in vitro suppressor mechanism. There was a wide variety of immune-mediated abnormalities that included autologous and/or allogeneic cell mediated inhibition as well as humoral suppression of hemopoiesis. Some of these effects were also seen with only one of the committed progenitors. Table 7 shows autologous, but not allogeneic cell-mediated inhibition of granuloerythropoiesis, compared with Table 8 where humoral inhibition of both normal and patient's progenitors were seen. Table 9 compares the results of these assays in four of our patients. Humoral inhibition of CFU-GM was seen in one patient, whereas an untransfused patient's serum inhibited both CFU-GM and CFU-E. Patient K. K. had an autologous cellular inhibitor; this patient was treated with ATG, with good response (*see* Table 10). On this table, the results shown are of immunosuppressive therapy of three patients with aplastic anemia and a patient with pure red cell aplasia (F. G.). Patients K. K. and G. B. were

Table 5
Clinical-Laboratory Characteristics of Patients with Cytopenias

	Aplastic Anemia	Erythroid Aplasia	Refractory Anemias	Neutropenias
# of patients	32	5	2	9
Age	23	31	42	45
Sex	M-14, F-17	M-1, F-4	M-1, F-1	M-7, F-2
Duration	8.4 mo	29 mo	6 mo	1d–4y
Prior therapy	Pred (12) Andr (13)	Pred (5)	Pred	None
Transfusion History	RBC's (17) Plts (16)	RBC's	RBC's Plts	None
Blood Counts				
WBC	2300	5900	3900	1700
Hgb	6.7	7	10.9	11.8
Retic. percent	.8%	.8	2.7	–
Plts	27,000	244,000	38,000	209,000

Table 6
Composite Analysis of Immune Mechanisms in Aplasia

	Patients studied	# Exhibiting immune-based inhibition of marrow growth
Aplastic anemia	32	9 (29%)
Neutropenia	9	1
Refractory anemia	2	2
Erythroid aplasia	5	3
Total	48	15 (31%)

Table 7
Lymphocyte-Mediated Inhibition of Autologous,
but Not Allogeneic Marrow Growth In Vitro

| | Colonies/10^5 Cells[a] | | | |
| | Normal Marrow | | Patient Marrow | |
Additions	CFU-E	CFU-GM	CFU-E	CFU-GM
Ep/CSF	295 ± 12	79 ± 5	77 ± 10	22 ± 7
+ Nl PBL	259 ± 10	71 ± 3	90 ± 6	19 ± 2
+ Pt PBL	339 ± 16	91 ± 5	28 ± 4	5 ± 1

[a]Mean ±SD.

treated with a standard course of ATG, patient S. C. with high dose steroids, and patient F. G. failed steroids initially, but responded dramatically to cyclophosphamide. Some of our other patients underwent bone marrow transplantation, so we could not evaluate their response to immunosuppressive therapy. From these studies, we confirmed prior observations on

Table 8
Suppression of Autologous and Allogeneic CFU-GM
and CFU-E Growth InVitro

| | Normal | | Patient's | |
	CFU-GM[a]/CFU-E[a]		CFU-GM/CFU-E	
Marrow	45 ± 2	17 ± 3	18 ± 3	8 ± 2
Marrow + Nl. serum	26 ± 2	21 ± 3	16 ± 1	12 ± 6
Marrow + Pt's serum	18 ± 2	3 ± 1	3 ± 2	1 ± 1

[a]Mean ±SD.

the detection of low numbers of hemopoietic progenitors in the majority of patients with aplastic anemia. This decrease could be owing to immune suppression in about 29% of the patients; this inhibition was seen occasionally only in autologous systems and required the use of both erythroid and myeloid clonal assays for its detection. The etiopathogenetic mechanisms in the remaining patients have not been identified.

Other groups have used the methods described above and, in addition, included the removal of T-cells by rosetting with sheep red blood cells,[91] readdition of T-cells to T-depleted marrow,[92] and incubation with ALG[93] or methylprednisolone.[94] In one study,[95] the inhibitory activity was directed only against autologous targets and was removed by treatment with corticosteroids. The inhibitory cells have been shown to be of phenotype T3+ and Ia+, but no definite subset has been identified in AA. The incidence of immune-mediated inhibition in vitro, ranged from 16 to 100% (averaging 25–30%), this latter study using coculture assays of transfused patients with random targets.[89] This is lower than the incidence of response to immunosuppressive therapy, which is around 50%, and sug-

Table 9

Effect of Patients' Serum or Lymphocytes on Patients' Autologous
Bone Marrow Growth In Vitro

	E. L.		A. B.[a]		K. K.		V. N.	
	CFU-GM[b]	CFU-E[b]	CFU-GM	CFU-E	CFU-GM	CFU-E	CFU-GM	CFU-E
BM	36±2	112±18	18±3	16±2	22±14	144±20	14±1	110±11
BM + Nl PBL	34±2	–	nd[c]		19±4	180±24	14±2	134±17
BM + Pt PBL	36±1	132±24	nd[c]		5±2	56±8	12±1	132±14
BM + Nl Serum	64±2	–	16±1	24±6	nd[c]	142±16	–	–
BM + Pt Serum	19±1	148±4	3±2	2±1	nd[c]	184±20	–	442±30

[a]Untransfused.
[b]Mean ±SD/10^5 cells.
[c]Not done.

Table 10

Analysis of Laboratory Parameters Before and After Immunosuppressive Therapy

Patient	Hgb		WBC		Platelets	
	Pre Rx	Post Rx	Pre Rx	Post Rx	Pre Rx	Post Rx
S. C.	5.0	13.1	1,400 (26)[a]	4.600 (71)	11,000	129,000
G. B.	11.1	14.4	3,000 (24)	5,700 (67)	1,000	224,000
F. G.	6.5	14.8	10,000	12,000	230,000	242,000
K. K.	5.0	10.0	1,000	8,000	100,000	210,000

[a]The numbers in brackets reflect the percentage of PMNs.

Table 11
Pathogenesis of Marrow Aplasia

Stem cell defects
Fanconi's anemia
Some cases of congenital hypoplastic anemia (CHA)
Stem cell deficiency
Toxic damage, chemicals, chemo Rx, radiation
Folate/B12 deficiency
Viral-induced damage
Microenvironmental alterations
Radiation damage
Rare cases of CHA
Accessory cell–aberrant function
Defective helper function
Enhanced suppressor function
T-lymphocytes
? Monocytes
? NK cells
Antibody-mediated inhibition

gests that: (1) the assays used may not be sensitive enough to detect all cases of suppressor-cell mediated aplasia; (2) the presence of inhibitory T-cells is an epiphenomenon; or (3) that the effect of immunosuppression is more broad and may benefit patients other than those identified by in vitro testing.[96] A tentative scheme for the classification of AA, based on in vitro parameters, is shown in Table 11. Other clinical evidence for immunemediated aplasia comes from bone marrow transplant studies in which rejection of a syngeneic graft was followed by recovery of autologous hemopoiesis.[92] A prognostic value for these tests has been postulated in these cases since rejection of grafts has occurred in patients with demonstrable cell-mediated suppression.[92] A time period has been defined (4 mo from date of diagnosis) for administration of immunosuppressive therapy beyond which recovery of hemopoiesis is not seen.[98] It may be that exhaustion of the stem cell compartment occurs during this period of time, pluripotent stem cells are damaged, or an underlying defect of stem cells occurs in these patients. The appearance of circulating small erythroid cells or cell fragments in patients with AA has been shown to correlate positively with response to ATG.[99] What these cells represent in the context of this disease has yet to be elucidated. Suda et al.[100] found that removal of adherent cells significantly increased the numbers of CFU-GM in cultures of aplastic marrows. However, other laboratories have failed to confirm these observations.[101,102]

It is also possible that some of these effects are mediated by NK cells, although direct evidence is still lacking. A few studies have demonstrated decreased killer cell activity in the peripheral blood and bone marrow patients with AA[103] that correlated with the severity of the AA. It was felt by these authors that reduction of K-cell activity was owing to the hypoproduction of these cells by the marrow.

Exciting new observations have been made in some cases of AA. Gamma-interferon may cause hemopoietic failure in vitro;[36,104] the addition of anti-γ-IF antibodies enhanced colony growth, [105] and γ-IF production by lymphocytes was decreased following successful therapy with ATG;[106] these patients have an increase in circulatory-activated suppressor cells[36] that are of the T8+, Ia+, and Tac+ (IL2+) phenotypes. These findings may explain the occurrence of AA following mononucleosis.[107] Another viral infection (parvovirus), known to cause "Fifth disease" in children, has been associated with 'aplastic crisis' in thalassemics or patients with sickle cell disease.[108] The inhibition of erythropoiesis appears to be exerted exclusively at the level of the erythroid progenitor and results from interaction of the virus with progenitor cells.[109] A better understanding of the altered immunological states seen in aplastic anemia will require serial studies particularly in the patients treated with immunosuppressive therapy.

Acknowledgments

We thank Gail Price, Virginia Corvino, and Rosemarie Ambrose for their help in the preparation of this manuscript. This research was supported, in part, by funds granted by the Charles H. Revson Foundation to J. L. Ascensao.

References

[1]Trentin, J. J. (1970) *Regulation of Hematopoiesis* (Gordon, A. S., ed.), Appleton-Century-Crofts, New York, p. 159.

[2]Quesenberry, P. and Levitt, L. (1979) *N. Engl. J. Med.* **301,** 755–760, 819–823, 868–872.

[3]Zanjani, E. D. and Kaplan, M. (1979) *Progress in Hematology* (Brown, E. B., ed.) Grune & Stratton, New York, p. 173.

[4]Ascensao, J. L., Vercellotti, G. M., Jacob, H. S., and Zanjani, E. D. (1984) *Blood* **63,** 553–558.

[5]Lipton, J. M. and Nathan, D. G. (1983) *Br. J. Haematol.* **53,** 361–367.

[6]Cline, M. J. and Golde, D. W. (1979) *Nature* **277,** 177–181.

[7]Iscove, N. N. (1978) *ICN–UCLA Symposium*, pp. 37–82.

[8]Hoffman, R., Zanjani, E. D., Lutton, J. D., Zalusky, R., and Wasserman, L. R. (1977) *N. Engl. J. Med.* **296,** 10–13.

[9]Aye, M. T. (1977) *J. Cell Physiol.* **91,** 69–77.

[10]Eaves, C. J., Humphries, R. K., Krystal, G., and Eaves, A. C. (1981) *Hemoglobins in Development and Differentiation* (Stamatoyannopoulos, G. and Nienhuis, A. W., eds.) Liss, New York, p. 63.

[11]Meytes, D., Ma, A., Ortega, J. A., Shore, N. A., and Dukes, P. P. (1979) *Blood* **54,** 1050–1070.

[12]Banisadre, M., Ash, R. C., Ascensao, J. L., Kay, N. E., and Zanjani, E. D. (1981) *Experimental Hematology Today* (Baum, S. J., Ledney, G. D., and Kahn, A., eds.) Karger, New York, p. 151.

[13]Ascensao, J. L., Kay, N. E., Banisadre, M., and Zanjani, E. D. (1981) *Exp. Hematol.* **9,** 473–478.

[14]Bacigalupo, A., Podesta, M., Mingari, M. C., Moretta, L., Piaggio, G., Van Lint, M., Durando, A., and Marmont, A. (1981) *Blood* **57**, 491–496.

[15]Nakao, S., Harada, M., Kondo, K., Odaka, K., Veda, M., Matsue, K., Mori, T., and Hattori, K. (1984) *J. Immunol.* **132**, 160–164.

[16]Sakamaki, H., Hamaguchi, H., Furusawa, S., and Shishido, H. (1985) *Br. J. Hematol.* **61**, 633–640.

[17]Harada, M., Okada, K., Kondo, K., Nakao, S., Veda, M., Matsue, K., Mori, T., and Matsuda, T. (1985) *Exp. Hematol.* **13**, 963–967.

[18]Linch, D. C. (1984) *Immunol. Today* **5**, 14 (abstract).

[19]Nathan, D. G., Chess, L., Hillman, D. G., Clarke, B., Breard, J., Merler, E., and Housman, D. (1978) *J. Exp. Med.* **147**, 324–339.

[20]Nomdedeu, B., Gormus, B. J., Banisadre, M., Rinehart, J. J., Kaplan, M. E., and Zanjani, E. D. (1980) *Exp. Hematol.* **8**, 845–859.

[21]Zuckerman, K. S. (1981) *J. Clin. Invest.* **67**, 702–709.

[22]Mangan, K. F., Chikkappa, G., Bieler, L. Z., Scharfman, W. B., and Parkinson, D. R. (1982) *Blood* **59**, 990–996.

[23]Haq, A. V., Rinehart, J. J., and Balcerzak, S. P. (1983) *J. Lab. Clin. Med.* **101**, 53–57.

[24]Lipton, J. M., Reinherz, E. L., Kudisch, M., Jackson, P. L., Schlossman, S. F., and Nathan, D. G. (1980) *J. Exp. Med.* **152**, 350–360.

[25]Ascensao, J. L., Vallera, D., and Zanjani, E. D. (1984) *Exp. Hemat.* **12**, 379 (abstract).

[26]Sieff, C. A., Emerson, S. G., Mufson, A., Gesner, T. G., and Nathan, D. G. (1986) *J. Clin. Invest.* **77**, 74–81.

[27]Verma, D. S., Spitzer, G., Zander, A. R., Fisher, R., McCredie, K. B., and Dicke, K. A. (1979) *Blood* **54**, 1376–1383.

[28]Herrmann, F., Cannistra, S. A., and Griffin, J. D. (1986) *J. Immunol.* **136**, 2856–2861.

[29]Bagby, G. C., McCall, E., and Layman, D. L. (1983) *J. Clin. Invest.* **71**, 340–344.

[30]Torok-Storb, B. and Hansen, J. A. (1982) *Nature* **298**, 473, 474.

[31]Lipton, J. M., Nadler, L. M., Canellos, G. P., Kudisch, M., Reiss, C. S., and Nathan, D. G. (1983) *J. Clin. Invest.* **72**, 694–706.

[32]Hoffman, R., Kopel, S., Hsu, S. D., Dainiak, N., and Zanjani, E. D. (1978) *Blood* **52**, 255–260.

[33]Bagby, G. C., Lawrence, H. J., and Neerhout, R. C. (1983) *N. Engl. J. Med.* **309**, 1073–1078.

[34]Mamus, S. W., Schroder-Beck, S., and Zanjani, E. D. (1985) *J. Clin. Invest.* **75**, 1496–1503.

[35]Torok-Storb, B. and Johnson, G. G. (1985) *Blood* **66**, 137a (abstract).

[36]Zoumbos, N. C., Gascon, P., Djeu, J. Y., Trost, S. R., and Young, N. S. (1985) *N. Engl. J. Med.* **312**, 257–265.

[37]Zoumbos, N. C., Djeu, J. Y., and Young, N. S. (1984) *J. Immunol.* **133,** 769–774.

[38]Santoli, D., Tweardy, D. J., Ferrero, D., Kreider, B. L., and Rovera, G. (1986) *J. Exp. Med.* **163,** 18–40.

[39]Broxmeyer, H. E., Lu, L., Platzer, E., Feit, C., Juliano, L., and Rubin, B. Y. (1983) *J. Immunol.* **131,** 1300–1305.

[40]Mamus, S. W., Oken, M. M., and Zanjani, E. D. (1986) *Exp. Hematol.* **14,** 1015–1022.

[41]Pestka, S., Kelder, B., Rehberg, E., Ortaldo, J. R., Heberman, R. B., Kempner, E. S., Moschera, J. A., and Tarnowski, S. J. (1983) *The Biology of the Interferon System* (Maeyer, E. and Schellekens, H., eds.), Elsevier, Amsterdam, p. 535.

[42]Blalock, J. E., Georgiades, J. A., Langford, M. P., and Johnson, H. M. (1980) *Cell. Immunol.* **49,** 390–394.

[43]Dianzani, F., Salter, L., Fleishmann, W. R., Jr., and Zucca, M. (1978) *Proc. Soc. Exp. Biol. Med.* **159,** 94–97.

[44]Pace, J. L., Russell, S. W., LeBlanc, P. A., and Murasko, D. M. (1985) *J. Immunol.* **134,** 977–981.

[45]Kelso, A. (1986) *J. Immunol.* **136,** 2930–2937.

[46]Cline, M. J., and Golde, D. W. (1974) *Nature* **248,** 703, 704.

[47]Hesketh, P. J., Sullivan, R., Valeri, C. R., and McCarroll, L. A. (1984) *Blood* **63,** 1141–1146.

[48]Broxmeyer, H. E., Lu, L., and Bognacki, J. (1983) *Blood* **62,** 37–50.

[49]Platzer, E., Rubin, B. Y., Lu, L., Welte, K., Broxmeyer, H. E., and Moore, M. A. S. (1985) *J. Immunol.* **134,** 265–271.

[50]Bacigalupo, A., Podesta, M., Mingari, M. C., Moretta, L., Van Lint, M. T., and Marmont, A. (1980) *J. Immunol.* **125,** 1449–1453.

[51]Pelus, L. M., Broxmeyer, H. E., and Moore, M. A. S. (1981) *Cell Tissue Kinet.* **14,** 515–526.

[52]Aglieta, M., Piacibello, W., and Gavosto, F. (1983) *Acta Haematol.* **69,** 376–381.

[53]Taetle, R. and Mendelsohn, J. (1980) *Blood Cells* **6,** 701–718.

[54]Kurland, J. I., Broxmeyer, H. E., Pelus, L. M., Bockman, R. S., and Moore, M. A. S. (1978) *Blood* **52,** 388–407.

[55]Kurland, J. and Moore, M. A. S. (1977) *Exp. Hematol.* **5,** 357–373.

[56]Kunkel, S. L., Chensue, S. W., and Phan, S. H. (1986) *J. Immunol.* **136,** 186–192.

[57]Broxmeyer, H. E., Moore, M. A. S., and Ralph, P. (1976) *Exp. Hematol.* **5,** 87–102.

[58]Bagby, G. C., Dinarello, C. A., and McCall, E. (1986) *Clin. Res.* **34,** 654a (abstract).

[59]Newton, R. C. (1986) *Immunology* **56,** 441–449.

[60]Moore, R. N., Oppenheim, J. J., Farrar, J. J., Carter, C. S., Waheed, A., and Shadduck, R. K. (1980) *J. Immunol.* **125**, 1302–1305.

[61]Bessis, M., Lessin, L. S., and Beutler, E. (1983) *Hematology* (Williams, W. J., Erslev, A. J., Beutler, E., and Rundles, R. W., eds.), McGraw-Hill, New York, p. 257.

[62]Iscove, N. N. and Guilbert, N. J. (1978) *In Vitro Aspects of Erythropoiesis* (Murphy, M. J., ed.), Springer-Verlag, New York, p. 3.

[63]Gordon, L. I., Miller, W. J., Branda, R. F., Zanjani, E. D., and Jacob, H. S. (1980) *Blood* **55**, 1047–1050.

[64]Reid, C. D. L., Baptista, L., and Chanarin, I. (1981) *Br. J. Hematol.* **48**, 155–164.

[65]Rinehart, J. J., Zanjani, E. D., Nomdedeu, B., Gormus, B. J., and Kaplan, M. E. (1978) *J. Clin. Invest.* **62**, 979–986.

[66]Mangan, K. F. and Desforges, J. F. (1978) *Exp. Hematol.* **8**, 717–727.

[67]Ascensao, J. L., Kay, N. E., Earenfight-Engler, T., and Zanjani, E. D. (1981) *Hemoglobins in Development and Differentiation* (Stamatoyannopoulos, G. and Nienhuis, A. W., eds.), Liss, New York, p. 103.

[68]Ascensao, J. L. and Mickman, J. K. (1984) *Exp. Hematol.* **12**, 177–182.

[69]Chan, H. S. L., Saunders, E. F., and Freedman, M. F. (1980) *J. Lab. Clin. Med.* **95**, 125–132.

[70]Zanjani, E. D., Schulman, J. C., and Lasky, L. C. (1986) *Future Developments in Blood Banking* (Smith-Sibinga, C. Th., Das, P. C., and Greenwald, T. J., eds.), Matinus-Nijhoff, Boston, p. 131.

[71]VanZant, G. and Goldwasser, E. (1979) *Blood* **53**, 946–965.

[72]Leary, A. G., Ogawa, M., Strauss, L. C., and Civin, C. I. (1984) *J. Clin. Invest.* **74**, 2193–2197.

[73]Lim, B., Jamal, N., and Messner, H. A. (1984) *J. Cell. Physiol.* **212**, 291–297.

[74]Kay, N. E. (1986) *CRC Crit. Rev. Clin. Lab. Sci.* **22**, 343–359.

[75]Pistoia, V., Ghio, R., Nocera, A., Leprini, A., Perata, A., and Ferrarinni, M. (1985) *Blood* **65**, 464–472.

[76]Hansson, M., Beran, M., Anderson, B., and Kiessling, R. (1982) *J. Immunol.* **129**, 126–132.

[77]Degliantoni, G., Perussia, B., Mangoni, L., and Trinchieri, G. (1985) *J. Exp. Med.* **161**, 1152–1168.

[78]Matera, L., Santoli, D., Garbarino, G., Pegoraro, L., Bellone, G., and Pagliardi, G. (1986) *J. Immunol.* **136**, 1260–1265.

[79]Degliantoni, G., Murphy, M., Kobayashi, M., Francis, M. K., Perussia, B., and Trinchieri, G.(1985) *J. Exp. Med.* **165**, 1512–1530.

[80]Bordignon, C., Daley, J. P., and Nakamura, I. (1985) *Science* **230**, 1398–1401.

[81]Gale, R. P. and Moran, C. R. (1979) *Nature* **281**, 220–222.

[82]Camitta, B. M., Storb, R., and Thomas, E. D. (1982) *N. Engl. J. Med.* **306**,

645–652, 712–718.

[83]Kagan, W. A., Ascensao, J. L., Fialk, M. A., Coleman, M., Valera, E. B., and Good, R. A. (1979) *Am. J. Med.* **66,** 444–449.

[84]Kern, P., Heimpel, H., Heit, W., and Kubanek, B. (1979) *Br. J. Hematol.* **35,** 613–623.

[85]Devergie, A., Gluckman, E., Faille, A., Boiron, M., and Bernard, J. (1980) *Blut* **41,** 171 (abstract).

[86]Ascensao, J., Pahwa, R., Kagan, W., Moore, M., Hansen, J., and Good, R. (1976) *Lancet* **1,** 669–671.

[87]Kagan, W. A., Ascensao, J. L., Pahwa, R., Hansen, J. A., Goldstein, G., Valera, E. B., and Good, R. A. (1976) *Proc. Natl. Acad. Sci. USA* **73,** 2890–2894.

[88]Hoffman, R., Zanjani, E. D., and Lutton, J. D. (1977) Unpublished observations.

[89]Singer, J. W., Brown, J. E., James, M. C., Doney, K., Warren, R. P., Storb, R., and Thomas, E. D. (1978) *Blood* **52,** 37–46.

[90]Singer, J. W., Doney, K. C., and Thomas, E. D. (1979) *Blood* **54,** 180–185.

[91]Amare, M., Abdou, N. L., Robinson, M. G., and Abdou, N. I. (1978) *Am. J. Hematol.* **5,** 25–32.

[92]Torok-Storb, B. J., Sieff, C., Storb, R., Adamson, J., and Thomas, E. D. (1980) *Blood* **55,** 211–215.

[93]Faille, A., Barrett, A. J., Balitrand, N., Ketels, F., Gluckman, E., and Najean, Y. (1979) *Br. J. Hematol.* **42,** 371–380.

[94]Bacigalupo, A., Podesta, M., and Van Lint, M. T. (1981) *Br. J. Hematol.* **47,** 423–432.

[95]Roodman, G. D., Ascensao, J. L., Banisadre, M., Bloom, P. M., and Zanjani, E. D. (1980) *Am. J. Med.* **69,** 325–328.

[96]Hunter, R. F., Mold, N. G., Mitchell, R. B., and Huang, A. T. (1985) *Proc. Natl. Acad. Sci. USA* **82,** 4823–4827.

[97]Royal Marsden Hospital Bone Marrow Transplantation Team (1977) *Lancet* **2,** 742.

[98]Hunter, R. F., Roth, P. A., and Huang, A. T. (1985) *Am. J. Med.* **79,** 73–78.

[99]Torok-Storb, B., Doney, K., Sale, G., Thomas, E. D., and Storb, R. (1985) *N. Engl. J. Med.* **312,** 1015–1022.

[100]Suda, T. Mizoguchi, H., Mura, Y., Kubota, K., and Takaku, F. (1980) *Exp. Hematol.* **8,** 659–665.

[101]Harada, T. and Abe, T. (1983) *Exp. Hematol.* **11,** 298–304.

[102]Kenyon, P. D., Ascensao, J. L., Ash, R. C., McGlave, P. B., Roodman, G. D., and Zanjani, E. D. (1980) *Clin. Res.* **28,** 729A (abstract).

[103]Voltarelli, J. C., Falcao, R. P., Carvalho, I. F., and Bottura, C. (1983) *Scand. J. Hematol.* **30,** 451–457.

[104]Linch, D. C. (1985) *Immunol. Today* **6,** 155 (abstract).

[105]Toretsky, J. A., Shahidi, N. T., and Finlay, J. L. (1986) *Exp. Hematol.* **14,** 182–186.

[106]Laver, J., Kernan, N. A., Levick, J., Moore, M. A. S., O'Reilly, R. J., and Castro-Malaspina, H. (1985) *Exp. Hematol.* **13,** 433 (abstract).

[107]Shadduck, R. K., Winkelstein, A., Ziegler, Z., Lichter, J., Goldstein, M., Michaels, M., and Rabin, B. (1979) *Exp. Hematol.* **7,** 264–271.

[108]Mortimer, P. P., Humphries, R. K., Moore, J. G., Purcell, R. H., and Young, N. S. (1983) *Nature* **302,** 426–429.

[109]Young, N. S., Harrison, M., Moore, J., Mortimer, P., and Humphries, R. K. (1984) *J. Clin. Invest.* **74,** 2024–2032.

Chapter 10

The Collagenous Hemopoietic Microenvironment

Renate E. Gay, C. W. Prince, K. S. Zuckerman, and S. Gay

Introduction

The collagens of the connective tissues serve to support a variety of tissue architectures throughout the body.[1] The various structural elements of the collagens preserve the physical and functional integrity of the various tissues. In general, the distribution as well as architectural disposition of collagens differ greatly from one connective tissue to another and may be correlated with specific roles. In this capacity, the collagenous hematopoietic stroma mechanically supports the blood cells and regulates the cellular migration. Blood cells follow circulatory pathways meticulously laid out in time and place.[2-4] Yet, it is only recently that our understanding of the complex role of collagen and cell–matrix interactions that influences cytodifferentiation, mitogenesis, and morphogenesis has truly come of age.[5-8] With respect to the regulation of hemopoiesis, it is known that the hemopoietic microenvironment influences the growth and differentiation of hematopoietic cells. Although still somewhat poorly defined, we shall see that this microenvironment contains structural well-defined extracellular collagenous components.

Prior to the last decade, the term "collagen" was used in a rather nebulous fashion to describe the cross-striated fibrils seen in various connective tissues when viewed with the electron microscope.[9] Indeed, it was used so often by classical morphologists to describe pathologic processes that "collagen" became the equivalent of "connective tissue," or the more modern term "matrix."[10] However, for several years, the term "collagens" has been most appropriately applied to a series of related, yet chemically-distinct macromolecular species.[9]

All collagen molecules are long, more or less stiff rods consisting of a triple helix of three polypeptide chains called a chains. Chemically, each collagen chain has unique primary structures and amino acid composition. Features of the collagen molecule, which are present in all species, are the presence of a repeating glycine-x-y amino acid triplet sequence in helical regions of each α chain that results in a $1/3$ glycine content for the helix and an amino acid content of 20–25%. Considerable variation is found for cysteine, the hydrophobic residues, and the basic amino acids. The significance of these differences is not totally understood, since no functional differences related solely to amino acid composition have been identified.

Exciting new information related to the discovery of additional genetically-distinct collagen molecules and considerable insight into the structure and location of the multiple genes for collagen synthesis have greatly facilitated acquisition of data on the structural features of the collagens.[11] Despite many chemical and structural similarities, sufficient diversity of physicochemical properties of the known collagens exists and provides the basis for their differentiation and division into different collagen types.[11] Currently, there are 11 known types of collagen molecules. The fibrils or aggregates derived from them are now recognized as distinct gene products. Table 1 lists the currently recognized types of collagens and presents information with respect to the molecular species formed by each chain and the cellular origin of the molecules.

Based on the fact that the most distinct feature of collagen chains is the presence of lengthy sequences of repeating Gly-X-Y amino acid triplets in which the X and Y positions are frequently occupied by prolyl and hydroxyprolyl residues, hydroxyproline has been widely used as a quantitative measure of collagen content in body fluids or in given tissues. However, there are varying levels of hydroxylation of the different chains. For example, the type III collagen molecule contains about 30% more hydroxyproline than type I. In addition, the presence of hydroxyproline in proteins like Clq seriously undermines the validity of using only determination of hydroxyproline for the quantitation of collagen content. Therefore, for both research and diagnostic evaluations, the combined use of chemical analysis, such as analysis of collagen type chains or peptides and the application of immuno(histo)-chemical techniques, are a necessity to evaluate the complexity of collagenous proteins in normal and pathologic tissues. In this regard, for example, a gel permeation, high-performance liquid chromatography system utilizing commercially-available silica-based gels has been developed for evaluation of the cyanogen bromide cleavage products derived from collagen α chains.[12] The high efficiency and precision of the system permits unequivocal identification of various chains by inspection of the peptide elution pattern and is sufficiently sensitive to permit analyses to be performed with as little as 1.0 µg of sample. On the other hand, based on the fact that each collagen molecule expresses a number of well-defined antigenic determinants,[13] antibodies

Table 1
Molecular Species and Cellular Origin of the Genetically-Distinct
Major and Minor Types of Collagen

Collagen type[a]	Molecular Species	Major Cellular Origin	Tissue for
I	$[\alpha1(1)]_2\alpha2(1)$	fibroblasts, osteoblasts	large crossbanded interstitial fibers
II	$[\alpha1(II)]_3$	chondroblasts	fibers of various size within collagenous matrices
III	$[\alpha1(III)]_3$	fibroblasts, reticulum cell	fine fibrillar reticular networks
IV	$[\alpha1(IV)]_2\alpha2(IV)$	epithelial and endothelial cells	basement membranes
V	$[\alpha1(V)]_2\alpha2(V)$ $[\alpha(1V)]$ $\alpha1(V)\alpha2^3(V)\alpha3(V)$	smooth muscle cells	pericellular and interstitial filaments
VI	$\alpha1(VI)\alpha2(VI)$ $\alpha3(VI)$	fibroblasts	interstitial filaments
VII	$[\alpha1(VII)]_3$	unknown	anchoring fibrils
VIII	unknown	endothelial cells	unknown
IX	$\alpha1(IX)\alpha2((IX)$ $\alpha3(IX)$	chondrocytes	filaments in cartilage
X	$[\alpha1(X)]_3$ (?)	hyperthrophied chondrocytes	filaments incartilage
XI	$1\alpha2\alpha3\alpha$	chondrocytes	fine fibrils of cartilage

[a]Several of these collagen types have been referred by an older terminology as follows: Type III—embryonic collagen; Type IV—basement membrane collagen; the $\alpha1(IV)$ chain has also been designated C-chain and the $\alpha2(IV)$ chain has been called D-chain; Type V—A-B collagen; the $\alpha1(V)$ chain was designated B-chain or αB, the $\alpha(V)$ chain has been called A-chain or αA, and the $\alpha3(V)$ chain has been termed αC; Type VI—intima or short chain (SC) collagen; Type VII—long chain (LC) collagen; Type VIII—endothelial cell (EC) collagen; Type IX—type M or HMW-LMW collagen; Type X—G collagen or short chain (SC) cartilage collagen; Type XI—K collagen or $1\alpha 2\alpha3\alpha$ collagen.

specific for globular procollagen determinants, amino- and carboxyterminal determinants as well as helical-conformational determinants (Fig. 1) have been produced[14,15] and used in refined immunohistochemical assays.[10]

Owing to the increasing complexity of the collagen family[11] and its associated noncollagenous components,[16] the use of monoclonal antibodies against the different molecular forms of the collagens has been extremely advantageous in structural and pathological studies. As such studies involve comparative studies on multiple tissue samples encompassing an extended period of time, a relatively large quantity of antibody that recognizes the same antigenic determinants in the various and multiple forms of collagens is essential. Consequently, specific criteria for the immunization, characterization, and isolation of poly- and monoclonal antibodies against collagens for use in immunohistochemistry have been developed[17] and comprehensive libraries of highly specific antibodies against the distinct types of collagen, their associated glycoproteins, and structural proteoglycans have been established.

The Genetically-Distinct Types of Collagen

In view of the complexity of the collagen family of proteins, it is advantageous to discuss them in terms of separate molecules and structural entities.

Type I Collagen

Type I collagen qualifies for designation as the prototype of all the collagens.[18] It is a heterotrimeric molecule comprised of two identical α1(I) chains and a similar, but clearly different α2(I) chain. These chains can be readily resolved by cation-exchange chromatography primarily owing to an elevated complement of basic amino acids in the α2(I) chain.[19] The

ANTIGENIC   DETERMINANTS

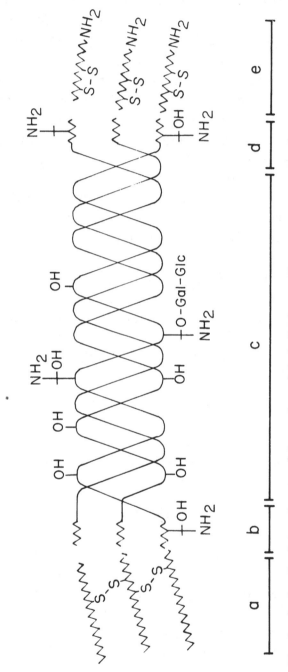

Fig. 1. Antigenic determinants of the native triple-helical procollagen and collagen molecules (modified after Timpl [13,15]: (a) COOH-terminal globular procollagen determinant; (b) COOH-terminal (nonhelical) collagen determinant; (c) Helical (conformational) collagen determinant; (d) NH$_2$-terminal (nonhelical) collagen determinant; and (e) NH$_2$-terminal globular procollagen determinant; reproduced with permission from (1983) Monographs in Pathology: Connective Tissue Diseases (Wagner, B. M., Fleischmajer, R., and Kaufman, N., eds.), William & Wilkins, Baltimore, p. 121.

structure of the gene for the α2(I) chain of type I collagen, the most abundant collagen in the human body, has been almost completely elucidated.[20] This gene comprises approximately 38 Kb, but only 10% of the DNA is involved in the coding sequence, which is divided into 51 exons. Using the R loop technique and electron microscopy, the distribution of these exons along the gene has been determined (Fig. 2). Sequence analysis data regarding the length of the individual exons and introns of the α2(I) gene, when compared with other collagen genes such as those of the α1(I) and α1(III) genes, show that the length of the noncoding introns varies to a large extent, whereas the length of the corresponding exons, at least those coding for the triple helical part of the molecule, is identical (for details, *see* K. Kühn[21]).

The correlation of exon size with the protein structural domains is not yet clear, but the 1014 residue-long triple helix appears to have evolved by repeated tandem duplication of a single ancestral exon 54 bp long. During evolution, fusion of individual exons into larger units may have led to the formation of functional and structural domains important for protein function that were subsequently conserved. Further, it appears that functionally important domains, such as the D units of the triple helix, force the molecules to aggregate in a parallel, staggered array that can evolve independently of the exon–intron organization of the gene.[21]

The biosynthesis of collagen type I molecules, as well as the other collagens, involves the regulated, concerted expression of the collagen structural genes and genes coding for posttranslational modification enzymes, as well as the intricate interactions between primary translation products and cotranslational and posttranslational modifying enzymes (review by Kivirikko and Myllyä[22]).

Type I molecules, similar to all the other molecular species of collagens, are assembled intracellularly through the inter-

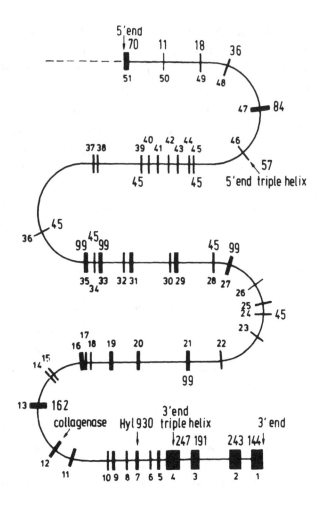

Fig. 2. Simplified rendition of the gene for a collagen α chain, compiled from studies on chick, mouse, and human α chains. Exons are represented by bars and are numbered from the 3′ end of the gene (small numerals 1–51). Unless indicated otherwise by large numerals, thin bars represent exons 54 bp long, thick bars have 108 bp. As indicated by arrows, the triple helical portion of the α chain is encoded in exons 4–49. The cleavage site for collagenase is apparently encoded by exon 12, and the arrow at exon 7 indicates the position of a hydroxylysine residue (Hyl 930) that is involved in crosslinking with adjacent collagen molecules. Exons outside those responsible for the triple helix are involved in formation of interchain bridges, globular and other nonhelical domains, signal propeptides, and linkage and cleavage sequences (reproduced with permission of the author and publisher from Kühn K (1984) *Collagen Rel Res* 4, 309).

action of precursors, so-called proα chains. The proα chains are considerably larger than α chains of the collagen molecule owing to the presence of extension sequences at both the NH_2-and COOH-termini of the chains (see Fig. 1). Both globular procollagen extension sequences are removed *en bloc* by two specific proteases, resulting in the loss of approximately one-third of the mol wt of the procollagen molecule and producing collagen molecules with chains of M_r 95,000.

The lengthy triplet regions in α1(I) and α2(I) chains extending over a sequence of 1014 amino acid residues plus the presence of prolyl and hydroxyprolyl residues in X and Y portions specify the triple-helical conformation and account largely for its stability.[18]

Although the precise nature of the interactions required for the formation of collagen fibers is not established, heterotrimers of type I collagen molecules aggregate laterally in a precise manner to create the abundant well-organized extracellular fibers of the dense connective tissue.

Fibrils sectioned longitudinally reveal a cross-banded pattern with a periodicity of about 68 nm. The fibrillar bundles occur either in compactly-bound parallel arrays that provide a structure of high tensile-strength as in tendons, or in an interwoven pattern allowing for a more pliable structure as in the dermis of the skin and fibrous capsules of various organs. Since the conversion of the procollagen type I molecules is nearly complete, only a few small fibrils containing type I procollagen molecules accompany the mass of the well-structured type I fibers (~ 45–180 nm in diameter). The intercellular organic matrix of bone is comprised predominantly of collagen fibers derived from type I molecules. The fibers show an acidophilic staining pattern owing to the presence of small amounts of proteoglycans. The collagen fibers in bone vary in arrangement and size, depending upon the age of the specimen studied. Fibers of infant bone are arranged less compactly and have a width ranging from about 20–60 nm. Fibers with diameters up to 150 nm are observed routinely in bones of mature individuals. The interaction of hydroxyapatite crystals with type I collagen within the dense collagenous matrix of bone adds to the enormous compressive strength of mineralized structures.

Type II Collagen

Collagen type II is the major interstitial component of hyaline cartilage and occurs also in the nucleus pulposus and the vitreous humor. The discovery of type II collagen initiated the era of research on collagen polymorphism.[23] Although the molecular composition of the triple helix of type II collagen chains is generally referred to as $[\alpha1(II)]_3$ (see Table 1), sequence data indicate microheterogeneity. At least two unique $\alpha1(II)$ chains differing in only a few amino acid residues have been identified.[24]

The isolation and partial characterization of the entire human $pro\alpha1(II)$ collagen gene have provided the molecular basis for studies of collagen type II gene expression in normal and diseased states.[25] Procollagen type II molecules are extracellularly processed resulting in molecules possessing a M_r of 95,000. Similarly to type I collagen, these molecules aggregate laterally to form fibrils. However, owing to varying levels of lysyl hydroxylation and glycosylation, as well as an intimate interaction with cartilagenous glycoproteins, a wide spectrum with respect to the diameter of fibers, e.g., 5–100 nm, is formed in the different zones of hyaline cartilage.[26]

Owing to the large amount of proteoglycan aggregates in cartilage, the collagen fibrils are largely masked[27] and require an enzymatic pretreatment with hyaluronidase prior to immunohistochemical staining.[28]

The chondrocyte phenotype is extremely sensitive to environmental changes with respect to collagen biosynthesis. For example, complete cessation of synthesis of type II collagen may sometimes occur in chondrocyte cultures,[29] or as in the case of the dedifferentiated hypertrophied chondrocytes of the epiphyseal growth plate, that have switched to type I collagen synthesis.[28] In analogy, the capacity of certain populations of chondrocytes in osteoarthritic cartilage to synthesize new cartilage specific type II collagen appears to be greatly diminished or lost and only partially substituted by synthesis of type I collagen.[28]

Type III Collagen

The chemical and structural features of the proα1(III) and α1(III) are likewise quite similar to proα1(I) and α1(I). However, a significant difference occurs in the extracellular processing of procollagen type III molecules. Initial observations on cultured fibroblasts suggested that the conversion of type III procollagen to collagen is incomplete[30] and that a substantial portion of the molecules deposited in the extracellular matrix of various tissues retain their N-terminal globular sequences.[31]

Type III collagen molecules are found in fine reticular networks of skin, liver, and spleen.[31] These fibers, described in the past by their argyrophilic properties as "reticulin," "immature collagen," or "precollagen," have a diameter that usually does not exceed 40 nm. The incomplete conversion of procollagen type III molecules most likely influences the growth of fibrils and results in a number of fine filaments surrounding the thin fibrils. Ultrastructural identification of amino propeptides of type III collagen in human skin has revealed a number of such structural entities.[32] This very special macromolecular tissue form of a fine reticular type III collagen network does not interfere with the metabolic exchange processes occurring between parenchymal cells, yet it provides a certain degree of cellular support and stability for parenchymal organs.

In histologic specimens, the fine fibrillar networks are often visualized by the silver "reticulin" stains. However, since these structures are associated with a variety of different glyco-proteins,[33] silver stains are highly variable with respect to intensity and are therefore not specific. Despite the fact that the fine fibrillar networks are largely comprised of procollagen and collagen type III molecules,[31,32,34] the anachronistic term "reticulin" should be avoided, especially since also the major basement membrane components, type IV collagen and laminin, may label when certain silver impregnation techniques are used.[35] Only the use of immunohistochemical techniques has made it possible to evaluate the complexity of collagenous and noncollagenous proteins in normal and pathological tissues.[10]

Since type III collagen is invariably found in tissues that also have a high complement of type I collagen and since the molecules are capable of forming aggregates of similar, if not identical, molecular architecture, questions have arisen concerning the potential of these molecular species to form co-aggregates.[11] In this regard, the identification of crosslinked peptides involving sequences from $\alpha 1(I)$ and $\alpha 1(III)$ chains[36] strongly supports the notion that, under certain circumstances, type I and III molecules may be present in the same fibrous element.

Type IV Collagen

Type IV collagen molecules are the major structural components of epithelial and endothelial basement membranes.[37] Investigations of basement membrane containing matrices have shown that type IV collagen has a completely different molecular and macromolecular structure from the fiber-forming collagen types I, II, and III. Integrity and mechanical resistance are generated by the formation of a large, regular network of type IV molecules.[38] The network is characterized by globular domains at one terminus that are responsible for the end-to-end interaction between two molecules, and by a short triple-helical segment at the opposite terminus that allows lateral alignment of four single molecules. Both interactions result in the formation of a web-like structure and explain the lack of cross-banded collagenous components in classical basement membranes.

The type IV collagen monomer molecules are comprised of proα1(IV) and proα2(IV) chains with M_r's of 185,000 and 170,000, respectively.[39] Interestingly, the molecules undergo little, if any, extracellular processing. The data strongly suggest that there are no chemical or structural differences between procollagen and collagen molecules in the type IV system and that molecules participating in aggregate formation have essentially the same characteristics as they possessed following assembly in intracellular compartments.[11] Sequence data account for a total of 1136 residues of the estimated 1700–1800 residues in the human α1(IV) chain.[40,41]

Type V Collagen

Type V collagen shares biochemical features of both basement membrane collagen and interstitial fibrillar collagen. Therefore, it is not surprising that type V collagen is not an integral component of basement membranes nor does it form regular cross-banded fibrils. As outlined in Table 1, molecules of the type V system contain three chains called α1(V), α2(V), and α3(V). The most common form appears to be a heterotrimer, with the chain composition $[\alpha1(V)]_2\alpha2(V)$, that occurs in dermis, blood vessels, bone, and placental membranes.[11] However, a homotrimeric form $[\alpha1(V)]_3$[42] and a molecule comprised of all three chains, namely $[\alpha1(V)\alpha2(V)\alpha3(V)]$, have been isolated from placental villi.[43] Type V collagen is synthesized in the form of a procollagen molecule that appears larger than the proα chains of type I, II, and III procollagen, but by rotary shadowing, resembles the general structural features of

these molecules.[44] Further special features of the type V collagen system include a quite slow extracellular processing, its
resistance to degradation by collagenases that cleave collagen
types I, II, and III into the typical three-quarter and one-quarter
fragments, and its cleavage by alternate proteolytic enzymes.[45]

Our initial data showing a cell surface association of type
V collagen[1] have been expanded by demonstrating that type V
collagen remains in the cell layer of cultured cells,[42] forms part
of the exocytoskeleton of smooth muscle cells and endothelial
cells,[46] and extends connecting filaments into the interstitial
matrix.[47-50] The latter observation confirms the concept that
type V collagen functions in part as an adhesive element.[1] In
addition, more recent data indicate that types I and V form hybrid fibrils in vitro[49] and are incorporated together in hetero-
typic fibrils.[50] Collagen types IV and V occur in close proximity
to each other, but are not codistributed in authentic basement
membranes.[46-50] This points to the necessity for a rigid protocol
for collagen purification and antibody characterization to overcome the association of macromolecular complexes in order to
ensure precise localization.[17]

Type VI Collagen

Type VI collagen is a large disulfide-bonded complex that
was initially called "intimal" collagen because of its isolation
in fragmented form from vascular endothelium.[51] Although
detectable in the vasculature,[52,53] it is also found in numerous
interstitial areas as large aggregates and differs radically in its
structure and macromolecular organization.[54] Type VI collagen probably represents less than 1% of the total collagenous
matrix in the body. The constituent polypeptide chains (M_r
110,000–140,000) consist of collagenous and noncollagenous
segments that assemble in a triple-stranded protomer of 105
nm in length flanked on each side by globular domains of
similar size.[54] Protomers are assembled to dimers by an anti-

parallel staggered alignment of triple-helical segments, and tetramers are formed from laterally aligned dimers that cross with their outer triple-helical segments in a scissors-like fashion.[54] Moreover, disulfide-linked collagen VI produced by cultured fibroblasts has a size similar to collagen VI found in tissue extracts. Microfibrillar structures comprised of type VI were found by immunoelectron microscopy of placenta.[48,54] Moreover, lateral aggregates of collagen VI microfibrils may exist in forms of "zebra collagen," and "Luse bodies."[54]

Type VII Collagen

Type VII collagen comprises a small proportion of the total tissue collagen with constituent chains of M_r 170,000.[55] It is expressed as an extended triple-helical domain with almost one and one-half times the length of the type I collagen triple helix.[56] Moreover, aggregates have been observed to occur as disulfide bond stabilized dimers formed by an antiparallel alignment of monomers with a 60 nm overlap. Ultrastructural data on laterally aggregated structures resemble features of anchoring fibrils observed in association with the basement membrane of skin.[56] Therefore, type VII collagen is currently considered to be the structural basis of anchoring fibrils.

Type VIII Collagen

Type VIII collagen has been identified as a product of transformed endothelial cells.[57] The biosynthetic products of these cells are highly sensitive to proteolytic degradation and have led initially to a model suggesting interruptions of the repetitive Gly-X-Y triplet structure. However, more recent data indicate a more conventional collagen model in which type VIII collagen is compared to three α1 chains of M_r 61,000 arranged in a predominantly helical structure with nonhelical domains at each end.[58]

Type IX Collagen

Type IX collagen was first isolated from hyaline cartilage, but only in a partially degraded form.[59] Subsequent investigations have shown that the low mol wt fragment was composed of three unique polypeptides α1(IX)α2(IX)α3(IX), indicating its derivation from a larger parent heterotrimeric molecule.[60] The gene for this type of collagen has been cloned and nucleotide sequencing suggests that the native molecule has a total length of at least 738 amino acid residues in which four relatively large nontriplet regions alternate with three Gly-X-Y triplet regions.[61] The results have further shown that α2(IX) is highly homologous to α1(IX) in both primary structure and the location of triplet and nontriplet regions. The covalent attachment of chondroitin sulfate and/or dermatan sulfate chains to certain chains of type IX collagen makes this collagen unique.[63] Immunohistological studies indicate a general distribution of type IX collagen throughout the cartilage matrix[64] at the intersection of type II collagen fibrils.[65]

Type X Collagen

Type X collagen is an additional cartilage-derived molecule,[66] synthesized only by hypertrophic chondrocytes[67] that contains a short helical domain (~150 nm) and a globular domain at one end of the molecule. The nature of the aggregates formed by probably three identical chains is presently unknown.

Type XI Collagen

Type XI collagen is likewise a quantitatively minor collagen, comprised of three α chains initially designated 1α2α3α with approximately the same size of α chains of collagen types I, II, and III. Type XI collagen, also designated as type K collagen,[11] containing the 3α chain, reveals a close relationship to type II collagen in that the 3α chain appears identical to α1(II) and is distinguished only with respect to elevated levels of hydroxylysine-linked carbohydrate moieties.[69] These data are confirmed by gene cloning showing that the gene for proα1(II) is present in only one copy number in the haploid vertebrate genome.[70] Figure 3 illustrates the polymorphism and structural features of the genetically distinct types of collagen.

Collagenous Bone Marrow Stroma

The various types of collagen occur throughout the hematopoietic environment in very distinct patterns of disposition (Fig. 4).

Type I collagen is found almost exclusively in bone osteoid. Type I collagen appears also in the single, well-structured fibers in the bone marrow.

Type II collagen is usually only found in articular hyaline cartilage; however, bone and marrow induction under the influence of decalcified bone matrix leads to a transient formation of a collagen type II containing matrix that eventually undergoes endochondral ossification.[71]

Type III collagen is restricted to the fine fibrillar network of the marrow stroma. Despite the fact that most of these fibers appear argyrophilic, they should not be referred to as "reticulin" fibers (*see* above). The thin fibrils of marrow stroma, comprised of type III collagen molecules, do not codistribute with the presence of type I collagen. Previous investigations based on paraffin-embedded, formalin-fixed sections have claimed a codistribution of both collagen types. However, as previously shown, peroxidase-labeled immunoglobulin, for example, has a strong nonspecific affinity for collagen in formalin-fixed, paraffin-embedded tissue sections.[72]

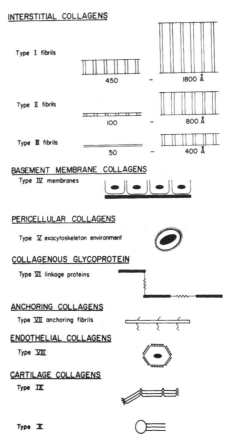

INTERSTITIAL COLLAGENS

Type I fibrils   450   —   1800 Å

Type II fibrils   100   —   800 Å

Type III fibrils   50   —   400 Å

BASEMENT MEMBRANE COLLAGENS
Type IV membranes

PERICELLULAR COLLAGENS

Type V exocytoskeleton environment

COLLAGENOUS GLYCOPROTEIN

Type VI linkage proteins

ANCHORING COLLAGENS
Type VII anchoring fibrils

ENDOTHELIAL COLLAGENS
Type VIII

CARTILAGE COLLAGENS
Type IX

Type X

Fig. 3. Polymorphism and structural features of the genetically-distinct types of collagen.

Type IV collagen is found normally, only quite sparsely, underlying the endothelium of marrow sinuses and may participate in the regulation of the entry of blood cells into the circulation. Probably owing to the interaction of cell surface receptors with extracellular matrices, the transit of some mature blood cells across this barrier appears possible, whereas it prevents developing, immature cell stages and other cells in the pool of mature blood elements from leaving the extravascular space.[73] In certain forms of marrow fibrosis, a deposition of basement membrane collagen type IV is found in an almost continuous, linear form. The latter results in continuous sheets

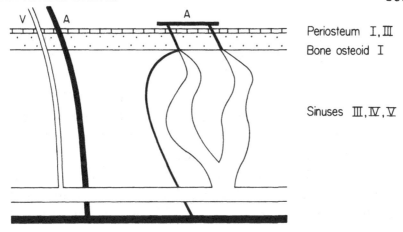

Periosteum I, III
Bone osteoid I

Sinuses III, IV, V

CELLULAR ORIGIN OF COLLAGENS IN BONE MARROW

SINUSES

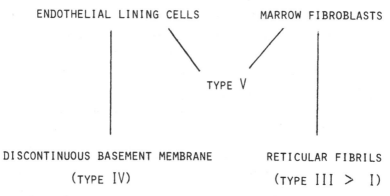

ENDOTHELIAL LINING CELLS   MARROW FIBROBLASTS

TYPE V

DISCONTINUOUS BASEMENT MEMBRANE   RETICULAR FIBRILS
(TYPE IV)   (TYPE III > I)

Fig. 4. Top: Collagens in vascular microcirculation of human bone marrow (modified after De Bruyn[2]). Bottom: Cellular origins of collagens in bone marrow. [Reproduced with permission from (1984) *Myelofibrosis and the Biology of Connective Tissue* (Berk, P. D., Castro-Malaspina, H., and Wasserman, L. R., eds.), Liss, New York, pp. 294, 295].

very similar to the "capillarization" of the sinusoids in the liver caused by an accelerated deposition of basement membrane collagen type IV in liver fibrosis.[74]

Type V collagen is restricted primarily to the larger vasculature in the marrow spaces. However, a pericellular staining of lymphocytic infiltrates has been observed in bone marrow from patients with acute lymphoblastic leukemia.[75] Similarly, in two cases of transformed cell lymphoma, there was a pericellular staining for type V collagen that was not seen in normal lymph nodes.[76] These data and biosynthesis studies on lymphocytic cell lines in vitro[77] suggest the possibility that certain cell clones of lymphoblastic origin participate in the synthesis and deposition of extracellular matrix.

Synthesis of Collagenous Matrix by Stromal Cells of the Bone Marrow

Endothelial cells, adipocytes, macrophages or phagocytic reticular cells, and fibroblasts or nonphagocytic reticular cells are the main cellular elements of the marrow stroma. The primary cell synthesizing collagen is the fibroblast found in the marrow parenchyma, often in close association with foci of granulopoiesis and near the marrow sinuses surrounding the endothelial cell layer as adventitial cells.[78]

A liquid culture system has been used to clone and characterize human bone marrow fibroblast colony-forming cells (CFU-F).[79] The linear relationship between the number of cells plated and the number of colonies formed suggests that fibroblast colonies originate in a single cell. Bone marrow CFU-F are adherent and nonphagocytic. Complement-mediated cytotoxicity using anti-Ia and antifactor-VIII antigen antisera did not inhibit fibroblast colony formation. Immunofluorescence staining was used to characterize the cells derived from CFU-F in vitro. No staining was observed after incubation of subconfluent cultures with anti-Ia and antifactor-VIII antigen antisera. A positive immunofluorescent staining was obtained when isolated antibodies against three of the main proteins of bone marrow matrix—type I collagen, type III collagen, and fibronectin—were used, supporting the conclusion that the colonies are of fibroblastic nature.

It is well established that maintenance of self-replication and differentiation of hematopoietic stem cells in long-term marrow cultures depends upon the formation of a heterogenous adherent cell layer. Employing specific antibodies to examine the adherent layer of long-term human marrow cultures fibroblasts can be recognized by staining with anti-type I collagen, anti-type III collagen, and antifibronectin; endothelial cells with antifactor VIII-antigen, anti-type IV collagen, antilaminin, and antifibronectin; and macrophages with antilysozyme, a monoclonal anti-Ia antigen, and a monoclonal anti-monocyte (Anti-Mac-1).[80] Adipocytes do not stain with any of the antibodies reacting with macrophages.

Similar observations were made in the adherent cell layer in long-term mouse bone marrow.[81-84] Moreover, it was shown that the inhibition of collagen deposition in the extracellular matrix by the proline analog *cis*-4-hydroxyproline prevents the establishment of a stroma supportive of hematopoiesis in long-term murine bone marrow cultures.[85] Therefore, formation of a collagen-containing matrix appears to be an essential prerequisite for proliferation and organization of stromal cells that are necessary for the maintenance of hemopoietic cell proliferation and differentiation.

Bone Marrow Collagen in Hematologic Disorders

The development of in vitro assay systems for cloning the progenitors of human blood cells and their application to the study of hematopoiesis in myeloproliferative disorders (MPD) have resulted in a better understanding of their pathophysiology.[86] Marrow fibroblasts from MPD patients with and without myelofibrosis (MF) displayed the same in vitro growth characteristics as fibroblasts from normal humans. Both types of fibroblasts exhibited anchorage and serum dependence, and contact inhibition of growth. Marrow fibroblasts were also characterized for the presence and distribution of fibronectin and collagen types by immunofluorescent staining, demonstrating that bone marrow collagen-producing cells from MPD patients with and without MF behave in vitro as do those from normal humans. These findings support the hypothesis that the marrow fibrosis observed in patients with MPD results from a reactive process rather than from a primary disorder affecting the marrow collagen-producing cells.[86]

Myelofibrosis

Despite the fact that histologists still describe two grades of bone-marrow fibrosis, namely "reticulin fibrosis" and "collagen fibrosis,"[87] the use of monoclonal or polyclonal antibodies directed against the different types of collagen allows a comparison of the collagen type distribution in normal bone marrow and various forms of myelofibrosis.[75] In this regard we have shown, for example, that under normal conditions type I collagen is almost exclusively restricted to the bone matrix and that very few fibrils occur in the bone marrow (Fig. 5). The reticular stroma of the marrow spaces and the endosteal lining of the bone trabeculae are found largely in a fine network formed by thin fibrils composed of collagen type III and procollagen type III molecules. Collagen types IV, V, and VI are associated with the vascular constituents of microcirculation.

The study of patients with Hodgkin's disease and fibrosis of the bone marrow revealed that marrow fibrosis is largely owing to excessive deposition of new type III collagen (Gay, R., Gay, S., and Prchal, J. T., in preparation). In contrast to other

FIBROPROLIFERATIVE DISORDERS

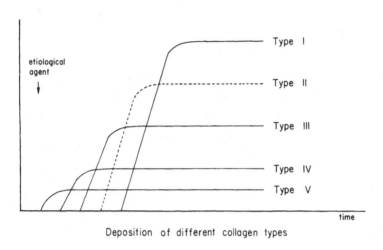

Fig. 5. A plot of the events in an inflammatory-fibroproliferative process as a function of time. [Reproduced with permission from (1983) *Monographs in Pathology: Connective Tissue Diseases* (Wagner, B. M., Fleischmajer, R., and Kaufman, N., eds.), Williams & Wilkins, Baltimore, p. 124].

myelofibrotic conditions, the proportion of newly formed stromal type I collagen is minimal. Moreover, considerable amounts of type III collagen (normally not detected as an integral constituent of bone osteoid) were found in certain parts of the bone matrix.

It has been previously demonstrated that successful therapy of Hodgkin's disease is associated with resolution of the marrow fibrosis. In this context, preliminary data support the notion that myelofibrotic conditions largely comprised of type III collagen are reversible following successful chemotherapy.

In general, by compiling data from our laboratory on over 100 bone marrow biopsies, it appears that type III collagen increases in the early stages of MF and type I in the latter stages

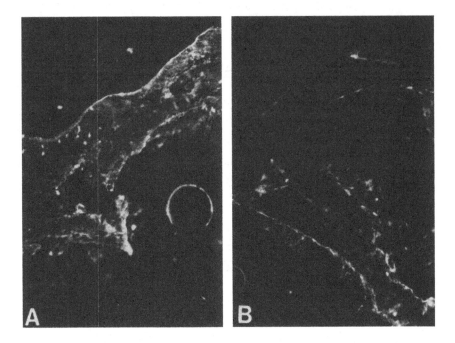

Fig. 6. Fresh frozen section from undermineralized normal human bone marrow (× 200): (A) Staining with antibodies against type I collagen shows staining over the mineralized bone osteoid. The relative weak labeling of the bone matrix is owing to the presence of hydroxyapatite crystals. Only few interstitial type I collagen fibers occur in the marrow stroma; and (B) Staining with antibodies against type III collagen reveals staining of the endosteal lining as well as few fine fibrils of the reticular stroma.

and follows the sequence similar to the inflammatory-reparative process[88] as illustrated in Fig. 5.

The connective tissue reaction to injury in wound healing or in fibroproliferative diseases is initially characterized by a neosynthesis of pericellular type V collagen and basement membrane type IV collagen by epithelial and/or endothelial cells and reflects the events of early embryonic development.[89] Eventually, synthesis and deposition of fine fibrillar type III collagen occur, closely followed by the formation of a matrix largely composed of interstitial type I collagen resembling scar tissue.

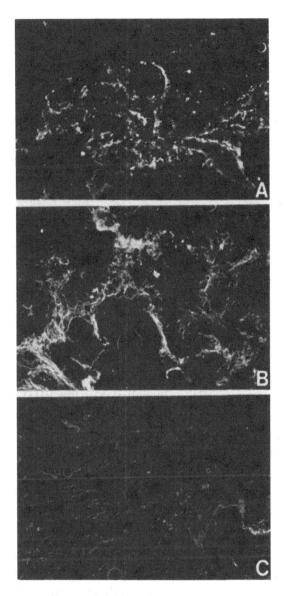

Fig. 7. Fresh frozen sections of bone marrow biopsies from patients with certain hematologic disorders (×200): (A) Staining with antibodies against type V collagen shows a pericellular staining of cellular infiltrates in acute lymphoblastic leukemia; (B) Bone marrow from a patient with idiopathic myelofibrosis reveals various degrees of focal marrow fibrosis characterized by a marked increase of fine reticular collagen fibrils stained with antibodies against type III collagen; and (C) Bone marrow from the same patient as described in (B) stained with antibodies against collagen type IV labels newly formed linear sheets of basement membrane throughout the marrow parenchyma.

The cellular origin of collagenous matrix in fibroproliferative disorders involves at least two different cell types. For example, in myelofibrosis the interstitial marrow fibers are produced by fibroblasts that are able to synthesize types I and III,
but the deposition of continuous sheets of basement membranes containing type IV collagen is derived from endothelial
cells (Figs. 4–7).

The procollagen III aminoterminal peptide immunoassay
has been utilized as a noninvasive means for assessment of a
degree of progression of bone marrow involvement and a
quantitative marker for myelofibrosis.[90–92]

Future Prospects

Collagens are complex macromolecules that occupy important positions in the extracellular interstitial matrix, the
basement membranes, and on the cell surface, especially where
most of the events involved in cell–cell interactions take place.
The different collagens are now recognized not as passive inert
macromolecules, but as essential components that influence
cell proliferation, cell recognition, and cytodifferentiation. In
this regard, it needs to be elucidated how the structural matrix
influences the physiology of the cell via plasma membrane
receptors, that alter the pattern of gene expression, resulting
from changes in the associations of the cytoskeleton with the
mRNA and the chromatin with nuclear components.[93]

References

[1]Gay, S. and Miller, E. J. (1978) *Collagen in the Physiology and Pathology of
    Connective Tissue,* Gustav Fischer, New York.
[2]De Bruyn, P. P. H. (1981) *Sem. Hematol.* **18**, 179–193.
[3]Tavassoli, M. and Friedenstein, A. (1983) *Amer. J. Hematol.* **15**, 195–203.
[4]Weiss, L. and Sakai, H. (1984) *Amer. J. Anat.* **170**, 447–463.

[5]Hay, E. D. (ed.) (1982) *Cell Biology of Extracellular Matrix*, Plenum, New York.

[6]Hewitt, A. T. and Martin, G. R. (1984) *The Biology of Glycoproteins* (Ivatt, R. J., ed.), Plenum, New York pp. 65–93.

[7]Ruoslahti, E., Hayman, E. G., and Pierschbacher, M. D. (1985) *Arteriosclerosis* 5, 581–594.

[8]Madri, J. A. and Pratt, B. M. (1986) *J. Histochem. Cytochem.* 34, 85–91.

[9]Gay, S. and Miller, E. J. (1983) *Ultrastruct. Path.* 4, 365–377.

[10]Gay, S. and Rhodes, R. K. (1986) *Applications of Histochemistry to Pathologic Diagnosis* (Spicer, S. S., Garvin, A. J., and Hennigar, G. R., eds.), Dekker, New York, pp. 755–789.

[11]Miller, E. J. and Gay, S. (1987) *Meth. Enzym.* 144, 3–41.

[12]Miller, E. J., Rhodes, R. K., and Furuto, D. F. (1983) *Collagen Rel. Res.* 3, 79–87.

[13]Timpl, R. (1984) *Extracellular Matrix Biochemistry* (Piez, K. A. and Reddi, A. H., eds.), Elsevier, New York pp. 159–190.

[14]Furthmayr, H. (1982) *Immunochemistry of the Extracellular Matrix* (Furthmayr, H., ed.), CRC, Boca Raton, Florida, pp. 143–178.

[15]Timpl, R. (1982) *Meth. Enzym.* 82A, 472–498.

[16]Zuckerman, K. S., Prince, C. W., and Gay, S., this volume.

[17]Gay, S. and Fine, J.-D. (1987) *Meth. Enzym.* 145, 148–167.

[18]Miller, E. J. (1985) *The Chemistry and Biology of Mineralized Tissues* (Butler, W. T., ed.), EBSCO Media, Birmingham, pp. 80–93.

[19]Miller, E. J. and Rhodes, R. K. (1982) *Meth. Enzymol.* 82A, 33–64.

[20]Boedtker, H., Fuller, F., and Tate, V. (1983) *Int. Rev. Connect. Tissue Res.* 10, 1–63.

[21]Kühn, K. (1984) *Collagen Rel. Res.* 4, 309–322.

[22]Kivirikko, K. I. and Myllyä, R. (1984) *Extracellular Matrix Biochemistry* (Piez, K. A. and Reddi, A. H., eds.), Elsevier, New York, pp. 83–118.

[23]Miller, E. J. and Matukas, V. J. (1969) *Proc. Natl. Acad. Sci. USA* 64, 1264–1268.

[24]Butler, W. T., Finch, J. E., and Miller, E. J. (1977) *J. Biol. Chem.* 252, 639–643.

[25]Sangiori, F. O., Benson-Chanda, V., de Wet, W., Sobel, M. E., Tsipouras, P., and Ramirez, F. (1985) *Nucleic Acids Res.* 13, 2207–2225.

[26]Weiss, C. (1973) *Fed. Proc.* 32, 1459–1466.

[27]Poole, A. R., Pidoux, I., Reiner, A., and Rosenberg, L. (1982) *J. Cell Biol.* 93, 921–937.

[28]Gay, S., Müller, P. K., Lemmen, C., Remberger, K., Matzen, K., and Kühn, K. (1976) *Klin. Wochenschrift* 54, 969–976.

[29]Miller, E. J. and Gay, S. (1980) *Internat. Rev. Cytol. Suppl.* 10, 93–101.

[30]Gay, S., Martin, G. R., Müller, P. K., Timpl, R., and Kühn, K. (1976) *Proc. Natl. Acad. Sci. USA* 73, 4037–4040.

[31]Nowack, H., Gay, S., Wick, G., Becker, U., and Timpl, R. (1976) *J. Immunol. Meth.* **12**, 117–124.

[32]Fleischmajer, R., Timpl, R., and Tuderman, L. (1981) *Proc. Natl. Acad. Sci. USA* **78**, 7360–7364.

[33]Unsworth, D. J., Scott, D. L., Almond, T. J., Beard, H. K., Holborow, E. J., and Walton, K. W. (1982) *Br. J. Exp. Path.* **63**, 154–166.

[34]Howard, P. S., Lally, E., and Macarak, E. J. (1985) *J. Cell Biol.* **101**, 93a.

[35]Apaja-Sarkkinen, M., Alavaikko, M., Karttunen, T., and Autio-Harmainen, H. (1986) *Histopathology* **10**, 295–302.

[36]Henkel, W. and Glanville, R. W. (1982) *Eur. J. Biochem.* **122**, 205–213.

[37]Martinez-Hernandez, A. and Amenta, P. S. (1983) *Lab. Invest.* **48**, 656–677.

[38]Timpl, R., Wiedemann, H., van Delden, V., Furthmayr, H., and Kühn, K. (1981) *Eur. J. Biochem.* **120**, 203–211.

[39]Kühn, K., Glanville, R. W., Babel, W., Qian, R.-Q., Dieringer, H.,Voss, T., Siebold, B., Oberbäumer, I., Schwarz, U., and Yamada, Y. (1985) *Ann. NY Acad. Sci.* **460**, 14–24.

[40]Brinker, J. M., Gudas, L. J., Loidl, H. R., Wang, S.-Y., Rosenbloom, J., Kefalides, N. A., and Myers, J. C. (1985) *Proc. Natl. Acad. Sci. USA* **82**, 3649–3653.

[41]Pihlajaniemi, T., Tryggvason, K., Myers, J. C., Kurkinen, M., Lebo, R., Cheung, M.-C., Prockop, D. J., and Boyd, C. D. (1985) *J. Biol. Chem.* **260**, 7681–7687.

[42]Haralson, M. A., Mitchell, W. M., Rhodes, R. K., Kresina, T. F., Gay, R., and Miller, E. J. (1980) *Proc. Natl. Acad. Sci. USA* **77**, 5206–5210.

[43]Rhodes, R. K. and Miller, E. J. (1981) *Collagen Rel. Res.* **1**, 337–343.

[44]Bächinger, H. P., Doege, K. J., Petschek, J. P., Fessler, L. I., and Fessler, J. H. (1981) *J. Biol. Chem.* **256**, 9640–9645.

[45]Mainardi, C. L., Seyer, J. M., and Kang, A. H. (1980) *Biochem. Biophys. Res. Comm.* **97**, 1108–1115.

[46]Gay, S., Martinez-Hernandez, A., Rhodes, R. K., and Miller, E. J. (1981) *Collagen Rel. Res.* **1**, 377–384.

[47]Martinez-Hernandez, A., Gay, S., and Miller, E. J. (1982) *J. Cell Biol.* **92**, 343–349.

[48]Amenta, P. S., Gay, S., Vaheri, A., and Martinez-Hernandez, A. (1986) *Collagen Rel. Res.* **6**, 125–152.

[49]Adachi, E. and Hayashi, T. (1986) *Connect. Tiss. Res.* **14**, 257–266.

[50]Fitch, J. F., Gross, J., Mayne, R., Johnson-Wint, B., and Linsenmayer, T. F. (1984) *Proc. Natl. Acad. Sci. USA* **81**, 2791–2795.

[51]Chung, E., Rhodes, R. K., and Miller, E. J. (1976) *Biochem. Biophys. Res. Comm.* **71**, 1167–1174.

[52]Furuto, D. K. and Miller, E. J. (1980) *J. Biol. Chem.* **255**, 290–295.

[53]Furthmayr, H., Wiedemann, H., Timpl, R., Odermatt, E., and Engel, J. (1983) *Biochem. J.* **211,** 303–311.

[54]Engel, J., Furthmayr, H., Odermatt, E., von der Mark, H., Aumailley, M., Fleischmajer, R., and Timpl, R. (1985) *Ann. NY Acad. Sci.* **460,** 25–37.

[55]Bentz, H., Morris, N. P., Murray, L. W., Sakai, L. Y., Hollister, D. W., and Burgeson, R. E. (1983) *Proc. Natl. Acad. Sci. USA* **80,** 3168–3172.

[56]Burgeson, R., Morris, N. P., Murray, L. W., Duncan, K. G., Keene, D. R., and Sakai, L. Y. (1985) *Ann. NY Acad. Sci.* **460,** 47–57.

[57]Sage, H., Pritzl, P., and Bornstein, P. (1980) *Biochemistry* **19,** 5747–5755.

[58]Benya, P. D., and Padilla, S. R. (1986) *J. Biol. Chem.* **261,** 4160–4169.

[59]Shimokomaki, M., Duance, V. C., and Bailey, A. J. (1980) *FEBS Lett.* **121,** 51–54.

[60]Mayne, R., van der Rest, M., Weaver, D. C., and Butler, W. T. (1985) *J. Cell. Biochem.* **27,** 133–141.

[61]Ninomiya, Y. and Olsen, B. R. (1984) *Proc. Natl. Acad. Sci. USA* **81,** 3014–3018.

[62]Ninomiya, Y., van der Rest, M., Mayne, R., Lozano, G., and Olsen, B. R. (1985) *Biochemistry* **24,** 4223–4229.

[63]Bruckner, P., Vaughan, L., and Winterhalter, K. H. (1985) *Proc. Natl. Acad. Sci. USA* **82,** 2608–2612.

[64]Irwin, M. H., Silvers, S. H., and Mayne, R. (1985) *J. Cell Biol.* **101,** 814–823.

[65]Müller-Glauser, W., Humbel, B., Glatt, M., Sträuli, P., Winterhalter, K. H., and Bruckner, P. (1986) *J. Cell Biol.* **102,** 1931–1939.

[66]Schmid, T. M. and Conrad, H. E. (1982) *J. Biol. Chem.* **257,** 12,444–12,450.

[67]Schmid, T. M. and Conrad, H. E. (1982) *J. Biol. Chem.* **257,** 12,451–12,457.

[68]Burgeson, R. E. and Hollister, D. W. (1979) *Biochem. Biophys. Res. Commun.* **87,** 1124–1131.

[69]Furuto, D. F. and Miller, E. J. (1983) *Arch. Biochem. Biophys.* **226,** 604–611.

[70]Sheffield, V. C. and Upholt, W. B. (1985) *Collagen Rel. Res.* **5,** 1–8.

[71]Reddi, A. H., Gay, R., Gay, S., and Miller, E. J. (1977) *Proc. Natl. Acad. Sci. USA* **74,** 5589–5592.

[72]Fan, K. (1980) *Stain Technol.* **55,** 307–311.

[73]De Bruyn, P. P. H., Michelson, S., and Thomas, T. B. (1971) *J. Morphol.* **133,** 417–438.

[74]Gay, S., Inouye, T., Minick, O. T., Kent, G., and Popper, H. (1976) *Gastroenterology* **71,** 907a.

[75]Gay, S., Gay, R. E., and Prchal, J. T. (1984) *Myelofibrosis and the Biology of Connective Tissue* (Berk, P. D., Castro-Malaspina, H., and Wasserman, L. R., eds.), Liss, New York pp. 291–306.

[76]McCurley, T. L., Gay, R., Gay, S., Glick, A., Haralson, M., and Collins, R. (1986) *Human Pathol.* **17,** 930–938.

[77]Chen-Kiang, S., Cardinale, G. J., and Udenfriend, S. (1978) *Proc. Natl. Acad. Sci. USA* **75,** 1379–1383.

[78]Castro-Malaspina, H., Ebell, W., and Wang, S.-Y. (1984) *Myelofibrosis and the Biology of Connective Tissue* (Berk, P. D., Castro-Malaspina, H., and Wasserman, L. R., eds.), Liss, New York pp. 209–236.

[79]Castro-Malaspina, H., Gay, R. E., Resnick, G., Kapoor, N., Mayers, P., Chiarieri, D., McKenzie, S., Broxmeyer, H. E., and Moore, M. A. S. (1980) *Blood* **56,** 289–301.

[80]Castro-Malaspina, H., Saletan, S., Gay, R. E., Oettgen, B., Gay, S., and Moore, M. A. S. (1981) *Blood* **58,** 107a.

[81]Bentley, S. A. and Foidart, J.-M. (1980) *Blood* **56,** 1006–1012.

[82]Castro-Malaspina, H., Gay, R. E., Saletan, S., Oettgen, B., Gay, S., and Moore, M. A. S. (1981) *Blood* **58,** 107a.

[83]Zuckerman, K. S. and Wicha, M. S. (1983) *Blood* **61,** 540–547.

[84]Zipori, D., Duksin, D., Tamir, M., Argaman, A., Toledo, J., and Malik, Z. (1985) *J. Cell. Physiol.* **122,** 81–90.

[85]Zuckerman, K. S., Rhodes, R. K., Goodrum, D. D., Patel, V. R., Sparks, B., Wells, J., Wicha, M. S., and Mayo, L. A. (1985) *J. Clin. Invest.* **75,** 970–975.

[86]Castro-Malaspina, H., Gay, R. E., Jhanwar, S. C., Hamilton, J. A., Chiarieri, D. R., Mayers, P. A., Gay, S., and Moore, M. A. S. (1982) *Blood* **59,** 1046–1054.

[87]Editorial (1980) *Lancet* **1,** 127–129.

[88]Gay, S.(1983) *Monographs in Pathology: Connective Tissue Diseases* (Wagner, B. M., Fleischmajer, R., and Kaufman, N., eds.), William and Wilkins, Baltimore, pp. 120–128.

[89]Sherman, M. I., Gay, R., Gay, S., and Miller, E. J. (1980) *Dev. Biol.* **74,** 470–478.

[90]Hochweiss, S., Fruchtman, S., Hahn, E. G., Gilbert, G., Donovan, P. B., Johnson, J., Goldberg, J. D., and Berk, P. D. (1983) *Amer. J. Hemat.* **15,** 343–351.

[91]Arrago, J. P., Poirier, O., and Najean, Y. (1984) *Presse Med.* **13,** 2429–2432.

[92]Hasselbalch, H., Junker, P., Lisse, I., and Bentsen, K. D. (1985) *Scand. J. Haematol.* **35,** 550–557.

[93]Bissell, M. J., Hall, H. G., and Parry, G. (1982) *J. Theor. Biol.* **99,** 31–68.

Chapter 11

The Hemopoietic Extracellular Matrix

Kenneth S. Zuckerman, Charles W. Prince, and Steffen Gay

Introduction

Despite the fact that hemopoietic progenitor cells circulate freely in the blood and are exposed to the microenvironments of virtually every organ of the body, hematopoietic cell proliferation and differentiation normally is confined to a limited number of organs that differ during various stages of ontogeny and in different species.[1-5] In humans, the yolk sac is the site of hemopoiesis in the early embryonic stages. The liver becomes the major hemopoietic organ during the end of the first trimester and through most of the second trimester, and the spleen has a minor hemopoietic role in the middle portion of fetal development. In the last trimester, the liver and spleen lose their capacity to support hemopoiesis.

The bone marrow subsequently becomes the almost exclusive site of hemopoiesis and remains so throughout development and adulthood. A similar sequence of events occurs in rodents, but the spleen retains its function as a hemopoietic (primarily erythropoietic) organ throughout the life of the animal. Other organs have the ability to support hemopoiesis in humans, but only in certain pathological conditions. Thus, since most organs of the body do not support hemopoiesis, there is strong presumptive evidence of specificity in the ability of the microenvironment of certain organs (i.e., bone marrow in humans and bone marrow and spleen in rodents) to support hemopoietic progenitor cell lodgement, proliferation, and differentiation. Furthermore, there is a good deal of evidence suggesting that the so-called hemopoietic inductive microenvironment (HIM) plays an important role in determining the lineage (e.g., erythropoietic vs granulocytopoietic) along which multipotent hemopoietic progenitor cells differentiate.[4–10]

Major microenvironmental/stromal cell types detected within hemopoietic tissues in vivo and in the adherent cell layer of long-term bone marrow cultures include fibroblasts, fat-containing cells, adventitial reticular cells, endothelial cells, and macrophages.[11–31] Although specific functions of each of these cell types within the hemopoietic microenvironment are not known, they presumably at least play roles in the attachment of hemopoietic progenitor cells and production of hemopoietic growth factors. Information that is known about the hemopoietic stromal cell populations is discussed in more detail in other chapters of this book.

It has only been within the last few years that any attention has been paid to the extracellular matrix that is found within the hemopoietic microenvironment. Histochemical staining studies done as early as 15 yr ago suggested that splenic glycosaminoglycans varied with stimulation and suppression of erythropoiesis and were different in genetically anemic mice as compared to normal mice.[32–41] However, further descriptive and physiologic studies of the extracellular matrix of hemopoietic tissues have been hampered by a lack of good model systems for studying the hemopoietic microenvironment and the slow development of immunologic and biochemical methods for assessing extracellular matrix materials. The availability of antibodies specifically reactive with individual collagen subtypes, laminin, fibronectin, and some types of proteoglycans, along with the development of biochemical techniques for the extraction and analysis of these and other less well characterized, quantitatively minor extracellular matrix components, has permitted small but significant advances in the state of knowledge at least about the composition of the hemopoietic extracellular matrix.

The Role of the Extracellular Matrix in Regulating Cell Growth and Differentiation

The extracellular matrix (ECM) is a highly organized structure of macromolecules that is capable of influencing cell proliferation and differentiation in vivo and in vitro. Possibly the most dramatic evidence for the ability of the ECM to influence cell proliferation and differentiation in vivo is found in the work of Urist[42] and Reddi.[19,43] These investigators have soundly demonstrated that devitalized extracts of bone ECM, implanted into soft tissue, are capable of inducing a well-defined developmental sequence that results in ectopic formation of bone and functional bone marrow (*see* below for further details).

Furthermore, supportive and perhaps inductive effects of ECM on cell differentiation have been shown in vitro. For example, endothelial cell-derived ECM coated on the surface of a culture vessel alters the growth of fresh endothelial cells and even permits cells inoculated at very low cell numbers, which fail to proliferate and eventually die when cultured in tissue culture dishes not coated with ECM, to grow to confluence.[44,45]

ECM extracted from liver promotes long-term growth, differentiation, and function of normal hepatocytes, and ECM prepared from mammary tissue supports the growth and function of mammary epithelial cells in vitro, although neither of these cell types will grow in culture for more than 3 wk in the absence of an ECM coating in the culture dish.[46,47] Moreover, the ECM derived from a given organ is specific in its ability to support the survival, growth, and function of cells from a given tissue in vitro.

In view of the important roles played by collagens, laminin, fibronectin, proteoglycans, and probably other extracellular matrix components in the development of a wide variety of tissues,[48–52] it seems reasonable to propose that the well-described and probably as yet uncharacterized extracellular matrix macromolecules are essential for normal lodgment, proliferation, and differentiation of cells involved in hematopoiesis. Since fibronectin, laminin, and most collagen subtypes are distributed widely in many organs of the body, they are most likely to play a necessary structural role, whereas yet uncharacterized, quantitatively minor ECM proteins probably play important tissue specific supportive functions.

Characterization of Noncollagenous Extracellular Matrix Macromolecules Found in Bone and Bone Marrow

It is beyond the scope of this chapter to review the literature on all of the known ECM macromolecules of various tissues, but it is appropriate to summarize the major features of those molecules previously demonstrated to be present in the hematopoietic microenvironment. Since the role of the collagens is discussed elsewhere in this volume, a brief description of noncollagenous matrix molecules is presented here.

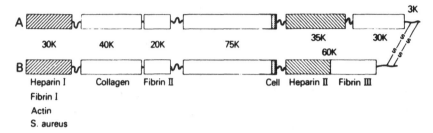

Fig. 1. Structural and functional domains of fibronectin. The molecule is composed of two or more disulfide-linked subunits. Each chain contains a similar linear sequence of modular domains that can be isolated by proteolytic cleavages. The apparent sizes of these domains for human plasma fibronectin are indicated by the numbers (K = Kilodaltons). The ligands that each of the domains bind are shown at the bottom. Note that there are two separate heparin-binding sites and three separate fibrin-binding sites that appear to differ in affinity for their ligands (Yamada, S. K., Akiyama, T., Hasegawa, E., Hasegawa, M. J., Humphries, Kennedy, D. W., Nagata, K., Urushihara, H., Olden, K., and Chen, W. T. (1985) *J. Cell Biochem.* **28**, 79–97, with permission).

Fibronectin

This large glycoprotein is present in plasma, basement membranes, and pericellular and intercellular matrices of most cells and tissues. The fibronectins from different sources within an organism are similar, but not identical, in amino acid composition, sequence, and glycosylation.[52,53] The major features of fibronectin are illustrated in Fig. 1. It has been determined that fibronectin is a macromolecule that is composed of two disulfide bonded subunits, each of 220,000–250,000 daltons. Intensive work over the past few years has resulted in the identification of several functional domains within the molecule. Thus, many of the biological activities ascribed to fibronectin, such as promoting cell adhesion and spreading, proteoglycan and collagen binding, and nonspecific opsonic activity, among others,[52-54] are beginning to be mapped to specific and separate structural sites on the molecule. Further

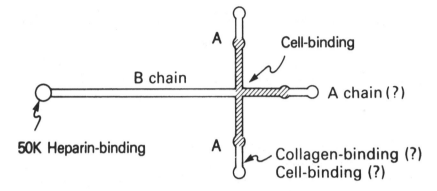

Fig. 2. Structural and functional domains of laminin. The molecule is a cruciform glycoprotein approximately 1,000,000 dalton in size, composed of two types of chains, termed A and B. There are three A chains and one B chain linked by disulfide bonds. The functional binding domains of laminin have not been mapped as conclusively as fibronectin. However, the best available evidence indicates that there is a 50,000 dalton globular heparin-binding domain at the end of the long arm of the molecule. Cell-binding (to unknown ligands) and collagen-binding regions have been postulated to exist on the short arms (Yamada, K. M., Akiyama, S. K., Hasegawa, T., Hasegawa, E., Humphries, M. J., Kennedy, D. W., Nagata, K., Urushihara, H., Olden, K., and Chen, W. T. (1985) *J. Cell. Biochem.* **28**, 79–97, with permission).

advances will lead to a clearer understanding of how fibronectin functions in organizing the ECM of various tissues, including bone and bone marrow.[48]

Laminin

Laminin is another large glycoprotein that is found in most body organs and in small amounts in the serum. As is true of fibronectin, several different structural sites on this molecule have been found to have specific functions. The cruciform structure and putative functional domains of this 850,000 dalton ECM glycoprotein are shown in Fig. 2. Laminin is generally found in basement membranes and functions primarily in the attachment of epithelial cells to Type IV collagen,[55] but other functions have been proposed, such as binding glycosaminoglycans,[56] promoting cell motility, and adhesion of cells to substrates.[57] Changes in laminin expression have been shown to occur during ECM-induced endochondral bone and bone marrow formation.[58]

Proteoglycans

These ECM macromolecules are composed of a core protein to which one or more glycosaminoglycans (polyanionic polysaccharides of various lengths composed of a repeating disaccharide unit that contains a hexosamine and, usually, a uronic acid residue) are attached by *O*-glycosidic linkages. This simple definition does not convey the enormous structural complexity that these molecules possess. Variations in core protein size and composition and in glycosaminoglycan number, size, and composition, as well as other modifications, e.g., phosphorylation, allow the biosynthesis of an enormous range of proteoglycans. Figure 3 illustrates the diversity of glycosaminoglycan structure by identifying the repeating disaccharides characteristic of each species. Such complexity of structure has hindered the analysis of proteoglycans, but in recent years methods have been developed that allow the extraction and purification of intact molecules.[59] Figure 4 depicts proposed structures for some of the recently described proteoglycans.

Because of their widespread distribution on cell surfaces, in basement membranes, and in the ECM of most tissues, particularly of connective tissues, and because of their unique physical and chemical properties, proteoglycans have been implicated in a wide spectrum of biological effects, including cell–substrate attachment, cell–cell interactions, cell migration, cell differentiation, and tissue morphogenesis.[50,60] Information obtained in our laboratories and elsewhere regarding proteoglycans of hematopoietic tissues is presented later in this chapter.

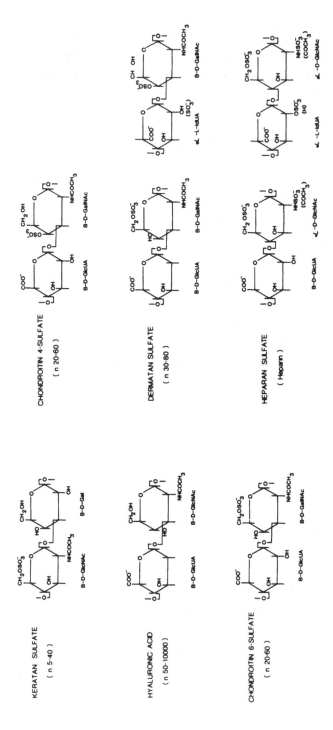

Fig. 3. Structures of the repeating disaccharides of the most common glycosaminoglycans of mammalian tissues: *n* = number of disaccharide units repeated in the molecule; GlcNAc = *N*-acetylglucosamine; Gal NAc = *N*-acetylgalactosamine; Gal = galactose; GlcUA = glucuronic acid; and IdUA = iduronic acid (Reprinted by permission of the publisher from Heinegård, D. and Paulsson, M. (1984) *Extracellular Matrix Biochemistry* (Piez, K. A., and Reddi, A. H., eds.), Elsevier, Amsterdam, pp. 277–328).

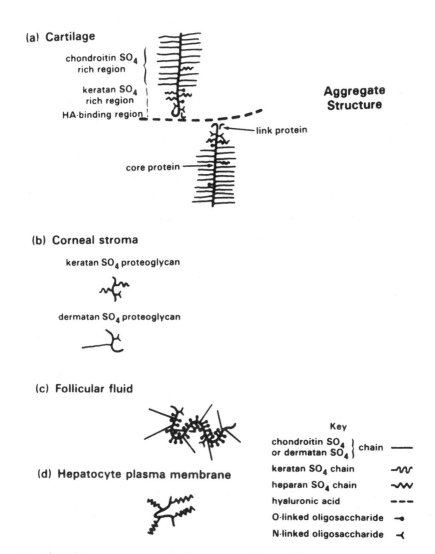

Fig. 4. Schematic diagrams of recently described representative proteoglycans from mammalian tissues. These few examples illustrate the wide diversity of structure and size that occur in proteoglycans. Other tissues also have unique proteoglycans. The proteoglycans of hemopoietic tissues have not been studied in enough detail to allow a description of their structure (*See* ref. 59, with permission).

Other Extracellular Matrix Proteins of Bone and Bone Marrow

Because of the intimate juxtaposition of the hematopoietic marrow with the surface of bone, it is reasonable to assume that the ECM of bone may have a role in maintaining a microenvironment supportive of hematopoiesis. Thus, a relatively brief review of the known proteins of bone ECM is included here. More extensive reviews have been published recently.[61-63]

About 90% of the extracellular matrix of bone is Type I collagen. Since this collagen is not unique to bone, it is probable that the noncollagenous proteins of bone ECM provide the tissue with its ability to mineralize in a spatially and temporally-defined manner. The noncollagenous bone proteins are a complex mixture of bone cell-derived proteins and their normal degradation products and a variety of serum derived proteins, including α_2-HS-glycoprotein, immunoglobulins, and transferrin,[64] which are adsorbed to the surfaces of the bone mineral. The functions in bone, if any, of these latter proteins are not known and they will not be discussed further. Only a few of the noncollagenous bone matrix proteins have been purified and characterized.

Two of the best characterized proteins of bone contain the unusual amino acid, gamma-carboxyglutamic acid (Gla), as the result of a vitamin K dependent posttranslational modification. Osteocalcin, also known as bone Gla protein, has 49–51 amino acids, including 3 Gla residues. It has a high affinity for hydroxyapatite, and its biosynthesis can be stimulated by 1,25-dihydroxyvitamin D_3. The structures of the protein and its gene are known. There is extensive homology among the osteocalcins of several species.[65] Another Gla-containing protein, matrix Gla protein, has recently been isolated and its amino acid sequence determined.[66] This protein has 79 amino acids and a calculated molecular weight of 9961. It is abundant in newly-formed bone and may play a role in osteogenesis.

Phosphoserine and phosphothreonine-containing proteins have been demonstrated in bone, but generally remain poorly characterized. However, Termine recently described a phosphate-containing acidic glycoprotein in bone. Termed osteonectin because of its affinity for hydroxyapatite and denatured collagen, this 29,000 dalton protein has been shown to promote mineral deposition in vitro,[67] and thus may play a role in regulating bone mineral formation. Our laboratory has recently isolated and characterized another bone phosphoprotein.[68] This 44,000 dalton protein is rich in aspartic acid, glutamic acid, and serine. It contains about 12 phosphoserine and 1 phosphothreonine residues/mol and also contains about 17% carbohydrate, including *N*- and O-linked oligosaccharides. Based on amino acid composition, this protein is similar to bone sialoprotein I, as described by Franzen and Heinegård.[69]

One of the first noncollagenous proteins isolated from bone was a sialic acid-rich protein of 23,000 dalton. More recently, a 70,000–80,000 dalton protein, bone sialoprotein II, probably represents the newly intact synthesized form of the protein isolated earlier, has been purified.[69,70] Indirect immunofluorescence on frozen, undemineralized sections showed the protein to be localized to newly formed osteoid. Rotary shadowing revealed it to have an extended rod-like shape.

The proteoglycans of bone are generally small, having a core protein of about M_r 38,000 with one or two chondroitin sulfate chains of M_r 35,000–40,000.[71,72] It has been suggested, based on differences in amino acid composition and immunoreactivity, that the form with one chain is a different gene product from the two chain form. A mechanism postulating different roles for these proteoglycans in bone matrix formation and mineralization has been presented.[61]

Finally, several proteins isolated from bone ECM or bone cells have been shown to have effects on cell growth or differentiation.[73] As previously mentioned, devitalized, demineralized bone matrix implanted in soft tissue can induce new bone and bone marrow formation. Urist[74] has succeeded in isolating a protein, bone morphogenetic protein (BMP) that has such a capability. BMP may act as a chemoattractant for undifferentiated mesenchymal cells and subsequently induce the sequence of events leading to bone formation. It is not known whether other factors are needed to allow the developmental sequence to proceed. Two small proteins, M_r 26,000, isolated from demineralized bone matrix, have recently been shown to induce differentiation of embryonic rat muscle mesenchymal cells into chondrocytes in vitro.[75] Originally termed cartilage-inducing factor (CIF)-A and CIF-B, it has been demonstrated that CIF-A is identical to transforming growth factor-β in biological activity and in the first 30 N-terminal amino acids.[76] Furthermore, cultures of fetal rat calvariae secrete a polypeptide with similar size and biologic activity.[73] Skeletal growth factor is another small protein, M_r 11,500, that has been isolated from demineralized bone matrix. This protein stimulates bone protein and DNA synthesis.

Summary of Extracellular Matrix Macromolecules Found in Bone and Bone Marrow

Although much remains to be learned about the composition of extracellular matrix of bone and bone marrow, several macromolecules that are distributed widely throughout many or most tissues, as well as a few apparent bone specific matrix proteins, have been isolated and biochemically characterized. Less is known about the functions of these macromolecules, but several have been found to promote mesenchymal cell differentiation and osteogenesis. Collagen appears to be the major structural protein of bone and bone marrow (as well as most other tissues). Some of the other matrix components apparently play an important role in promoting cell–cell adherence and interactions of cells with other components of the

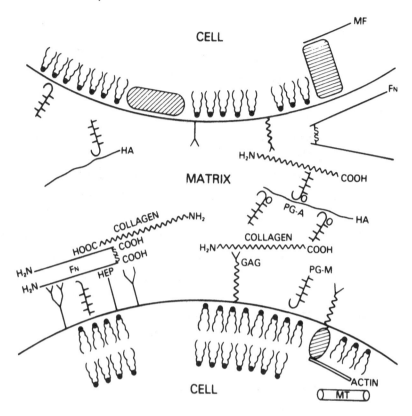

Fig. 5. A model for extracellular matrix–cell surface interactions. The cell surface glycosaminoglycans (GAG), proteoglycan monomers (PG-M), heparin, and heparan sulfates (HEP) interact with fibronectin (Fn) and collagen. Both specific molecular binding sites and electrostatic forces probably play a role in these interactions. The intracellular microfilaments (MF), microtubules (MT), and actin cables modulate and transduce external signals at the cell surface–matrix interface to the interior of the cell. This results in dynamic changes in cell shape, motility, and eventually, phenotype, as seen during embryonic development. Reprinted by permission of the publisher, Reddi, A. H. (1984) *Extracellular Matrix Biochemistry* (Piez, K. A., Reddi, A. H., eds.), Elsevier, Amsterdam, pp. 375–412.

organ stroma. A model of some of these relationships is shown in Fig. 5. Thus, the noncollagenous proteins of bone ECM may not only participate in providing the proper architecture for hematopoiesis, but they also may influence the metabolism of nearby cells and the interactions of hemopoietic progenitor cells with cellular and molecular components of the stroma.

Identification of Extracellular Matrix Proteins in the Stroma of Long-Term Bone Marrow Cell Cultures

The long-term bone marrow cell culture system, first developed by Dexter et al., has proven to be an excellent model for analyzing several aspects of the role of the bone marrow stromal microenvironment in regulating hemopoiesis.[20,23–31,77–82] This system is amenable to several types of analyses of the hemopoietic microenvironment that would be extremely difficult or impossible to study in the intact laboratory animal or human. Several investigators have shown that collagen types I, III, IV, and V (*see* preceding chapter), laminin, fibronectin, and proteoglycans (including chondroitin sulfates, heparan sulfate, and dermatan sulfate glycosaminoglycans, as well as hyaluronic acid) are produced by the stromal cells in murine and human long term bone marrow cultures in vitro.[20–26,77–82]

Fibronectin and Laminin

Antisera specific for given ECM components, such as fibronectin and laminin, have been used to identify the presence and distribution of these extracellular matrix proteins within the stroma of the long-term marrow cultures (Fig. 6). In addition, radioisotope labeling has been used to determine rates of synthesis of some ECM molecules during the life of the long-term marrow cultures. No direct studies of the fibronectin synthesis rate in these cultures have been reported. However, it is interesting that we have noted in our immunofluorescence studies that both intracellular and extracellular fibronectin are readily detectable from the first through third weeks of culture, but that no intracellular fibronectin is noted in marrow stromal cells after the fourth week.[20] This suggests, but does not prove, that cellular synthesis of fibronectin may be greatly diminished once a sufficient amount of this protein has been deposited in

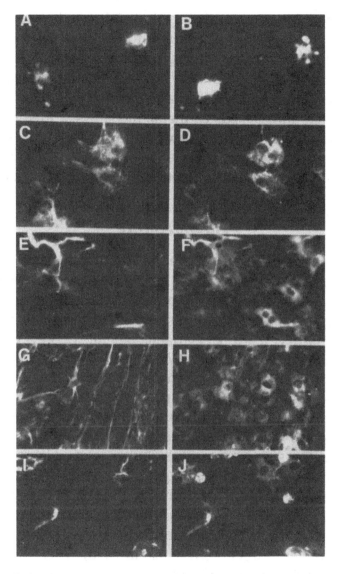

Fig. 6. Deposition of extracellular matrix components in the stroma of murine long-term bone marrow cultures. Sequential double-label immunofluorescent staining and photomicrography of the adherent stromal layer using FITC-bound antifibronectin antiserum and TRITC-bound antilaminin or antitype IV collagen antisera. (A) Fibronectin and (B) laminin in 4-d-old cultures; (C) fibronectin and (D) laminin in 2-wk-old cultures; (E) fibronectin and (F) laminin in 3-wk-old cultures; (G) fibronectin and (H) laminin in 4-wk-old cultures; (I) fibronectin and (J) type IV collagen in 3-wk-old cultures. Adapted from Zuckerman, K. S. and Wicha, M. S. (*See* ref. 20, with permission).

the extracellular matrix and that this could occur by a feedback inhibition mechanism. In contrast to the observations with fibronectin, laminin and collagen were detectable both intracellularly and extracellularly throughout the duration (at least 12 wk) of long-term bone marrow cultures (Fig. 6).[20] Using radiolabeled amino acids as metabolic labels, a low level of laminin synthesis has been detected in the first and second weeks of culture, with a marked increase from the third to fifth weeks, and a subsequent reduction in the synthesis rate to a steady-state level.[23]

Proteoglycans

The only components of the extracellular matrix of hemopoietic organs that have been implicated in alterations in hematopoiesis in vivo are the proteoglycans.[32-40] A series of histochemical and biochemical studies of hemopoietic tissues from normal mice made pancytopenic, anemic, or polycythemic or from congenitally anemic W/W^v or Sl/Sl^d mice, showed apparent alterations in the quantity of detectable neutral and acidic glycosaminoglycans and proteoglycans.[32-40] In particular, the results of these studies suggested that accumulation of proteoglycans and/or free glycosaminoglycans was associated with the suppression of erythropoiesis. However, no definite cause and effect relationship was established in those experiments. Subsequent studies by Ploemacher et al.[41] also indicated that colony formation by erythroid progenitors in vitro was suppressed by chondroitin and heparan sulfate, but not by keratan sulfate or hyaluronic acid, whereas colony formation by granulocyte–macrophage progenitors was not inhibited by any of these glycosaminoglycans.

Wight et al.[82] reported biochemical and structural studies of proteoglycans synthesized and secreted in human long-term bone marrow cell cultures. In these studies of 4–5-week-old cultures, proteoglycans bound to the stromal layer were very similar to those secreted into the medium. About 40% of ^{3}H-glucosamine was incorporated into hyaluronic acid, whereas the remaining 60% was incorporated almost exclusively into large proteoglycans containing predominantly chondroitin sulfate, with the glycosaminoglycans chains having a molecular weight of approximately 38,000 dalton. There also was a moderate proportion of dermatan sulfate and a small amount of heparan sulfate glycosaminoglycans. Electron micrographic studies showed a complex layer of hemopoietic cells adherent to the stromal cell layer and enmeshed in a dense, flocculent network of thin proteoglycans filaments. Removal of the proteoglycans by enzymatic treatment with chondroitinase ABC also resulted in the loss of many of the adherent hemopoietic cells, suggesting that the proteoglycans may have played an important role in keeping the hemopoietic cells in close contact with stromal microenvironmental cells.

Recently, our group has begun to examine the synthesis of glycosaminoglycans and proteoglycans in murine long-term bone marrow cell cultures over time. As shown in Table 1, proteoglycan and glycosaminoglycan synthesis increased progressively to a peak level in about the fourth week, then tapered off to a lower, but relatively stable baseline for the next 2 mo. Our preliminary results indicate that the alterations in glycosaminoglycans synthesis is a result of both changes in the number of stromal cells and the amount of material synthesized per cell. In our studies chondroitin sulfates, heparan sulfate, and to a lesser extent dermatan sulfate, were the major glycosaminoglycans synthesized. This is in basic agreement with the other reports, in which either murine or human long-term bone marrow cultures have been analyzed.

Summary of Extracellular Matrix Glycoproteins and Proteoglycans Produced in Long-Term Bone Marrow Cultures

It is interesting to note that all of these studies of the production of known extracellular matrix components, by the stromal cells in long-term bone marrow cell cultures, at least suggest the possibility of both positive and later negative feed-

Table 1
Proteoglycans/Glycosaminoglycans Synthesis
in the Stromal Layer of Murine Long-Term
Bone Marrow Cell Cultures

Weeks of Culture	Total Macromolecular CPM ($\times 10^{-3}$) per Dish	
	$^{35}SO_4$	^{3}H-Glucosamine
1	95.1	72.0
2	265.3	119.2
3	383.0	183.9
4	534.4	205.3
5	216.9	61.7
6	182.2	44.3
7	234.1	68.1
8	197.1	24.3
9	183.4	38.2
10	130.2	37.2
12	143.8	40.0

back control mechanisms that determine the rate of synthesis of
ECM components in these cultures. Unfortunately, very little
is known about the control of synthesis and secretion of extracellular matrix components in vivo or in vitro. Obviously, further work will be needed to characterize the regulatory factors
for ECM production.

The Role of Extracellular Matrix Components in Regulating Hemopoiesis in Long-Term Bone Marrow Cultures

Spooncer et al.[79] have reported that β-D-xylosides, which
selectively increase levels of free chondroitin sulfates by preventing their association with proteoglycans core proteins,
enhanced hemopoiesis in murine long-term bone marrow cell
cultures. Although these studies do not prove that glycosaminoglycans and proteoglycans are important in regulating

hemopoiesis, along with the known importance of these macro-molecules in morphogenesis, they support the hypothesis that proteoglycans may play an important role in modulating hemo-poiesis.

The only other studies of changes in hemopoiesis, after manipulation of levels of extracellular matrix component pro-duction in long-term cultures, are those described in the pre-vious chapter that demonstrated that inhibition of collagen synthesis prevents normal hemopoiesis from being estab-lished.[78] Thus, there is emerging evidence that perhaps several extracellular matrix components may be important in regu-lating hematopoiesis. Much more in depth study will be necessary to determine how the extracellular matrix interacts with hemopoietic stromal cells, as well as multipotent and unipotent hemopoietic progenitor cells.

Reconstitution of Bone and Bone Marrow In Vivo by Ectopic Implantation of Devitalized, Demineralized Bone Matrix

Although very little is known about the proteins and pro-teoglycans that comprise the extracellular matrix of bone and bone marrow, Reddi and colleagues demonstrated in a series of experiments over the last 15 yr that if coarsely ground particles of rat bone were decalcified and implanted subcutaneously in other rats, a sequence of events was initiated at the implanta-tion site that reproduced the ontogeny of osteogenesis.[19,43,48,49,83–91] The stages of development of the ectopic bone and bone marrow are shown pictorially in Fig. 7 and diagrammatically in Fig. 8. First, there is infiltration of the area of implanted matrix by fibroblast-like mesenchymal cells, followed by angiogene-sis, cartilage formation, production of new bone (detected mor-phologically and by ^{45}Ca incorporation and alkaline phosphatase synthesis), and finally, by the end of the third week, appear-ance of islands of hematopoiesis (detected morphologically

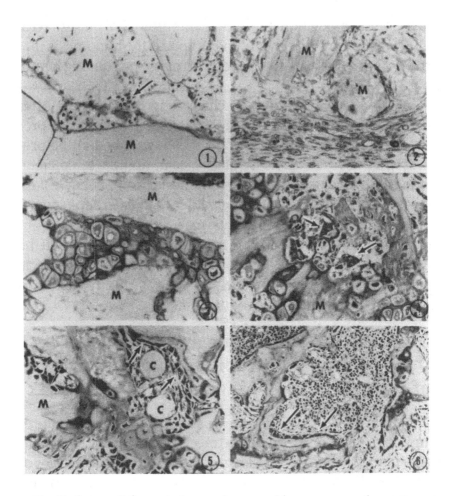

Fig. 7. Sequential events in new bone and bone marrow formation at ectopic sites of implantation of devitalized, demineralized rat bone matrix. (1) Day 1—Polymorphonuclear leukocytes (arrow) and fibrin around the matrix (M); (2) Day 3—Mesenchymal cells around implanted matrix (M); (3) Day 7—Chondrocytes in close apposition to the implanted matrix (M); (4) Day 9—Calcified cartilage matrix and early vascular invasion (Note the multinucleated chondroclasts [arrows] in relation to chondrolytic foci.); (5) Day 11—Early stages of bone formation (Observe the invading capillaries [c] and the location of basophilic osteoblasts [arrows] in relation to the blood vessels.); (6) Day 21—Hematopoietic bone marrow in the ossicle (Note the palisade of osteoblasts [arrows] and trabeculae of bone. (Reddi, A. H. and Kuettner, K. E. (1981) *Dev. Biol.* **82,** 217–223, with permission).

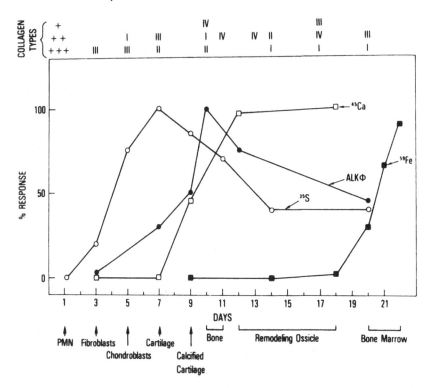

Fig. 8. Developmental sequence of extracellular matrix-induced cartilage, bone, and bone marrow formation. Changes in $^{35}SO_4$ incorporation into proteoglycans and ^{45}Ca incorporation into mineral phase indicate peaks of cartilage and bone formation, respectively. The ^{59}Fe incorporation into heme is an index of erythropoiesis, and is used as one quantitative measure of hematopoiesis as a whole. The increase in alkaline phosphatase activity indicates early stages of bone formation. The transitions in types of collagen being synthesized are summarized on top of the figure and are based on immunofluorescent localization studies. PMN = polymorphonuclear leukocytes, (Reddi, A. H. (1981) *Coll. Rel. Res.* 1, 209–226, with permission).

and confirmed by ^{59}Fe incorporation studies) that persist at least for many months. Reddi et al. have examined the course of synthesis of extracellular matrix materials during bone and bone marrow regeneration from demineralized bone matrix. Fibronectin formed a fibrillar network during the mesenchymal cell proliferation, became covered with proteoglycans during cartilage formation, extended in a "cottony" array around osteoblasts during osteogenesis, and was intimately associated with developing colonies of hematopoietic cells.[48] The species of proteoglycans synthesized during ectopic chondrogenesis and osteogenesis were quite similar to those synthesized by normal developing cartilage and bone.[90,91] By about 1 wk, when there was active chondrogenesis, the predominant proteoglycans were relatively large and contained 95% chondroitin-4-sulfate and very little keratan sulfate. At day 11, when osteogenesis had become active, synthesis of a smaller type of proteoglycans with longer chondroitin sulfate chains, typical of bone proteoglycans, predominated.

All the specific components of the demineralized bone matrix, essential for supporting or inducing the growth of new bone and bone marrow, have not yet been purified or well-defined biochemically. In addition to BMP isolated by Urist,[42,74] Sampath and Reddi[85–89] have found that dissociative extraction of the demineralized bone matrix with $4M$ guanidine HCl, $8M$ urea/$1M$ NaCl, or 1% $NaDodSO_4$ resulted in a residue that no longer supported new bone formation, but the activity could be reconstituted by mixing the soluble extracts with the inactive matrix residues. Furthermore, the soluble component(s) of bone matrix that was (were) capable of reconstituting induction of bone and bone marrow growth was (were) small (<50 kD), trypsin-sensitive protein(s) resistant to digestion by chondroitinase.[85] Whether this factor is similar to the cartilage-inducing factors isolated by Seyedin et al.[75,76] is unknown. Further studies have shown that the soluble-bone-inductive material is conserved evolutionarily in that there is homology among the bone-inductive proteins from human, monkey, bovine, and rat bone matrix.[87]

Another interesting finding is that the soluble bone-inductive activity was not detectable or present in very small quantities in bone matrix from vitamin D deficient, rachitic rats.[89]

The bone-inductive activity was reconstituted by adding the soluble low molecular weight fraction from normal rats to insoluble matrix residue from rachitic rats, but the addition of soluble extract from rachitic rat bone matrix to the insoluble residue from normal rat bone matrix did not support new bone/bone marrow formation. Reddi's group has reported the isolation of a single bone/bone marrow-inductive protein that they called osteogenin.[89a] It is obvious that there also are many other bone/bone marrow-specific extracellular matrix components,[64] some of which undoubtedly play critical roles in supporting and/or inducing normal bone and bone-marrow growth. Further characterization and purification of such proteins should be accomplished in the next few years.

Studies of the Abnormal Hemopoietic Microenvironment of Sl/Sl[d] Mice

The Sl/Sl[d] mouse is the only known useful animal model of a genetically abnormal hemopoietic microenvironment that is unable to support normal proliferation and differentiation of normal hemopoietic progenitor cells.[1,4,8–10,92–107] These mice have been shown by studies done in vivo and in vitro to have intrinsically normal hemopoietic stem cells and a defective hemopoietic microenvironment.[1,4,8–10,92–107]

In our laboratory, we have found that total hemopoietic cell and hemopoietic progenitor cell production by Sl/Sl[d] cells over several weeks to months in long-term bone marrow cultures never exceeds 10% of the levels of hematopoiesis observed in cultures of their congenic WCB6F1 (+/+) mouse marrow cells; and little, if any, significant hemopoietic cell production persisted in Sl/Sl[d] cultures after the first 4–5 wk.[104–107] These results are similar to the findings of several other groups.[100–103] Examination of +/+ and Sl/Sl[d] cultures by phase contrast microscopy during the first 10 wk of culture (Fig. 9)

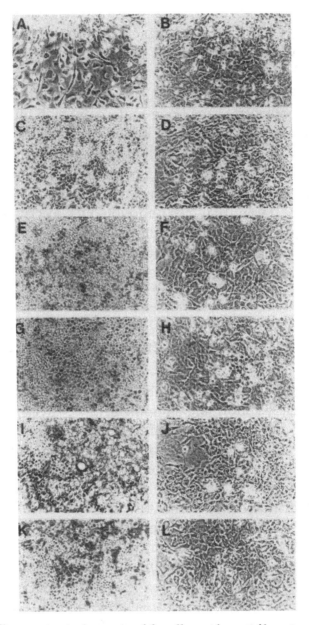

Fig. 9. Phase contrast microscopy of the adherent layers of long-term WCB6F1 +/+ and Sl/Sl^d mouse bone marrow cell cultures. Photographs were taken after 1 (A and B), 2 (C and D), 3 (E and F), 4 (G and H), 6 (I and J), and 10 (K and L) wk +/+ culture adherent layers are shown in panels A, C, E, G, I, and K. Sl/Sl^d culture adherent layers are shown in panels B, D, F, H, J, and L (*See* Ref. 105, with permission).

revealed only one striking and consistent difference—large numbers of small round hemopoietic cells adherent to and, in many cases, obscuring the stromal layer of +/+ culture, and very few detectable adherent hemopoietic cells in the Sl/Sl^d cultures. Neither we[104,105] nor others[100,101] have been able to detect any obvious difference in types or distribution of adherent marrow stromal cells between normal and Sl/Sl^d cultures, with the possible exception of a modest increase in the number of fat-containing cells in the stroma of Sl/Sl^d cultures. The stromal cell number increased at about the same rate and the stromal layer became confluent by about 4 wk in both +/+ and Sl/Sl^d cultures. These findings were corroborated by scanning electron microscopy of confluent stromal cell layers of 4-wk-old +/+ and Sl/Sl^d cultures (Fig. 10). The phase contrast and scanning electron micrographs revealed the presence of the same stromal cell populations described by other investigators, namely fibroblastic cells, endothelial-like cells, fat-containing cells, macrophages, and blanket cells (probable adventitial reticular cells). Finally, at a high magnification ($\times$ 20,000), we were able to discern a course, fibrillar, and sometimes globular-appearing extracellular matrix in both the +/+ and Sl/Sl^d cultures.

Since no obvious morphologic differences between the stromal cells of +/+ and Sl/Sl^d marrow cultures could be detected, a search has begun for differences in extracellular matrix products.[104,105] As shown in Fig. 11, there was no obvious difference in deposition of fibronectin, laminin, or collagen between long-term cultures of Sl/Sl^d and +/+ bone marrow cells. No other studies of these nearly ubiquitous extracellular matrix proteins in the bone marrow of Sl/Sl^d mice have been reported. Only very preliminary information is available to date on other quantitatively minor ECM components extracted from the stroma of the long term marrow cultures (Zuckerman, K. S., Prince, C. W., and Ribadeneira, M., unpublished data). Our laboratory group has observed several apparent differ-

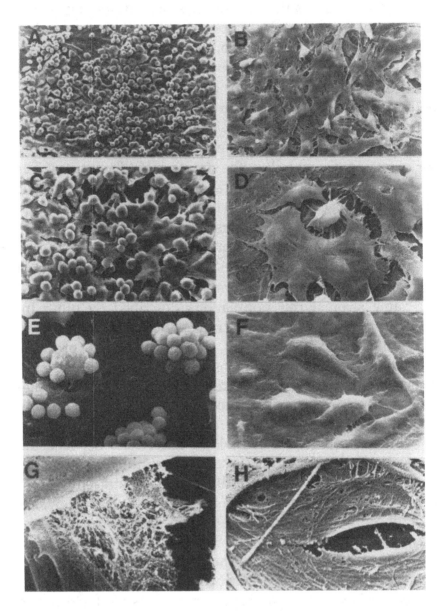

Fig. 10. Scanning electron microscopy of the adherent layers of long-term WCB6F1 +/+ and Sl/Sl^d bone marrow cell cultures. Photographs were taken after 4 wk of culture. (A) +/+ (500×); (B) Sl/Sl^d (500×); (C) +/+ (1000×); (D) Sl/Sl^d (1250×); (E) +/+ (2500×); (F) Sl/Sl^d (2500×); (G) +/+ (20,000×); (H) Sl/Sl^d (*See* Ref. 105, with permission).

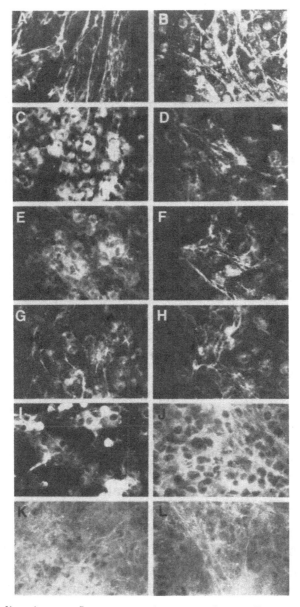

Fig. 11. Indirect immunofluorescence microscopy of extracellular matrix components in the adherent stromal layers of long term WCB6F1 +/+ and Sl/Sl[d] mouse bone marrow cell cultures. Fibronectin (A and B); laminin (C and D); collagen type I (E and F); collagen type III (G and H); collagen type IV (I and J); and collagen type V (K and L). +/+ culture adherent layers are shown in panels A, C, E, G, I, and K. Sl/Sl[d] culture adherent layers are shown in panels B, D, F, H, J, and L (*See* Ref. 105, with permission).

ences in protein elution patterns from gel filtration, ion exchange, and reverse phase HPLC columns, but these studies are not yet definitive.

In addition, we have used the methods of Sampath and Reddi[85-89] to extract cell-free ECM from bones and bone marrow of +/+ and Sl/Sl^d mice, as well as normal C57Bl/6J mice, and we have analyzed the noncollagenous ECM proteins by SDS-polyacrylamide gel electrophoresis (Fig. 12). We could not discern any obvious differences between normal WCB6F1 (+/+) and C57Bl/6J bone/bone marrow ECM in the nearly 30 protein bands that were detectable by Coomassie blue staining. However, there were definite differences between normal and Sl/Sl^d mice. In particular, there is an apparent missing 33 kD and a quantitatively decreased 24 kD protein in the Sl/Sl^d ECM, an extra 36 kD band in the Sl/Sl^d matrix, and probable missing or quantitatively decreased 42 and 51 kD proteins in the Sl/Sl^d matrix. These findings represent the first description of a specific abnormality in the hemopoietic microenvironment of Sl/Sl^d mice.

Considering the strong evidence indicating the importance of specific extracellular matrix components in the morphogenesis and differentiation of cells in other organs, it is not surprising to find that abnormalities in composition of the hemopoietic extracellular matrix may account for the defective hemopoietic progenitor cell proliferation and differentiation in Sl/Sl^d mice. These findings in a strain of mice in which a defective microenvironment is known to be responsible for impaired hematopoiesis, along with the findings of Reddi's group discussed above, provide very strong evidence for a critical role of the extracellular matrix in supporting and perhaps regulating hemopoiesis.

Summary

There is little doubt that the hemopoietic microenvironment as a whole is of major importance in supporting and regu-

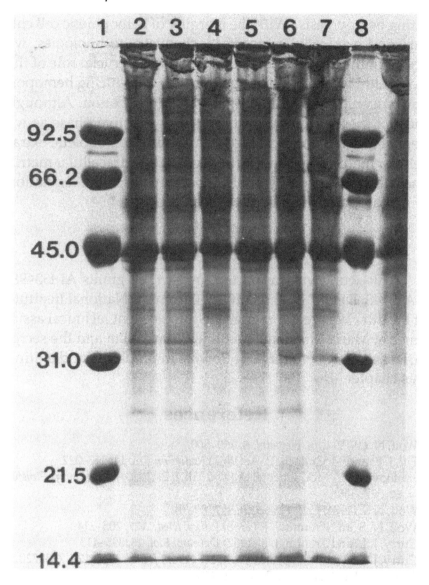

Fig. 12. SDS-12.5% polyacrylamide gel electrophoresis of noncollagenous extracellular matrix proteins extracted under denaturing and reducing conditions from bones and bone marrow of normal (C57B1/6J and WCB6F1 +/+) and Sl/Sl^d mice. Lanes 1 and 8 are gels of mol wt markers (labeled in kDa). Lanes 2 and 5 are gels of separate ECM preparations from C57B1/6J mice. Lanes 3 and 6 are gels of separate ECM preparations from WCB6F1 (+/+) mice. Lanes 4 and 7 are gels of separate ECM preparations from Sl/Sl^d mice (*See* Ref. 105, with permission).

lating hemopoiesis. With the merging of hemopoietic cell culture and extracellular matrix biochemistry technologies, we are beginning to understand the potentially crucial role of the extracellular matrix in supporting and/or inducing hemopoietic progenitor cell proliferation and differentiation. Although most of these studies are still in the descriptive phase as we begin to identify and characterize specific hemopoietic extracellular matrix proteins, the function of the extracellular matrix and the mechanisms by which it participates in the regulation of hematopoiesis will become clear.

Acknowledgments

This work was supported, in part, by grants AM33498, CA13148, DEO6739, and DEO2670 from the National Institute of Health. We greatly appreciate the excellent technical assistance of Maria Ribadeneira and Jan Marchman and the secretarial assistance of Margaret Powers in preparing and editing this chapter.

References

[1]Wolf, N. (1979) *Clin. Hematol.* **8,** 469–500.

[2]Till, J. E. and McCulloch, E. A. (1961) *Radiation Res.* **14,** 213–222.

[3]Siminovitch, L., McCulloch, E. A., and Till, J. E. (1963) *J. Cell. Comp. Physiol.* **62,** 327–336.

[4]Wolf, N.S. (1974) *Cell. Tissue Kinet.* **7,** 89–98.

[5]Wolf, N. S. and Trentin, J. J. (1968) *J. Exp. Med.* **127,** 205–214.

[6]Curry, J. L. and Trentin, J. J. (1962) *Develop. Biol.* **15,** 395–413.

[7]Curry, J. L., Trentin, J. J., and Wolf, N. (1967) *J. Exp. Med.* **125,** 703–720.

[8]Trentin, J. J. (1971) *Am. J. Pathol.* **65,** 621–628.

[9]Trentin, J. J. (1978) *Transplant. Proc.* **10,** 77–82.

[10]Tavassoli, M. (1975) *Exp. Hematol.* **3,** 213–226.

[11]Lichtman, M. A. (1981) *Exp. Hematol.* **9,** 391–410.

[12]Gordon, M. Y., King, J. A., and Gordon-Smith, E. C. (1980) *Br. J. Haematol.* **46,** 151–152.

[13]LaPushin, R. W. and Trentin, J. J. (1977) *Exp. Hematol.* **5,** 505–522.

[14]Westen, H. and Bainton, D. F. (1979) *J. Exp. Med.* **150,** 919–937.

[15]Friedenstein, A. J., Chailakhyan, R. K., Latsinik, N.V., Panasuk, A. F., and Keiliss-Borok, I.V. (1974) *Transplantation* **17**, 331–340.

[16]Friedenstein, A. J., Latsinik, N. V., Grosheva, A. G., and Gorskaya, U. F. (1982) *Exp. Hematol.* **10**, 217–277.

[17]Chertkov, J. L., Drize, N. J., Gurevitch, O. A., and Udalov, G. A. (1983) *Exp. Hematol.* **11**, 231–242.

[18]Patt, H. M., Maloney, M. A., and Flannery, M. L. (1982) *Exp. Hematol.* **10**, 738–742.

[19]Reddi, A. H. and Huggins, C. B. (1975) *Proc. Natl. Acad. Sci. USA* **72**, 2212–2216.

[20]Zuckerman, K. S. and Wicha, M. S. (1983) *Blood* **61**, 540–547.

[21]Bentley, S. A. and Foidart, J. M. (1980) *Blood* **56**, 1006–1012.

[22]Keating, A., Singer, J. W., Killen, P. D., Striker, G. E., Salo, A. C., Sanders, J., Thomas, E. D., and Fialkow, P. J. (1982) *Nature* **298**, 280–283.

[23]Zuckerman, K. S. (1984) *Long Term Bone Marrow Culture* (Wright, D. G. and Greenberger, J. S., eds.), Liss, New York, pp. 157–178.

[24]Zuckerman, K. S. and Rhodes, R. K. (1985) *Hematopoietic Stem Cell Physiology*, (Cronkite, E. P., Dainiak, N., McCaffrey, R. P., Palek, J., and Quesenberry, P. J., eds.), Liss, New York, pp. 257–266.

[25]Castro-Malaspina, H., Gay, R. E., Saletan, S., Oettgen, B., Gay, S., and Moore, M. A. S. (1981) *Blood* **58**, 107a.

[26]Castro-Malaspina, H., Saletan, S., Gay, R. E., Oettgen, B., Gay, S., and Moore, M. A. S. (1981) *Blood* **58**, 107a.

[27]Allen, T. D. and Dexter, T. M. (1976) *Differentiation* **6**, 191–194.

[28]Dexter, T. M., Allen, T. D., and Lajtha, L.G. (1977) *J. Cell. Physiol.* **91**, 335–344.

[29]Dexter, T. M. (1978) *Clin. Haematol.* **8**, 453–468.

[30]Dexter, T. M., Spooncer, E., Tosoz, D., and Lajtha, L. G. (1980) *J. Supramol. Struct.* **13**, 513–524.

[31]Dexter, T. M., Testa, N. G., Allen, T. D., Rutherford, T., and Scolnick, E. (1981) *Blood* **58**, 699–707.

[32]McCuskey, R. S., Meineke, H. A., and Townsend, S. F. (1972) *Blood* **39**, 697–712.

[33]McCuskey, R. S., Meineke, H. A., and Kaplan, S. M. (1972) *Blood* **39**, 809–813.

[34]Schrock, L. M., Judd, J. T., Meineke, H. A., and McCuskey, R. S. (1973) *Proc. Soc. Exp. Biol. Med.* **144**, 593–595.

[35]McCuskey, R. S. and Meineke, H. A. (1973) *Am. J. Anat.* **137**, 187–198.

[36]McCuskey, R. S. and Meineke, H. A. (1977) *Proc. Soc. Exp. Biol. Med.* **156**, 181–185.

[37]McCuskey, R. S. and Meineke, H. A. (1977) *Kidney Hormones. II. Erythropoietin* (Fisher, J. W. ed.), Academic, New York, NY, pp. 311–327.

[38]Tavassoli, M., Eastlund, D. T., Yam, L. T., Neiman, R. S., and Finkel, H. (1976) *Scand. J. Haematol.* **16**, 311–319.

[39]Noordegraaf, E. M. and Ploemacher, R. E. (1979) *Scand. J. Haematol.* **22**, 327–332.

[40]Noordegraaf, E. M., Erkens-Versluis, E. A., and Ploemacher, R. E. (1981) *Exp. Hematol.* **9**, 326–331.

[41]Ploemacher, R. E., van't Hull, E., and van Soest, P. L. (1978) *Exp. Hematol.* **6**, 311–320.

[42]Urist, M. R. (1965) *Science* **150**, 893–899.

[43]Reddi, A. H. and Huggins, C. B. (1972) *Proc. Natl. Acad. Sci. USA* **69**, 1601–1605.

[44]Gospodarowicz, D. and Ill, C. (1980) *J. Clin. Invest.* **65**, 1351–1364.

[45]Gospodarowicz, D., Delgado, D., and Vlodavsky, I. (1980) *Proc. Natl. Acad. Sci. USA* **77**, 4094–4098.

[46]Rojkind, M., Gaitmaitan, Z., Mackensen, S., Giambrone, M. A., Ponce, P., and Reid, L. M. (1980) *J. Cell Biol.* **877**, 255–263.

[47]Wicha, M. S., Lowrie, G., Kohn, E., Bagavandoss, P., and Mahn, T. (1982) *Proc. Natl. Acad. Sci. USA* **79**, 3213–3217.

[48]Weiss, R. E. and Reddi, A. H. (1981) *J. Cell Biol.* **88**, 630–636.

[49]Reddi, A. H. (1984) *Extracellular Matrix Biochemistry* (Piez, K. A. and Reddi, A. H., eds.), Elsevier, New York, pp. 375–412.

[50]Toole, B. P. (1981) *Cell Biology of Extracellular Matrix* (Hay, E. D., ed.), Plenum, New York, pp. 259–294.

[51]Hay, E. D., (ed.) (1981) *Cell Biology of Extracellular Matrix* Plenum, New York, pp. 379–409.

[52]Hynes, R. O. (1981) *Cell Biology of Extracellular Matrix* (Hay, E. D., ed.) Plenum, New York, pp. 295–334.

[53]Yamada, K. M. (1983) *Ann. Rev. Biochem.* **52**, 761–799.

[54]Yamada, K. M., Akiyama, S. K., Hasegawa, T., Hasegawa, E., Humphries, M. J., Kennedy, D. W., Nagata, K., Urushihara, H., Olden, K., and Chen, W.-T. (1985) *Cellular Biochem.* **28**, 79–97.

[55]Terranova, V. P., Rohrbach, D. H., and Martin, G. R. (1980) *Cell* **22**, 719–726.

[56]Del Rosso, M., Cappelletti, R., Viti, M., Vannucchi, S., and Chiarugi, V. (1981) *Biochem J.* **199**, 699–704.

[57]Couchman, J. R., Höök, M., Rees, D. A., and Timpl, R. (1983) *J. Cell Biol.* **96**, 177–183.

[58]Foidart, J. -M. (1980) *Dev. Biol.* **75**, 130–136.

[59]Hascall, V. C. and Kimura, J. H. (1982) *Methods in Enzymology*, vol. 82, part A, (Cunningham, L. W. and Frederickson, D. W., eds.), Academic, New York, pp. 769–802.

[60]Lindahl, U. and Höök, M.(1978) *Ann. Rev. Biochem.* **47**, 385–417.

[61]Fisher, L. W. and Termine, J. D. (1985) *Clin. Orthop.* **200**, 362–385.

[62]Butler, W. T. (1984) *Coll. Rel. Res.* **4**, 297–307.

[63]Boskey, A. (1981) *Clin. Orthop.* **157**, 226–257.

[64]Delmas, P. D., Tracy, R. P., Riggs, B. L., and Mann, K. G. (1984) *Calcif. Tissue Intl.* **36**, 308–316.

[65]Price, P. A. (1985) *Vitamins and Hormones* **42**, 65–108.

[66]Price, P. A. and Williamson, M. K. (1985) *J. Biol. Chem.* **260**, 14,971–14,975.

[67]Termine, J. D., Kleinman, H. K., Whitson, S. W., Conn, K. M., McGarvey, M. L., and Martin, G. R. (1981) *Cell* **26**, 99–105.

[68]Prince, C. W., Oosawa, T., Butler, W. T., Tomana, M., Bhown, A. S., and Schrohenloher, R. E. (1987) *J. Biol. Chem.* **262**, 2900–2907.

[69]Franzen, A. and Heinegård, D. (1985) *Biochem. J.* **232**, 715–725.

[70]Fisher, L. W., Whitson, S. W., Avioli, L. V., and Termine, J. D. (1983) *J. Biol. Chem.* **258**, 12,723–12,727.

[71]Fisher, L. W., Termine, J. D., Dejter, S. W. Jr., Whitson, S. W., Yanagashita, M., Kimura, J. H., Hascall, V. C., Kleinman, H. K., Hassell, J. R., and Nilsson, B. (1983) *J. Biol. Chem.* **258**, 6588–6594.

[72]Franzen, A. and Heinegård, D. (1984) *Biochem. J.* **224**, 59–66.

[73]Centrela, M. and Canalis, E. (1985) *Endocrine Rev.* **6**, 544–551.

[74]Urist, M. R., Huo, Y. K, Brownell, A. G., Hohl, W. M., Buyske, J., Lietze, A., Tempst, P., Hunkapiller, M., and DeLange, R. J. (1984) *Proc. Natl. Acad. Sci. USA* **81**, 371–379.

[75]Seyedin, S. M., Thomas, T. C., Thompson, A. Y., Rosen, D. M., and Piez, K. A. (1985) *Proc. Natl. Acad. Sci. USA* **82**, 2267–2271.

[76]Seyedin, S. M., Thompson, A. Y., Bentz, H., Rosen, D. M., McPherson, J. M., Conti, A., Siegel, N. R., Galluppi, G. R., and Piez, K. A. (1985) *J. Biol. Chem.* **261**, 5693–5695.

[77]Bentley, S. A. (1982) *Br. J. Haematol.* **50**, 491–497.

[78]Zuckerman, K. S., Rhodes, R. K., Goodrum, D. D., Patel, V. R., Sparks, B., Wells, J., Wicha, M. S., and Mayo, L. A. (1985) *J. Clin. Invest.* **75**, 970–975.

[79]Spooncer, E., Gallagher, J. T., Krizsa, F., and Dexter, T. M. (1983) *J. Cell Biol.* 510–514.

[80]Kirby, S. L. and Bentley, S. A. (1985) *Exp. Hematol.* **13**, 373 (abstract).

[81]Zuckerman, K. S., Rhodes, R. K., Sparks, B., and Wells, J. (1985) *Clin. Res.* **33**, 358A (abstract).

[82]Wight, T. N., Kinsella, M. G., Keating, A., and Singer, J. W. (1986) *Blood* **67**, 1333–1343.

[83]Reddi, A. H., Gay, R., Gay, S., and Miller, E. J. (1977) *Proc. Natl. Acad. Sci. USA* **74**, 5589–5592.

[84]McCarthy, K. F., Weintroub, S., Hale, M., and Reddi, A. H. (1984) *Exp. Hematol.* **12**, 121–129.

[85]Sampath, T. K. and Reddi, A. H. (1981) *Proc. Natl. Acad. Sci. USA* **78**, 7599–7603.

[86]Sampath, T. K. and Reddi, A. H. (1984) *Biochem. Biophys. Res. Commun.* **119,** 949–954.

[87]Sampath, T. K. and Reddi, A. H. (1983) *Proc. Natl. Acad. Sci. USA* **80,** 6591–6595.

[88]Sampath, T. K. and Reddi, A. H. (1984), *J. Cell Biol.* **98,** 2192–2197.

[89]Sampath, T. K., Weintroub, S., and Reddi, A. H. (1984) *Biochem. Biophys. Res. Commun.* **124,** 829–835.

[89a]Sampath, T. K., Muthukumuran, N., and Reddi, A. H. (1987) *Proc. Natl. Acad. Sci. USA* **84,** 7109–7113.

[90]Reddi, A. H., Hascall, V. C., and Hascall, G. K. (1978) *J. Biol. Chem.* **253,** 2429–2436.

[91]Tian, M., Yanagishita, M., Hascall, V. C., and Reddi, A. H. (1986) *Arch. Biochem. Biophys.* **24,** 221–232.

[92]Bernstein, S. E., Russell, E. S., and Keighley, G. (1968) *Ann. NY Acad. Sci.* **149,** 475–485.

[93]Bernstein, S. E. (1970) *Am. J. Surg.* **119,** 448–451.

[94]Russell, E. S. (1979) *Adv. Genetics* **20,** 357–459.

[95]Harrison, D. W. (1979) *Clin. Haematol.* **8,** 239–262.

[96]McCulloch, E. A., Siminovitch, L., Till, J. E., Russell, E. S., and Bernstein, S. E. (1965) *Blood* **26,** 399–410.

[97]Altus, M. S., Bernstein, S. E., Russell, E. S., Carsten, A. L., and Ypton, A. C. (1971) *Proc. Soc. Exp. Biol. Med.* **138,** 985–988.

[98]Trentin, J. J., McGarry, M. P., Jenkins, V. K., Gallagher, M. T., Spiers, R. S., and Wolf, N. S. (1971), *Morphological and Functional Aspects of Immunity* (Lindahl-Kiessling, K., Alm, G., and Hanna, M. G., eds.), Plenum, New York, pp. 289–298.

[99]Fried, W., Chamberlin, W., Knospe, W. H., Husseini, S., and Trobaugh, F. E., Jr., (1973) *Br. J. Haematol.* **24,** 643–650.

[100]Dexter, T. M. and Moore, M. A. S. (1977) *Nature* **269,** 412–414.

[101]Wiktor-Jedrzejczak, W., Prasznik, A., Ahmed, A., and Szczylik, C. (1983) *Exp. Hematol.* **11,** 63–72.

[102]Keller, G. M. and Phillips, R. A. (1984) *Exp. Hematol.* **12,** 822–824.

[103]Oblon, D. J. and Vellis, M. K. (1986) *Exp. Hematol.* **14,** 492.

[104]Zuckerman, K. S., Rhodes, R. K., Sparks, B., Chenier, B., Gay, R., and Denys, F. (1985) *Clin. Res.* **33,** 358A (abstract).

[105]Zuckerman, K. S., Prince, C. W., Gay, R., and Denys, F. *Humoral and Cellular Regulation of Erythropoiesis* (Zanjani, E. D., Tavassoli, M., and Ascensao, J., eds.), Spectrum, New York (in press).

[106]Zuckerman, K. S., Prince, C. W., Rhodes, R. K., and Ribadeneira, M. (1986) *Exp. Hematol.* **14,** 1056–1062.

[107]Zuckerman, K. S., Prince, C. W., and Ribadeneira, M. (1986) *Blood* **68,** 1201–1206.

Chapter 12

Bone Marrow Microenvironment
Clinical Observations

N. T. Shahidi and W. B. Ershler

There is now ample evidence that regulation of hemopoietic stem cell proliferation is controlled by bone marrow microenvironment. The localization of hematopoietic cells to specific sites,[1] the establishment of bone marrow stroma prior to appearance of hemopoietic cells in bone marrow or splenic tissue implanted in ectopic sites,[2,3] and failure of the bone marrow to recover after destruction of the stroma by radiation[4] are a few examples. The concept of local control of hemopoietic cell proliferation has been further strengthened by demonstration that partial body radiation results in active proliferation of the pluripotent stem cells (CFU-S) only in the irradiated area.[5] Various investigations have suggested that factors controlling the replication of the hemopoietic stem cells are short range humoral stimulators and inhibitors.[6-12] Such factors have been isolated from murine bone marrow extracts and have been shown to be specific to CFU-S population. It has been further demonstrated that the effect of these factors, both inhibitor and stimulator, are reversible.[8,9] Although both factors are present simultaneously, their relative concentration depends on the proliferative stage of CFU-S in a given cell population.[10]

Long term bone marrow culture studies have lent further support to the occurrence of these molecules within the bone marrow microenvironment.[13] It is well known that in long-term liquid culture of the bone marrow, the maintenance and differentiation of hemopoietic stem cells are dependent on the establishment of a foundation of adherent cells. Upon removal of nonadherent cells, including stem cells suspended in culture medium, the stem cell lodged within the adherent layer are triggered into DNA synthesis. This proliferative activity gradually declines and reaches a steady state until the next removal of nonadherent cells. The regulation of stem cell proliferation by modulation of inhibitor/stimulator levels has been further substantiated by examination of culture medium at different periods. Indeed, low levels of inhibitor and high levels of stimulator have been found on d 1 post feeding media and a reverse situation has been observed on d 7 post feeding media.[13]

Clinical Implications

Until recently, it was widely held that human bone marrow failure syndromes, such as aplastic anemia, are the result of a defect in stem cells caused by viral agents or environmental toxins. The basis for such an assumption was successful bone marrow engraftment in some of the patients. Further evidence was provided by complete hemopoietic recovery following isogeneic bone marrow transplantation without prior conditioning. However, it was soon discovered that not all identical twins with aplastic anemia recover following isogeneic bone marrow transplantation, and prior conditioning is required in some of the patients. A recent report[14] indicates that only about 50% of patients receiving bone marrow from identical twins show evidence of hemopoietic recovery. The majority of the nonresponders, however, recover after a second transplant conditioned with immunosuppressive agents. The nature of the hostile bone marrow microenvironment in these patients remains obscure. Indeed, bone marrow culture studies in three patients, who exhibited hemopoietic recovery after a second isogeneic bone marrow transplant following conditioning with immunosuppressive agents, failed to reveal any in vitro evidence of cellular or humoral inhibition.[14] In view of the recent experimental evidence for the presence of local stimulator and inhibitor, one might speculate that in these patients a disturbance in the hemopoietic microenvironment resulted in excessive production of the local inhibitor.

The first conclusive evidence for a defective bone marrow microenvironment in humans was provided by hematologic and biochemical studies in a young woman with congenital hypoplastic anemia.[15] The bone marrow cells from this patient, obtained by means of aspiration, showed exuberant erythroid growth in vitro despite marked erythroid hypoplasia in bone marrow aspirate. In contrast, when whole bone fragments were similarly cultured, no appreciable hemoglobin synthesis was observed.

Functional Abnormalities of Cellular Components of Bone Marrow Microenvironment

Unfortunately because of limitations of the in vitro techniques, functional dissection of bone marrow microenvironment in normal individuals and particularly in pathologic states has been difficult. Because of hemopoietic recovery in a large number of patients with aplastic anemia, following the administration of anti-thymocyte and anti-lymphocyte globulins[16,17] and other immunosuppressive agents,[18,19] an immunological mechanism implicating T-cells has been suggested. In other instances, an abnormality in bone marrow adherent cells has been incriminated. Since T-lymphocytes, like bone marrow macrophages, are both anatomically and physiologically a part of bone marrow microenvironment, a brief discussion of their role in bone marrow failure syndromes is warranted.

T-Lymphocytes

Numerous reports employing various techniques, such as bone marrow cocultures, T-cell depletion, and T-cell addition, have suggested that T-suppressor lymphocytes may play role in the pathogenesis of certain types of bone marrow failure syndromes.[20,21] However, as recently pointed out by Young,[22] the interpretation of the data remains difficult and clinical correlates are scarce. In addition, the exact mechanism whereby the suppressor cytotoxic lymphocytes result in the destruction of hemopoietic stem cells remains unknown. In a recent study by Zoumbos and associates,[23] a significant number of circulating activated lymphocytes were found in 10 of 12 patients with aplastic anemia. The same investigators reported[24] abnormalities in interferon production by lectin-stimulated lymphocytes and elevated levels of interferon in the sera of their patients with aplastic anemia. It is well known that the administration of interferon results in granulocytopenia, thrombocytopenia, and/or anemia.[25,26] It has also been shown that interferon inhibits proliferation of hemopoietic cells in vitro.[27] However, in a more recent report using a radioimmunoassay technique, Torok-Storb et al.[28] could not detect any significant levels (>10μ/mL) in 50 patients with aplastic anemia. Furthermore, it should be pointed out that cytopenias occasionally seen following the administration of pharmacologic doses of interferon are usually dose dependent and reversible. These findings make the possibility of endogenous production of interferon an unlikely pathogenic mechanism. It is possible, however, that activated T-lymphocytes may exert their effect on hemopoietic stem cells indirectly by stimulating the production of local inhibitors, or directly by producing short range inhibitors. In any event, to exert their effect, the lymphocytes must enter the extravascular compartment of the bone marrow where hemopoietic stem cells and progenitors reside.

Animal studies have indicated that there exists, in the lymphocyte pool within the bone marrow extravascular compartment, a small fraction (less than 10%) of mature T-lymphocytes.[29,30] Similar observations have been made by Fauci[31] using human bone marrow. In 22 normal subjects, ranging in age from 19 to 25 yr, the percent of T-cells was estimated at 8.6 ± 1.7 SEM. In addition, it was found that there are definite differences between peripheral blood and bone marrow lymphocytes in their responsiveness to mitogens.[31]

The circulating T-lymphocytes can migrate freely into and out of the lymphoid compartment. It has been shown that the migration of the small lymphocytes to the lymph nodes across the vascular endothelium is facilitated by anatomical adaptation of the venules columnar epithelium[32] and their homing is determined by cell surface carbohydrate composition.[33] The bone marrow microenvironment, however, is devoid of lymphatic circulation, and the extent and mechanism of accessibility of the bone marrow extravascular compartment to the traffic of circulating mature T-lymphocytes remains unknown. The quantitative and qualitative differences between the peripheral blood and bone marrow lymphocytes in normal individuals, suggest that the traffic of the cells across the sinusoidal endothelium must be under local control. It is thus conceivable that certain drugs, toxins, or viral agents may jeopardize such a control mechanism, and may as a result increase the permeability of the endothelial lining of the bone marrow sinusoids to cytotoxic lymphocytes. In this connection, Mangan et al.[34] recently reported a patient with lymphoma who developed a progressive and irreversible pancytopenia with marrow aplasia following the administration of alpha interferon in conventional antitumor dose. The patient's bone marrow contained a large number of T-suppressor cytotoxic lymphocytes (above 36% of total nucleated cells) that were found to be inhibitory to bone marrow erythroid progenitor cells in vitro. The activation of T-suppressor cytotoxic lymphocytes (OKT8+) by interferon is well documented[35,36] and these T-cells are found in increased numbers in the blood of patients treated with interferon.

The occurrence of high numbers of cytotoxic lymphocytes within the patient's bone marrow, following interferon therapy associated with irreversible aplastic anemia, is highly unusual. It is interesting that prior to interferon therapy the patient had received cytoxan, vincristine, and prednisone every 4 wk and marrow recovery had been prompt after each cycle. It is possible that the above chemotherapeutic agents resulted in the disruption of local control allowing greater influx of cytotoxic lymphocytes within the bone marrow extravascular compartments.

Bone Marrow Macrophages

The intimate association of macrophages and erythroblasts in the bone marrow and spleen has been known for many years.[37,38] Within the bone marrow extra vascular compartment, a central macrophage surrounded by erythroblasts is a distinct anatomical unit known as erythroblastic ilet. These anatomical units have been the subject of extensive studies. Unfortunately, however, the biological significance of this association and the role of the central macrophage in the erythropoietic process remain obscure. It has been suggested that the central cells provide the surrounding erythroblasts with ferritin.[39] A sudden surge of these erythroblastic islands in the bone marrow of a patient with Fanconi anemia and hypotrans-ferrenemia during transition into acute erythroleukemia provided further support to this concept.[40] Since macrophages are known to produce a variety of hemopoietic factors,[41] it is highly likely that, through cell–cell interaction, these hemopoietic factors may be transferred to the surrounding erythroblasts. In many ways the anatomical and functional relationship between the central macrophage and the surrounding erythroblasts resemble that between Sertoli and germ cells in testes. The juxtaposition of Sertoli and germ cells has led many investigators to believe that Sertoli cells play an important regulatory role in spermatogenesis.[42]

Using clonal culture techniques, it has been shown that normal human bone marrow macrophages influence the growth of both early (BFU-E) and late erythroid progenitors (CFU-E).[43-45] It has been further found that bone marrow macrophages modulate erythropoiesis both by synthesis of soluble factors and through cell–cell interaction.[46,48] Although at low concentrations the macrophages exert a stimulatory effect, they are inhibitory at high concentrations. Similar observations have been made using soluble factors present in the condition media of cultured macrophages.[46,48] There are reasons to believe that the effect of bone marrow macrophages on hemopoietic progenitors is different from that exerted in the peripheral blood macrophages.[46]

On clinical grounds, macrophages have been implicated in the pathogenesis of chronic refractory anemias[49] and anemias associated with chronic infection[50,51] and cancer.[51] It has been found that macrophages from patients with the above condition significantly inhibit both early and late erythroid progenitors. A soluble inhibitor seems to be involved; for, conditioned media from these cells and feeder layer experiments have both yielded similar results.

It should be pointed out, however, that in all these experiments bone marrow macrophages have been removed by adherence. The effect of other adherent cells such as natural killer cells on erythroid progenitors should also be considered. Indeed such an effect in patients with viral or bacterial infection is a likely possibility. In a study by Suda and associates,[52] the removal of bone marrow macrophages by Carbonyl iron method resulted in a significant increase in the number of CFU-C in the bone marrow of their patients with aplastic anemia. Such a finding is not surprising for macrophages may cooperate with T-lymphocytes in suppressing CFU-C.

Bone Marrow Fibroblasts

There have been several reports examining the effect of bone marrow stroma on the growth of hemopoietic progenitors in vitro. Unfortunately, however, because of the diversity of methodology, the nature of cellular elements involved remains uncertain. The studies by Castro-Malaspina et al.,[53] using human bone marrow, have identified the bone marrow fibroblasts as nonphagocytic adherent cells. Fibroblasts are unable to phagocytize carbonyl iron or latex particles; in contrast to endothelial cells, they do not contain Weibel-Palade bodies or factor VIII antigen. They produce, however, Type I and III collagen and fibronectin.

Using a liquid culture system, Greenberg and associates[54] found that the fibroblasts obtained from normal human bone marrow stimulated the growth of myeloid colony, whereas fibroblasts from patients with myelocytic leukemia (AML) generally did not. Furthermore, the bone marrow fibroblasts from two of their patients with AML stimulated the myeloid colonies (CFU-C) during remission, but not during relapse. Since the fibroblasts are not derived from the leukemic clone, a defective interaction between leukemic progenitors and stromal cells was implicated in the pathogenesis of relapse and maturation arrest. Similar to the above observation, the ability of bone marrow macrophage to produce CSA is impaired in patients with AML.[55] In studies by Blackburn and Goldman,[56] it was found that the fibroblasts from human bone marrow enhanced the growth of both CFU-C and BFU-E. Furthermore, it was reported that conditioned media from human bone marrow fibroblasts increased the survival of murine CFU-S. It is interesting to note that in the studies by Greenberg and associates,[54] the conditioned media from normal bone marrow fibroblasts inhibited the growth of CFU-C in marrow containing a large number of endogenous CFU-C. This finding suggested the release of inhibitory factors in condition media by fibroblasts. The above observation indicates that bone marrow fibroblasts may exert a dual regulatory role upon myelopoiesis. In this connection, in vivo studies have described fibroblastic stromal cells morphologically similar to the in vitro fibroblasts that are intimately associated with granulopoietic regions in the bone marrow[57] and spleen.[58]

Several attempts have also been made to explore the possibility of quantitative and qualitative alterations in bone marrow fibroblasts in patients with aplastic anemia. It has been repeatedly demonstrated that fibroblast colonies can be normally grown from bone marrow of the patients with this disorder. Several studies, however, have detected various functional abnormalities in marrow fibroblasts in aplastic anemia. For instance, Juneja and associates[59] have found an abnormal response to dexamethasone and a lack of contact inhibition in bone marrow fibroblasts from patients with aplastic anemia. Studies by Gordon and Gordon-Smith[60] have revealed that normal bone marrow fibroblasts enhance the effect of colony stimulating factor on CFU-C. These investigators further found that, under similar culture conditions, the bone marrow fibroblasts from patients with aplastic anemia failed to exhibit this property. More recently, Hotta et al.[61] have found that marrow stromal cells from some of their patients with aplastic anemia were functionally defective in their ability to sustain normal CFU-C in long-term cultures.

Despite the diversity of the techniques used, failure to obtain a homogenous population of cells and limitations inherent to the in vitro culture techniques, the above studies collectively suggest that a disturbance in the function of the bone marrow microenvironment is often present in a variety of bone marrow failure syndromes. Such a disturbance, whether primary or secondary, would lead to the disruption of normal regulatory mechanisms.

References

[1]Till, J. E. and McCulloch, E. A. (1961) *Radiat. Res.* **14,** 213–222.

[2]Tavassoli, M. and Crosby, W. H. (1968) *Science* **161,** 54–56.

[3]Tavassoli, M. and Crosby, W. H. (1970)*Science* **169,** 291.

[4]Knospe, W. H., Blom, J., and Crosby, W. H. (1966) *Blood* **28,** 398–415.

[5]Croizat, H., Frindel, E., and Tubiana, M. (1970) *J. Radiat. Biol.* **18,** 347–358.

[6]Frindel, E., Croizat, H., and Vassort, F. (1976) *Exp. Hematol.* **4,** 56–61.

[7]Frindel, E. and Guigon, M. (1977) *Exp. Hematol.* **5,** 74–76.

[8]Lord, B. I., Mori, K. J., Wright, E. G., and Lajtha, L. G. (1976) *Br. J. Haematol.* **34,** 441–445.

[9]Lord, B. I., Mori, K. J., and Wright, E. G. (1977) *Biomedicine* **27,** 223–226.

[10]Wright, E. G. and Lord, B. I. (1980) *Leuk. Res.* **3,** 15–22.

[11]Wright, E. G. and Lord, B. I. (1978) *Biomedicine* **28,** 156–160.

[12]Dexter, T. M., Allen, T. D., and Lajtha, L. G. (1977) *J. Cell. Physiol.* **91,** 335–344.

[13]Toksoz, D., Dexter, T. M., Lord, B. I., Wright, E. G., and Lajtha, L. G. (1980) *Blood* **55,** 931–936.

[14]Gale, R. P., Champlin, R. E., Feig, S. A., and Fitchen, J. H. (1981) *Ann. Intern. Med.* **95,** 477–494.

[15]Ershler, W. B., Ross, J., Finlay, J. L., and Shahidi, N. T. (1980) *N. Engl. J. Med.* **302,** 1321–1327.

[16]Champlin, R., Ho, W., and Gale, R. P. (1983) *N. Engl. J. Med.* **308,** 113–118.

[17]Speck, B., Gratwohl, A., Nissen, C., Osterwalder, B., Wursh, A., Techelli, A., Lori, A., Reusser, P., Jeannet, M., and Signer, E. (1986) *Exp. Hematol.* **14,** 126–132.

[18]Marmont, A. M., Bacigalupo, A., Van Lint, M. T., Frassoni, F., Podesta, M., Reali, G., and Piaggio, G. (1984) *Prog. in Clin. Biol. Res.* **148**, 271–287.

[19]Finlay, J. L. and Shahidi, N. T. (1984) *Blood* **64**, 109a (abstract).

[20]Ascensao, J., Kagan, W., Moore, M., Pahwa, R., Hansen, J., and Good, R. (1976) *Lancet* **1**, 669–671.

[21]Hoffman, R., Zanjani, E. D., Lutton, J. D., Zalusky, R., and Wasserman, L. R. (1977) *N. Engl. J. Med.* **296**, 10–13.

[22]Young, N. (1981) *Hematol.* **12**, 227–274.

[23]Zoumbos, N. C., Gascon, P., Djeu, J. Y., Trost, S. R., and Young, N. S. (1985) *N. Eng. J. Med.* **312**, 257–265.

[24]Zoumbos, N. C., Gascon, P., Djeu, J., and Young, N. S. (1985) *Proc. Natl. Acad. Sci. USA* **82**, 188.

[25]Borden, E. C. and Ball, L. A. (1981) *Progress in Hematology*, vol. XII (Brown, E. B., ed.), Grune & Stratton, New York, pp. 299–339.

[26]Urbaniak, S. J., Halliday, I. M., Beveridge, G. W., and Kay, A. B. (1978) *Lancet* **1**, 553,554.

[27]Toretsky, J. A., Shahidi, N. T., and Finlay, J. L. (1986) *Exp. Hematol.* **14**, 182–186.

[28]Torok-Storb, B., Johnson, G., Bowden, R., and Storb, R. (1987) *Blood* **69**, 629.

[29]Rosse, C. (1972) *Blood J. Hematol.* **40**, 90–97.

[30]Ropke, C. and Everett, N. B. (1974) *Cell Tissue Kinet.* **7**, 137–150.

[31]Fauci, A. S. (1975) *J. Clin. Invest.* **56**, 98–110.

[32]Schoefl, G. I. (1972) *J. Exp. Med.* **136**, 568–588.

[33]Gesner, B. M. and Ginsburg, V. (1964) *Proc. Natl. Acad. Sci. USA* **52**, 750–755.

[34]Managan, K. F., Zidar, B., Shadduck, R. K., Zeigler, Z., and Winkelstein, A. (1985) *Am. J. Hematol.* **19**, 401–413.

[35]Rosenblatt, M. H., Kronenberg, L. H., Rosenblatt, H. M., Bryson, Y., and Merigan, T. C. (1982) *Interferon: Immunobiology and Clinical Significance. Ann. Intern. Med.* **96**, 80.

[36]Mittelman, A., Krown, S. E., Cirrinclone, C., Safai, B., Oettgen, H. F., and Koziner, B. (1983) *Am. J. Med.* **75**, 966–972.

[37]Bessis, M. (1958) *Rev. Hematol.* **13**, 8–11.

[38]Bessis, M. and Breton-Gorius, J. (1959) *Rev. Hematol.* **14**, 165–175.

[39]Policard, A. and Bessis, M. (1958) *CR Acad. Sci.* **246**, 3194.

[40]Taher, A., Gilbert, E., and Shahidi, N. T. (1981) *Am. J. Ped. Hematol./Oncol.* **3**, 121–125.

[41]Rich, I. N. (1986) *Exp. Hematol.* **14**, 738–745.

[42]Tindall, D. J., Rowley, D. R., Murthy, L., Lipshultz, L. I., and Chang, C. H. (1985) *Intern. Rev. of Cytology* **94**, 127.

[43]Rhinehart, J. J., Zanjani, E. D., Nomdedeu, B., Gormus, B. J., and Kaplan, M. E. (1978) *J. Clin. Invest.* **62**, 979–986.

[44]Mangan, K. F. and Desforges, J. F. (1980) *Exp. Hematol.* **8,** 717–727.

[45]Zuckerman, K. S. (1980) *Exp. Hematol.* **8,** 924–932.

[46]Gordon, L. I., Miller, W. J., Branda, R. F., Zanjani, E. D., and Jacob, H. S. (1980) *Blood* **55,** 1047–1050.

[47]Zuckerman, K. S. (1981) *J. Clin. Invest.* **67,** 702–709.

[48]Hanada, T., Nagasawa, T. and Abe, T. (1982) *Exp. Hematol.* **10,** 561–567.

[49]Bjornson, G., Martin, J., MacKinney, A. A., and Shahidi, N. T. (1981) *Blood* **58,** 339a(abstract).

[50]Zanjani, E. D., McGlave, P. B., Davies, S. F., Banisadre, M., Kaplan, M. E., and Sarosi, G. A. (1982) *Br. J. Haematol.* **50,** 479–490.

[51]Roodman, G. D., Horadam, V. W., and Wright, T. L. (1983) *Blood* **62,** 406–412.

[52]Suda, T., Mizoguchi, H., Miura, Y., Kubota, K., and Takaku, F. (1980) *Exp. Hematol.* **8,** 659–665.

[53]Castro-Malaspina, H., Gay, R. E., Resnick, G., Kapoor, N., Meyers, P., Chiarieri, D., McKenzie, S., Broxmeyer, H. E., and Moore, M. A. S. (1980) *Blood* **56,** 289–301.

[54]Greenberg, B. R., Wilson, F. D., and Woo, L. (1980) *Blood* **58,** 557–564.

[55]Greenberg, P. L., Mara, B., and Heller, P. (1978) *Blood* **52,** 362–378.

[56]Blackburn, M. J. and Goldman, J. M. (1980) *Exp. Hematol.* **8,** 79 (abstract).

[57]Western, H. and Bainton, D. F. (1979) *J. Exp. Med.* **150,** 919–937.

[58]La Pushing, R. W. and Trentin, J. J. (1977) *Exp. Hematol.* **5,** 505–522.

[59]Juneja, H. S., Gardner, F. H., Minguell, J. J., and Helmer, R. E., III (1984) *Exp. Hematol.* **12,** 221–230.

[60]Gordon, M. Y. and Gordon-Smith, E. C. (1985) *Br. J. Haematol.* **53,** 65–69.

[61]Hotta, T., Kato, T., Maeda, H., Yamao, H., Yamada, H., and Saito, H. (1985) *Acta Haematol.* **74,** 65–69.

Index

A

Adherent layer cell types,
256
adipocytes, 261
endothelial cells, 259–261
function, 262, 263
interactions, 261, 262
macrophage and epithe-
loid cell, 256–259
Association of hematopoi-
esis and bone forma-
tion, 209, 210

B

Bone
role of in modulation of
hemopoiesis, 160–163
Bone marrow, 88, 385–390
adventitial reticular cells,
97–99
blood circulation, 88, 89
cell release, 100–104
disorders, 389
endothelial cells, 91–97
coated pits, 92–94

endocytosis, 92
fat cells, 99
myelofibrosis, 390
nerves, 99, 100
sinuses, 90
Bone marrow
fatty involution, 157–187
red and yellow mar-
row, 157–160
distribution
normal and abnor-
mal, 159, 160
Neuman's Law, 159
Temperature gradi-
ent hypothesis, 160
Bone marrow adipocyte,
170–181
characteristics in long-
term bone marrow cul-
ture, 180, 181
development, 170, 171
distinction from extra-
medullary adipocyte,
174–178
functional differences,
176–178
function, 172–174
heterogeneity, 178–180

structure, 171, 172
Capacity of cloned stromal
    cell lineages to support
    hematopoiesis in vivo,
    214, 215
Clonigenic hematopoietic
    stem cells developing
    on CEM enriched with
    stromal cells, 194–198,
    211
Collagen, 369
    measurement, 371
    role, 369
    structure, 370
    types
        I, 373–378, 385, 390
        II, 378, 379, 385
        III, 379, 380, 385, 390
        IV, 380, 381, 386, 390
        V, 381, 382, 388, 390
        VI, 382, 383
        VII, 383
        VIII, 383
        IX, 384
        X, 384
        XI, 384
Collagenous matrix, 388
    origin, 394
    synthesis, 388
Components of bone mar-
    row stroma
    cellular, 219–246
        fibroblastic reticular

cells in vitro, 225–230
    fibroblastic reticular
    cells in vitro
        blanket cell, 227
        fat cells, 226
        fibroblasts, 225
    macrophages, 230–244
        central macrophage,
            231–243
        erythroblastic island,
            231
        macrophages dis-
            persed in hemato-
            poietic cord, 243,
            244
        perisinal macro-
            phage, 243
    other cellular compo-
        nents, 246, 247
        stromal cell recog-
            nized by lantha-
            num uptake, 246,
            247
    reticular cells in vivo,
        220–225
        advential reticular
            cells, 221–224
        fibroblastic reticular
            cells, 224, 225
        intercellular matrix,
            224
        monoclonal antibody
            ER-HR 1, 224

D

Dexter, 272
Dexter stem cells, 254

E

Ectopic implantation of
bone marrow, 163–169
Effect of membrane compo-
sition and pore size on
hematopoiesis devel-
oping on stromal cell
enriched CEM, 198–201
cellulose acetate
(Celotate™), 199
cellulose ester (nitrates
and acetates) mem-
branes, 198
marrow stromal cells,
199-201
polycarbonate (Nucle-
pore™), 199
polyethylene linear, 199
polytetrafluoroethylene
(Teflon™ or Mitex™),
199
polyvinyl chloride mem-
brane (Polyvic™), 199
Egress from marrow

anatomy of leukocyte,
121, 122
anatomy of pathological
states, 130, 131
anatomy of platelet,
123–130
anatomy of reticulocyte,
111–120
cell releasing factors,
107–111
Electron microscopy of
hematopoietic stromal
cells developing on en-
riched CEM, 195–198
Extracellular matrix
hemopoietic, 399–432
matrix molecules,
402–410
bone Gla protein, 408
bone morphogen-
etic protein (BMP),
410
collagen, 408–411
fibronectin, 403, 404
laminin, 404, 405
osteocalcin, 408
ostrogenesis, 420
osteogenin, 419
proteoglycans,
405, 409
regulation of cell
growth and differen-
tiation, 401, 402

G

Growth factor production,
264–267

H

Hematopoiesis on CEM
implanted in Sl/Sl^d
mice, 193, 194
Hematopoiesis on ip im-
planted CEM enriched
or coated with hemato-
poietic stromal cells,
194–198
bone stromal cells, 195
marrow stromal cells, 195
regulation of stromal
cells, 194–198
splenic stromal cells, 196
stromal cells from Dexter
layers (LTMC), 212
stromal cells from regen-
erating endosteum, 195
Hematopoiesis on uncoated
ip implanted CEM,
189–194
endothelial cells, 190
fibroblasts, 190
macrophages–monocytes,
190

types of stromal cells
identified on falt CEM,
194
Hemopoiesis
abnormal, 354–363
aplastic anemia,
354–363
comparison with
immunodefi-
ciency, 354, 355
immunosuppressive
therapy, 358–363
in vitro suppressor
mechanisms
cell mediated,
355–357
humoral, 355–359
pathogenesis of
marrow aplasia,
361
role of NK cells, 362
Hemopoiesis
control of, 68–77
stochastic model, 68–77
normal, 335–354
role of T-lymphocytes
BPA
production of, 336,
337
in growth of BFU-E,
337–348

interferon (α and γ)
mediation of T-cell
effects, 348–350
production of CSF,
350, 351
ricin-antibody
depletion of,
340–348
role in granulopoi-
esis, 350
T-cell markers,
338–344
role of monocytes,
351–353
roles of monocytes
BPA, 352
in erythroid islets,
352
MRA, 351
production of IL-1,
tumor necrosis
factor, intereron,
352, 353
prostaglandins, 351
role of NK cells, 353,
354
graft rejection, 353
LAK cells, 353, 354
NK cell-derived
colony inhibiting

activity (NA-
CIA), 353
regulation of, 335–368
cellular interactions,
335–368
Hemopoietic cells
biophysical properties,
104
cell chemotaxis, 106
cell deformability, 105,
106
cell motility, 104, 105
cell surface features,
107
Hemopoietic inductive
microenvironment
(HIM), 28–40
evidence, 29-39
bone marrow colonies,
29, 30
"cure" of Sl/Sl^d, 33–36
marrow stroma trans-
plantation, 32, 33
rat CFU-S in mouse
microenvironment,
36–38
tetanus toxoid sensiti-
zation, 38, 39
whole spleen trans-
plantation, 30–32

cellulose acetate mem-
  branes, 42
CFU-S heterogeneity,
  42–46
hemopoietic hormone
  receptors, 50, 51
hypothesis, 28–39
mast cell differentiation,
  39, 40
roles of marrow, spleen,
  thymus stroma, 40, 41
Hemopoietic microenviron-
  ment, 287–297
nature of stromal cells,
  290–293
definition, 292
primary stromal cell
  cultures, 293–296
  Dexter cultures, 293
  other systems, 294–296
putative functions,
  287–290
  hemopoietic inductive
    microenvironment
    (HIM), 288
  stochastic model of
    stem cell self-re-
    newal, 288–290
Hemopoietic microenviron-
  ments
  concept of, 1–4
    homing, 5–9
      effect of erythropoi-

etin deprivation,
  18–23
lineage decision,
  23–28
primary spleen
  colonies
    types of, 9–18
  secondary spleen
    colonies, 14–18
radiation protection, 4
spleen colony assay
  definition, 5
Hemopoietic microenviron-
  ments
  historical perspectives,
    1–78
Hemopoietic stromal cell
  lines, 297–326
  adipogenesis, 306, 307
  cell surface markers, 309
  classification, 309-311
    endothelial–adipose
      cell, 309, 310
    endothelial-like cell,
      310
    fibroblast of advential
      reticulum cell, 310
    fibroendothelial cell,
      311
  long-term maintenance
    of hemopoiesis,
    311–313
  macrophage, 311

CSF, 313–316
  other soluble regula-
    tors of hemopoiesis,
    316, 317
  cytoplasmic enzymes, 307
  derivation and growth,
    297–304
  extracellular matrix, 308,
    309
  interactions between
    components of stroma,
    324, 325
  leukemia cell inhibitory
    activity (LCIA), 317–
    321
  list of human and murine
    stromal cell lines,
    298–301
  morphology, 304–306
  promotion of leukemia
    cell growth, 321–323
  transplantation, tumori-
    genesis, 323, 324
Hodgkin's disease, 390–392

L

Long-term bone marrow
    cultures, 55–59, 434
  matrix proteins, 412–416
  regulation by matrix

components, 416, 417
Lymphoid inductive
  microenvironments,
  51–55
Lymphoid long-term cul-
  ture, 272–274

M

Matrix proteins secreted by
    hematopoietic stromal
    cells, 201–207
  bone matrix powder
    (demineralized),
    202–207
  collagen I, 203
  collagen II, 203
  collagen IV, 203
  glycosaminoglycans, 201
  proteoglycans, 201
  tooth matix powder
    (demineralized),
    203–207
Microenvironment
  bone marrow, 433–444
    cellular components,
      435–442
    fibroblasts, 440–442
    functional abnor-
      malities, 435, 436
    macrophages, 438–
      440

T-lymphocytes, 436–
438
clinical implications,
434, 435
aplastic anemia, 434,
435
Microenvironments in
malignancy, 77, 78
Microscopic methods
in vivo, 142–146
basic methods, 142, 143
perfused prepara-
tions, 142, 143
surgically-exposed
organs *in situ*, 142
visualization
through windows
contained within
chambers im-
planted in ectopic
sites, 143
Epi-illumination
methods, 146
methods to study
hemopoietic tissue,
147–154
erythropoietin as a
vasoactive media-
tor, 147–150
other vasoactive
substances, 150,
151

role of prostaglan-
dins, adenosine,
153
sources of vasoactive
substances, 150,
151
transillumination
methods, 143–146
compound trinocular
microscope, 144,
145
quartz, glass, plastic
light rods, fiber
optic light guides,
143, 144
use of specific wave-
lengths of mono-
chromatic light,
145, 146
Microvasculature within
hemopoietic tissue, 141
Model of stromal regula-
tion, 278–280
Myelofibrosis, 390

O

Origin of hematopietic
stromal cells (donor or
host), 207, 208

P

Proliferation
  hemopoietic stem cell,
    433, 434
    inhibitors and stimula-
      tors
    humoral, 435
    regulation by the
      marrow microenvi-
      ronment, 433, 434

R

Radiation sensitivity of
    hematopoietic stromal
    cells, 207, 208

S

Serum supplement, 254
Stem cells
  circulation, 131, 132
  reentry into marrow, 131,
    132
Stromal cell lines
    from other times, 325,
    326

Stromal cells, 59–68
  of erythroid colonies,
    59–64
  of granuloid colonies, 64,
    65
Studies in different species,
    267–272

T

TC-1 cell line, 274–278

W

Whitlock-Witte, 273
Wound healing, 392